ECONOMIC ANALYSIS IN HEALTH CARE

Second Edition

ECONOMIC ANALYSIS IN HEALTH CARE

Second Edition

Stephen Morris
Nancy Devlin
David Parkin and
Anne Spencer

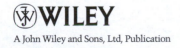

A John Wiley and Sons, Ltd, Publication

This edition first published 2012

© 2012 John Wiley & Sons, Ltd

Registered office

John Wiley & Sons Ltd, The Atrium, Southern Gate, Chichester, West Sussex, PO19 8SQ, United Kingdom

For details of our global editorial offices, for customer services and for information about how to apply for permission to reuse the copyright material in this book please see our website at www.wiley.com.

The right of Stephen Morris, Nancy Devlin, David Parkin and Anne Spencer to be identified as the authors of this work has been asserted in accordance with the Copyright, Designs and Patents Act 1988.

Wiley publishes in a variety of print and electronic formats and by print-on-demand. Some material included with standard print versions of this book may not be included in e-books or in print-on-demand. If this book refers to media such as a CD or DVD that is not included in the version you purchased, you may download this material at http://booksupport.wiley.com. For more information about Wiley products, visit www.wiley.com.

Designations used by companies to distinguish their products are often claimed as trademarks. All brand names and product names used in this book are trade names, service marks, trademarks or registered trademarks of their respective owners. The publisher is not associated with any product or vendor mentioned in this book. This publication is designed to provide accurate and authoritative information in regard to the subject matter covered. It is sold on the understanding that the publisher is not engaged in rendering professional services. If professional advice or other expert assistance is required, the services of a competent professional should be sought.

Library of Congress Cataloging-in-Publication Data
Economic analysis in health care / Stephen Morris . . . [et al.].—2nd ed.
   p. ; cm.
  Rev. ed. of: Economic analysis in health care / Stephen Morris, Nancy Devlin, David Parkin. c2007.
  Includes bibliographical references and index.
  ISBN 978-1-119-95149-0 (paper : alk. paper)
 I. Morris, S. (Stephen), 1971- II. Morris, S. (Stephen), 1971- Economic analysis in health care.
  [DNLM: 1. Delivery of Health Care—economics. 2. Costs and Cost Analysis. W 84.1]
  338.4'73621—dc23

                                                                    2012002906

A catalogue record for this book is available from the British Library.

Set in 10/12.5pt Palatino-Roman by Thomson Digital, India

Printed in Great Britain by TJ International Lts, Padstow, Cornwall

This book is for our lovely children:
from Steve to Eve and Stella;
from Nancy to Sophie, Molly and Hugh;
from Dave to Susannah, Eleanor, Laura and Stephen;
from Anne to Adam and Zoë

CONTENTS

PREFACE

Each of us has, for many years, taught health economics courses to both masters and undergraduate students in the UK (and, in Nancy's case, New Zealand) and our objective here was to write the sort of book we always wished was available for our students.

As health economics has grown as a subdiscipline, so too have the number of textbooks that are available. The many fine textbooks from the USA in this subject are inevitably influenced by the particular system for funding and provision of health care in that country; the focus of these is not always appropriate for the principal concerns and issues in *other* health care systems. And while there are textbooks on health economics in the UK, for example, these generally either aim to provide an easy-to-understand, non-technical introduction to health economics for those with no economics background, or focus on one particular aspect of health economics, such as economic evaluation or health care financing. While some of these books are excellent, their objectives limit their usefulness as a teaching tool for a more general course in health economics.

This book is written to provide (we hope!) a useful balance of theoretical treatment, description of empirical analyses and breadth of content for use in undergraduate modules in health economics for economics students, and for students taking a health economics module as part of their postgraduate training. Although we are writing from a UK perspective, we have attempted to make the book as relevant internationally as possible by drawing on examples, case studies and boxed highlights, not just from the UK, but from a wide range of countries including Australia, Canada, Finland, Iran, Ireland, Italy, Namibia, New Zealand, Norway, Sweden, Tanzania, Thailand, USA and the Vietnam, plus multinational sources including the OECD, the WHO and the World Bank.

There are other things about this book that we hope will be of particular value to students. First, we have paid special attention to explaining key elements of theory in health economics – for example, the contributions of Arrow (1963) and a full account of the Grossman (1972) model, both of which we view as critical to any account of health economics. We have not shied away from presenting and explaining the technical aspects of the theory, but have endeavoured to do so in as user-friendly a manner as possible. Secondly, we have been careful to link the practice of economic evaluation to underlying concepts in production, costs and efficiency. This reflects our own view that, as the practice of economic evaluation has come to be dominated by increasingly sophisticated statistical and modelling techniques, the underlying economics concepts (and, incidentally, a remaining rich research territory) are sometimes overlooked.

We very much hope that this book will serve to provoke thought and stimulate a deep interest in health economics, in the same way as earlier writers, particularly Alan Williams, Victor Fuchs and Tony Culyer, served to inspire us in our careers.

In this edition we have incorporated helpful suggestions made to us by readers of the first edition. We have also added a new chapter on the economics of health care labour markets, justified by the size of this sector and its importance to health care production. We have updated the boxed examples and case studies, and also used more of these, and from a wider range of countries.

As well as revising the book, we have improved the companion website. We have added to the depth and breadth of material available. It contains a wide range of complementary teaching and learning resources, such as practical exercises, animated slides, and study questions, including a new series of more technical questions that will be of particular interest to economics students.

Lastly, we would like to say thank you to a number of people who have helped us: Steve Hardman, Jennifer Edgecombe and Nicole Burnett from our publishers, John Wiley & Sons, for their careful advice and understanding; several anonymous reviewers for their constructive criticism; Laura Vallejo-Torres for her comments on Chapter 7; Augustin de Coulon for his input into Chapter 8; Stephen Pollock for his help with notation; and Aki Tsuchiya for her extensive and invaluable feedback. To these people as well as the many readers who contacted us with comments about the first edition, thank you for your helpful advice and kind words.

Stephen Morris, Nancy Devlin, David Parkin, Anne Spencer

CHAPTER 1

Introduction to economic analysis in health care

1.1 Life, death and big business: why health economics is important

You may come to this book knowing a great deal about economics, but not about health care, other than your personal experience of ill health and its treatment. Alternatively, you may come to this book with experience in the health care sector, but no training in economics. Whatever background you bring to it, we are confident that you will find the study of health economics fascinating. Learning to look at health and health care issues through the distinctive lens of the economist will forever change the way you think about them.

Understanding health care economics is important for a number of reasons. First, health is important to us as individual people and as a society. Health care is one, though not the only, way to modify the incidence and impact of ill health. The availability of health care can determine the quality of our lives and our prospects for survival. Economic analysis offers a unique and systematic intellectual framework for analysing important issues in health care, and for identifying solutions to common problems. Health economics is literally a matter of life and death.

Secondly, the health care sector of the economy is very large. The US Centers for Medicare and Medicaid Services (CMS) reported that health spending in the USA approached US$2 500 billion by 2009, accounting for around 17.6% of Gross Domestic Product (CMS, 2011). They also forecast that by 2020 health spending will account for over US$4 600 billion – nearly one-fifth of all US economic activity. Other forecasts suggest that this will reach one-third by the middle of the century (Hall and Jones, 2007) and plausibly even one-half by 2082 (US Congressional Budget Office, 2007). In the UK, where health care is predominantly funded by general taxation, spending on health care comprises 17% of all government spending (HM Treasury, 2011). Health care is therefore a major consideration in fiscal management of the UK economy. Indeed, health care is a major component of spending, investment and employment in every developed economy, so the economic performance of the health care system is crucially linked to the overall economic well-being of a country and its citizens.

The size of health spending is not just important in countries where it is large. In many countries, the issue is how low it is. For example, data from the World Bank show that in 2009 Eritrea and Myanmar spent around 2% of their GDP on health care. A starker contrast is that per person this amounts to around $US10, compared with $US7 400 in the USA. Table 1.1 shows the international scale of health care spending, its contrasts and how it has changed over time.

TABLE 1.1   International health expenditure, 1995 and 2009

	Per person ($US)		% Gross Domestic Product		% Public spending	
	1995	2009	1995	2009	1995	2009
World	$ 457	$ 864	8.8	10.0	62.1	60.8
High income	$2 364	$4 457	9.6	11.8	63.5	62.5
North America	$3 557	$7 110	13.2	15.7	46.3	49.8
European Union	$1 664	$3 371	8.7	10.3	78.0	76.1
Low & middle income	$ 52	$ 168	5.0	5.6	48.6	51.8
Latin America & Caribbean	$ 243	$ 543	6.5	7.7	48.3	51.7
Europe & Central Asia	$ 78	$ 387	4.8	6.0	70.4	66.0
Middle East & North Africa	$ 57	$ 183	4.4	5.3	46.9	50.7
East Asia & Pacific	$ 25	$ 148	3.3	4.4	47.4	50.4
Sub-Saharan Africa	$ 32	$ 76	5.8	6.6	39.0	43.9
Upper middle income	$ 90	$ 316	5.3	6.0	51.5	54.3
Lower middle income	$ 21	$ 61	3.8	4.3	36.3	40.6
Low income	$ 10	$ 25	4.1	5.1	38.2	39.4

Source: The World Bank website, www.data.worldbank.org. Income groups defined by 2010 Gross National Income per person in $US: low income, $1 005 or less; lower middle income, $1 006 – $3 975; upper middle income, $3 976 – $12 275; and high income, $12 276 or more.

Thirdly, decisions about how health care is funded, provided and distributed are strongly influenced by the economic environment and economic constraints. Global, national and local policy responses to health issues are increasingly being informed by economics ideas and methods of analysis. One good reason for understanding health economics, even if you do not intend ultimately to practise as an analyst yourself, is to be able to engage in policy debates as an informed critic. As Joan Robinson commented: 'the purpose of studying economics is not to acquire a set of ready-made answers to economic questions, but to learn how to avoid being deceived by economists' (Robinson, 1980). Less cynically, for those working in the health services, familiarity with the theory and methods of economic analysis is becoming essential, both to understand the context of professional practice and because evidence on productivity, efficiency and value for money are increasingly the norm in modern health care systems.

Health economics is the application of economic theory, models and empirical techniques to the analysis of decision making by people, health care providers and governments with respect to health and health care. It is a branch of economic science – but it is not merely the *application* of standard economic theory to health and health care as an interesting topic. Health economics is solidly based in economic theory but it also comprises a body of theory developed specifically to understand the behaviour of patients, doctors and hospitals, and analytical techniques developed to facilitate resource allocation decisions in health care. Health economics has evolved into a highly specialised field, drawing on related disciplines including epidemiology, statistics, psychology, sociology, operations research and mathematics in its approach. It may also be regarded as an essential part of a set of analytical methods applied to health, which are usually labelled *health services research*.

Chapters 2–8 deal with central economic topics such as demand, supply, efficiency, equity, and market and non-market approaches to resource allocation. Chapters 9–13 are devoted to a comprehensive treatment of a special topic, economic evaluation, including its theoretical foundations, principles, practice and uses. The rest of this chapter provides a gentle introduction to some basic economics concepts that underpin the more detailed and rigorous treatment of health economics in the remainder of the book.

1.2 Health care as an economic good

Economics is a social science. Its central concern is the study of the behaviour of economic agents – people, firms, governments and other organisations – when confronted with scarcity. Underpinning economic analysis are two general observations:

- resources are limited
- potential uses of those resources are unbounded.

Economic analysis focuses on decisions and choices about the production and consumption of *economic goods*. These are defined as any goods or services that are scarce relative to society's wants for them. Health care is therefore an economic good. The resources that are used to produce health care services, such as human resources, capital and raw materials, are finite. Society can only devote more of these resources to the production and consumption of health care by diverting them from other uses. Society's wants for health care have no known bounds. There is no known limit to what we would choose to consume in the absence of constraints on our ability to pay for it as a nation or as a consumer. No health care system, anywhere in the world, has achieved levels of spending sufficient to meet *all* of its clients' wants for health care.

The implications of regarding health care as an economic good are profound. Choices must be made about what quantity and mix of health care to produce, how to produce it, who pays for it and how it is distributed. These basic economic questions are unavoidable. Health care is not available in endless supply, and the more health care we choose, the more of something else must be sacrificed. And because health care is so important to human beings' welfare, these choices are particularly difficult and contentious.

The nature of choice, and the inevitable tradeoffs encountered in making these choices, is captured in what is probably the most fundamental notion in economics – *opportunity cost*. The opportunity cost of committing resources to produce a good or service is the benefits forgone from those same resources not being used in their next best alternative.

Each action taken by patients, health care providers or governments with respect to the use of health care involves the sacrifice of the benefits that would have been enjoyed by other, alternative uses of the resources used to provide that care. The concept of opportunity cost lies at the heart of *all* economic analysis. When economists refer to cost, we mean opportunity cost, not an accounting category. For example, weighing up the costs and benefits of a decision to make beta-interferon available to all multiple sclerosis patients means comparing the benefits gained by those patients from that treatment to the benefits that would have been gained by using the same resources to treat patients suffering from other conditions. Box 1.1 illustrates the concept of opportunity cost in relation to a 2004 recommendation by the UK National Institute for Health and Clinical Excellence that the NHS should fund *in vitro* fertilisation (IVF) services for infertility (NICE, 2004).

BOX 1.1   The opportunity cost of *in vitro* fertilisation (IVF)

To provide one course of IVF treatment, the UK's National Health Service pays around £3 300 in 2010/11 prices. If each patient received, on average, three courses of IVF, the benefit, for women less than 40 years of age, is an increase in the probability of a successful pregnancy, defined as a live birth, of 0.3. Is this good value for money? Answering this question requires us explicitly to weigh up this benefit against the opportunity cost (Devlin and Parkin, 2003). The resources devoted to each IVF patient could instead be used to provide:

In the UK health care sector:

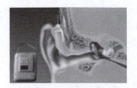

One-half of a cochlear implant

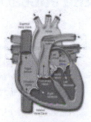

One heart bypass operation

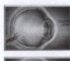
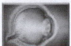

Nine cataract removals

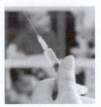

Three hundred vaccinations for
measles, mumps and rubella (MMR)

Elsewhere in the UK public sector:

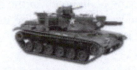

One-four-hundreth of a Challenger 2
military tank

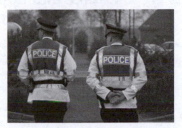

One-third of a police constable
for a year

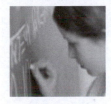

Three-quarters of a school teaching
assistant for a year

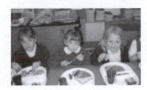

Five thousand school dinners

Sources:

Costs of IVF: National Institute for Clinical Excellence (2004) *Costing clinical guidelines: fertility (England)* 23 February 2004. Updated to 2010/11 prices using Curtis, L. *Unit Costs of Health & Social Care, 2010*. Personal Social Services Research Unit, University of Kent, Canterbury.

National average costs for cochlear implants, heart bypass operations and cataract removals: National Schedule of Reference Costs.

Costs for MMR: British National Formulary and Curtis (*op cit*).

Challenger 2 price estimates: www.armedforces.co.uk/army/listings/l0023.html.

Police Officer salary estimates: www.police-information.co.uk/policepay.htm.

Salary for teaching assistants: www.teaching-assistants.co.uk.

Cost of school dinners: www.jamieoliver.com/.

Focusing on opportunity cost provides a powerful way of sharpening thinking about decision making at all levels of the health care system. Table 1.2 represents these decisions as a series of choices, identifying the opportunity costs associated with each.

TABLE 1.2	Choice and opportunity cost in the allocation of health care resources

iel Implications to other areas.

We face choices about:	If we decide to:	The opportunity cost is:
How much should we spend on health care as a country?	Increase public spending on health care by increasing taxes/social insurance contributions	Lower net incomes for consumers, so benefits of private consumption are forgone. Higher taxes for firms either lowers profits, reducing incentives to invest and creating incentives to cut costs, including labour costs, or results in increased prices where taxes can be 'passed on' to consumers
	Increase public spending on health care by spending less on other government services	The benefits forgone from lower education, social welfare or defence spending
	Increase public spending on health care by running a fiscal debt	Economy-wide consequences of public sector debt and borrowing
How much of the health care budget is allocated to each state/region/health care purchaser?	Increase the share of the total health care budget devoted to one geographical area/health care purchaser	The health and other benefits forgone from reduced health care services in other areas
What share of the purchaser's budget should we devote to each type of health care service or product?	Increase the resources devoted to one set of services or products	The health and other benefits forgone from reduced resources for other services and products

Which patients should get access to the treatments we have decided to fund?	Ensure patients with particular characteristics, for example those who have been waiting the longest, get access to services	The health and other benefits forgone as a result of those same services not being made available to other patients, with different characteristics
How much of our limited income as consumers should be spent on health-related versus non-health-related goods and services?	Spend more of our income on health-related goods and services	The utility forgone from our consumption of other goods and services

In a predominantly tax-funded health care system such as those in New Zealand and the UK, where the government fixes the budget at the start of each period, these choices are effectively a 'top-down' hierarchy of decisions, implemented in roughly the order shown. In other health care systems, such as Germany's social insurance system, or the complex mix of private insurance and federal- and state-funded programmes in the USA, there is no hierarchy. For example, how much is spent on health care overall is partly determined 'bottom-up', by decisions of individual insurers and patients.

Regardless of how the health care system is organised, the key point is this: the production and consumption of health care incurs real, human costs, as well as creating real, human benefits.

1.3 Health and health care

We have referred to the subject matter of this book as health economics, but we have so far mainly discussed health care. This is an important point: *health* economics is not shorthand for *health care* economics. Although health economists are interested in health care as a sector of the economy, they are equally interested in its ultimate aim, which is to improve health. Health economics studies not only the provision of health care, but also how this impacts on patients' health. Other means by which health can be improved are also of interest, as are the determinants of ill-health. Health economics studies not only how health care affects population health, but also the effects of education, housing, unemployment and lifestyles.

This is not to say that improving health is the only characteristic of health care that health economics takes into account. Many types of health care may impact on other aspects of a person's welfare. For example, it may provide reassurance or increased anxiety about their health state, whether or not their health itself is changed. Some services offered by health professionals and health care organisations may be intended only to have such an impact, by simply providing information about health. And even when the main or sole purpose of health care is to improve health, the way in which it is provided may also be important. For example, the quality of meals that are provided during a stay in hospital may be important to people even if that aspect has no impact on health. But for most types of health care, their most important and interesting characteristic is that they are intended to alter health, not that they are services provided by the health care industry.

Given the importance of thinking about health itself, how is it to be conceptualised so that we can apply economic reasoning to it? The most powerful and important insight is that in addition to health care being an economic good, health itself can be thought of as a good, albeit one with special characteristics. It can be regarded as a 'fundamental commodity', one of the true objects of people's wants and for which other more tangible goods and services such as health care are simply a means to create it. This theory originates from the work of Becker (1965) and Grossman (1972), but can be traced to eighteenth-century economists, principally Jeremy Bentham, who wrote of 'the relief of pain' as a 'basic pleasure' (Bentham, 1780). Economically relevant characteristics of health are that it can be manufactured by people and households; that it has an impact on people's welfare; that it is wanted and people are willing to pay for improvements in it; and that it is scarce relative to people's wants for it. Obviously, it is less tangible than conventional goods, though it may manifest itself in tangible ways such as sickness episodes. It also cannot be traded because it is intrinsic to people and cannot normally be transferred to others. Nevertheless, it is possible to derive important analytical insights by applying to it economic analysis tools such as demand and production theory, as will be demonstrated in Chapters 2 and 3. But in each case, as we discuss below, this application is not straightforward.

1.4 Wants, demands and needs

If we accept that health is a 'fundamental commodity', we can analyse the demand for improvements in health in very similar ways to the analysis of demand for other goods and services. A key difference is that, because health cannot be traded, it is not possible to analyse it in the context of a market. Improvements in health cannot be purchased directly. Instead, we focus on the production of health as the key means by which people express their demand for it. This may involve the purchase of goods such as health care, thereby indirectly purchasing health improvements. Health care therefore has a 'derived demand' from the demand for health. Of course, such analysis can be used for almost any goods or services but it is particularly important in health because health care consumption is usually not in itself pleasurable. Indeed it is often the opposite. It is undertaken simply to improve health.

In analysing the demand for most goods and services, economics distinguishes between a *want*, which is simply the desire by someone to consume something, and *effective demand*, which is a want backed up by the willingness and ability to pay for it. Although these concepts can easily be applied to the analysis of the demand for health care, there is a complication. There is a widespread view that what matters in health care is not wants or demands, but *needs*. 'Need' is a far less precise concept than demand and is open to a number of different definitions. (See, for example, Bradshaw, 1972). However, health economists generally interpret the need for health care as the *capacity to benefit* from it, that is, to obtain a valued improvement in health from it. It follows, therefore, that not all wants are needs and vice versa. For example, many women opt to give birth by caesarean section. It is one of the most commonly performed surgical procedures amongst women in the UK and in 2009/10, 40% of these procedures were elective (NHS Information Centre, 2010). Clearly many women *want* caesareans, but sometimes for reasons which are not related to health; indeed, the procedure entails some risks. Further, some needs are not wants. For example, a person may experience pain and discomfort relating to their teeth and recognise that they would benefit from seeking dental treatment, but they may not *want* to seek care.

As we will see, the implications of basing the allocation of health care resources on needs rather than demands are profound. They call into question some of the most deeply-held assumptions and convictions held in economics, such as the primacy of the consumer's viewpoint in assessing their own welfare and the reliability of market forces to create efficient outcomes.

1.5 The production of health and health care

Like any good or service, health care is produced, and an understanding of many important issues in health economics requires knowledge of production theory. It is important in analysing health care costs and supply, discussed in more detail in Chapter 3. It is also a key input to the understanding and practice of economic evaluation, which is the subject of Chapters 9–13 of this book. It underlies some of the analysis of efficiency, which is, as discussed below, a key evaluative criterion. Moreover, as explained above, production is an important element of the theory of demand for health, so again some knowledge of concepts and tools of production analysis is required. It is therefore worthwhile considering briefly here the key elements and how they are applied in health economics.

Analysis of production is based on the concept of a *production function*. This is simply a relationship between the inputs to a productive process and the outputs of that process. Inputs are resources such as personnel, equipment, buildings and raw materials. Outputs might, for example, be an amount of health care of a given quality. A production function focuses on analysing the relationship between quantities of inputs and quantities of outputs. It is not, however, a detailed description of the production process itself. Indeed, the production process is often regarded as a 'black box' into which resources disappear and out of which outputs emerge, as illustrated in Figure 1.1. There may of course be other factors that affect the relationship between inputs and outputs, for example market conditions, so the production function also takes account of 'mediating factors' as the figure shows.

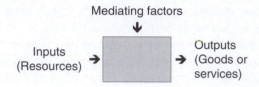

Figure 1.1 Production function

This model is valuable because it can be used to analyse many different issues in the same framework. This flexibility arises because we can measure inputs and outputs in different ways, and look at different aspects of the relationships between them. For example, we can measure inputs as quantities of physical resources or weight them according to prices or costs. Similarly, outputs can be measured in physical quantities or in terms of prices, costs or other values. By varying all inputs by the same amount and looking at the impact on output, we can look at economies of scale: is it more efficient to have large or small hospitals? By looking at the impact on output of changing one input, we can look at productivity: if we add an extra nurse to a hospital, how much does it raise the number of treatments that the hospital provides? By looking at how different combinations of inputs can produce the same level of output, we can analyse substitution between different resources: is it more efficient for nurses to replace doctors in undertaking certain tasks?

Application of this model to the production of health by individual people, which will be covered in detail in Chapter 2, uses very similar kinds of analysis. For example, what combination of prevention, self care and professional care would most efficiently produce a desired level of health?

At the other extreme, it has been proposed (for example Evans *et al.*, 1994; Parkin and Devlin, 2003; Mullahy, 2010) that such models might be used to study the health of populations and its production. This provides a distinctive economics contribution to the study of the *social determinants of health*, which is a key element of global public health initiatives to improve equity in health (CSDH, 2008). An example is the *pathways to health* model described by Birch *et al.* (2000).

1.6 Deciding who gets what in health care

As noted, to state that health care is an economic good is not to suggest that it is the same as other consumer goods and services in every relevant respect. Indeed, a considerable part of past and current research in health economics is concerned with the questions of whether or not health care is 'different', if so, in what ways it differs and what the implications are for how society organises its production and consumption. Economics is concerned with *what* is produced, *how* it is produced and *for whom* it is produced. Should these issues be decided differently for health care?

One way in which such decisions might be made is to allow market forces to determine who gets what. This is precisely the way in which production and consumption decisions are

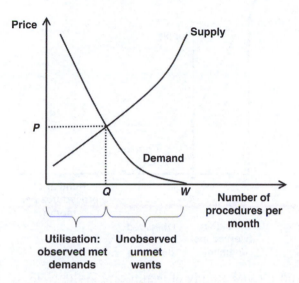

Figure 1.2 The demand for and supply of liposuction

made about most economic goods and services – clothes, domestic insurance, MP3 players, industrial fork-lift trucks, books, wine, estate agencies, cinemas. In the absence of government intervention, firms decide how much to produce and how to produce it, guided by the profit motive. Consumers decide how much to purchase and from where to purchase it, guided by their own view of their interests. Simple economic models of supply and demand predict how firms and consumers behave in such markets, and in some cases these will be relevant to health care.

For example, in most countries, cosmetic surgery, such as liposuction, is bought and sold in private markets. A simple model is illustrated in Figure 1.2. The demand and supply curves are explained in more detail in Chapters 2–4. Briefly, the demand curve slopes downward from left to right, indicating that as the price of liposuction falls the demand for it increases. The supply curve is upward sloping from left to right, indicating that as the price rises, the supply of liposuction also rises. The model suggests that market forces will establish an equilibrium price, marked as P, where the number of services demanded equals the number of services supplied, marked as Q. In a private market such as this, not everyone who wants cosmetic surgery receives it. People who obtain such services are those who are both willing and able to pay for them. We can readily observe these effective demands. However, potential consumers who are not willing and able to pay the market price are invisible. If liposuction were free (price $= 0$), the demand for it would be as high as the point marked W. But the market does not generate information about W and we do not observe wants that are *not* satisfied (W-Q).

However, in most countries and for most health care services and products, a reliance on unfettered market forces is rare. Typically, governments intervene in health care markets to a far greater degree than most other economic goods. They regulate who may provide services, what providers can charge or what profits they may earn. They subsidise health care either partially or fully, funded via various types of taxes. In some cases, they directly provide health

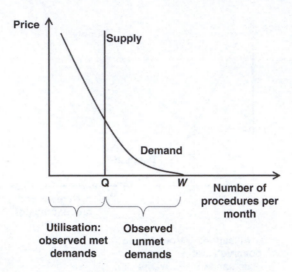

Figure 1.3 The demand for and supply of health care in the NHS

care, such as public hospitals. In the case of the UK National Health Service (NHS), the government dominates funding and provision of health care, so supply is essentially fixed in each time period by political decisions. Moreover, most health care is fully subsidised, so that nothing is charged at the point of consumption. Effective demand is therefore higher than it would be if patients had to pay. Figure 1.3 shows a highly stylised economic model of the NHS, treating all health care services as measurable in some comparable units on the horizontal axis. The demand curve is defined analogously to that in Figure 1.2. Because price = 0, effective demand is now at W. The supply curve is vertical, because supply is fixed at the level Q. Without a price system to reconcile supply and demand, demand exceeds supply by W-Q. Who obtains health services is determined by factors other than price, for example, by waiting lists. A crucial difference with the market model of Figure 1.2 is that W-Q can be observed. Because there is no distinction between wants, demands and needs, free care may generate observed unmet needs.

Figures 1.2 and 1.3 show two extreme cases: a complete reliance on private markets and a complete reliance on public provision. In each case, not everyone who wants health care gets it. Health care is rationed, either by price or by some other mechanism. In practice, most health care systems are a complex mix of private and public sector activities. Why are governments so often involved in health care? What is it that makes health care 'special'?

1.7 Is the market for health care special?

In a seminal paper, which is still requisite reading for any serious student of health economics, Arrow (1963) analysed the characteristics that make health care different to other goods and services. He concluded that 'taken together, they do establish a special place for medical care in economic analysis'.

Arrow asserted that the principal characteristic of medical care is uncertainty and that 'the special economic problems of medical care can be explained as adaptations to the existence of uncertainty'. Uncertainty arises in two ways. First, we do not know when we will become ill, or what health care we will require when ill, or at what cost. Whereas the demand for most goods, for example food, is regular and predictable, ill health occurs randomly and its consequences can be severe. Secondly, there is uncertainty about how any given state of ill health will respond to health care. Recovery from a disease is as uncertain as its incidence.

Arrow noted the following key characteristics of consumer and provider behaviour in medical markets.

Patients Do Not Behave in the Same Way as Consumers

- They cannot 'test' the product before consuming it. Indeed, they often have difficulty gauging the quality of care even *after* experiencing it. Consumers of health care find it difficult to 'shop around' to get the best deal.
- It is difficult for patients to obtain information about what medical care is appropriate for their condition – medical knowledge is complex. As consumers, patients know considerably less than sellers, and place trust in the provider of care.
- There are interdependencies between consumers' actions. The health care seeking behaviour of one consumer may affect the outcome of others, for example immunising against an infectious disease decreases the likelihood of others becoming infected. In a more general sense, this interdependency extends to people caring about the health of others.

Doctors Do Not Behave in the Same Way as Firms

- Their entry into this 'industry' is restricted by medical licensing regulations.
- Advertising and overt competition are virtually absent in medical markets.
- Advice given by physicians is supposed to be completely divorced from self-interest. Treatment is, or at least is claimed to be, dictated by clinical need, not by the financial interests of the provider.
- Providers with goals other than profit maximisation dominate provision. Profit maximisation is unlikely to be the sole or principal motivation of providers. Social and ethical factors are likely to be as important in determining their behaviour.
- Doctors sometimes charge different fees to different people: high fees to high-income people, and low fees to people with low incomes including, sometimes, charging no fees to very poor people.

The central tenet of Arrow's work is that *all* of these special economic features of medical care stem from uncertainty. Entry to the medical profession is limited to those who have met certain medical training requirements, because consumers cannot judge quality for themselves and need to be protected. And, because patients are poorly informed about what treatment is best for them, trust is the key feature in the doctor–patient relationship. If doctors were perceived to be behaving in a commercially aggressive manner, or their decisions to be influenced by pecuniary gain, this trust would quickly break down.

Finally, Arrow also noted that while the uncertainty element of ill health can be partly addressed through insurance markets, this too is problematic. Insurance markets work best where there is a given probability of an insured event arising, but for many illnesses demand is certain, because they are pre-existing chronic conditions. There will therefore be gaps in coverage. Many people will not be able to purchase health care insurance. Further, insurance works well if the person insured is unable to modify the probability of making a claim. In many cases, the demand for medical care will increase as a result of being insured, as consumers seek, and doctors provide, more and higher-quality care.

Arrow was careful not to claim that these characteristics are unique to medical care markets. Many markets for professional services share these characteristics. However, taken together, they suggest that health care is a special case. The behaviours of consumers and providers of medical care are very different from the norm of a competitive market in standard economic theory. This has two implications.

First, economic analysis of health and health care behaviours requires specialised theoretical approaches that acknowledge these differences. Arrow's paper marked the intellectual beginnings of health economics. Since then, theoretical and empirical research on these issues, detailed in subsequent chapters, has considerably improved our understanding of medical markets.

Secondly, a reliance on unregulated private markets for medical care is unlikely to produce outcomes that are socially optimal. Private markets are efficient where consumers are well informed and choose firms that deliver high-quality goods at competitive prices over poor-quality, high-price firms. In such markets, the consumer's strategy is represented by the phrase *caveat emptor* – let the buyer beware. In medical care, the roles of consumers and providers are very different, and the behaviours of each are affected by the incentives created by third-party payment for care by private or social insurance or by government.

1.8 Describing versus evaluating the use of health care resources

We have established that, although health care is an economic good, the ways in which consumers and producers of health care behave are often fundamentally different from those observed in other markets. Economic analysis plays a valuable role in *describing* these behaviours and *predicting* the outcomes of market interactions, in terms of prices, quantities traded and the distribution of services between people. However, economic analysis frequently goes beyond description and prediction and is concerned with *evaluating* how resources are used. Much of economics, including health economics, is concerned with whether or not one set of arrangements is preferable to another.

Analysis that is restricted to the description or prediction of behaviours and outcomes is called *positive economics* (Friedman, 1953). Positive economics investigates the relationship between economic variables, by both theoretical and empirical analyses. For example, we might describe the market for dental care in the UK as regulated private practices that provide services to patients who pay a price for care that is subsidised by the state. We might construct a theoretical model that predicts that as price rises, demand falls. We could then obtain data on prices, use of services and other relevant factors and use statistical analysis to test this theory. Examples of evidence of this kind are the studies by Beazoglou *et al.* (1993) and Stahlnacke *et al.* (2005). We might conclude from the first of these studies that an increase in the price of dental services by 10% will, controlling for other factors, lead to a reduction in the number of dental services demanded by about 6%. Such an analysis provides useful information for dentists and those concerned with oral health policy. But it does not judge the desirability of prices increasing, decreasing or staying the same. It simply tells us the consequences.

In principle, economic analysis establishes facts in the same way as other sciences do, by describing theoretical relationships tested by real-world data. Positive economic statements, whether derived empirically or from theoretical analysis, are in principle testable. However, many economists' statements take the form of *stylised facts*. These are simplifications and generalisations of empirical findings, without precise scientific details. For example, a precise estimate of the response of demand for dental care to price changes is valid only for the conditions under which the data were collected, such as the place and the time. Stahlnacke *et al.* (2005) found that changes in price did not affect utilisation appreciably. But if a similar estimate was found in many other places and at many different times, we might state a stylised fact that dental care demand is not very responsive to price changes. Any theory of the demand for dental care would then have to be consistent with this finding.

Unfortunately, stylised facts are prone to misuse and to interpretation beyond the scientific goals of positive economics. As an example, Newhouse (1998) reported a survey of health economists in the USA and the UK, in which participants were asked whether or not they agreed with various propositions. One of these was that 'technological change is responsible for most of the medical care cost increase', which is a positive statement because it can be tested by reference to evidence. The vast majority (81%) of economists from the USA agreed, but only around half (51%) of UK health economists agreed. Newhouse regarded agreement as a 'correct' answer, although this is not surprising, as he is from the USA! The problem here is that the evidence may be very different in each country. In the USA, market forces largely drive technological change. However in the UK, increases in health spending are politically determined and responses to technology are a matter of choice (Dolan, 1999). So this statement is context dependent and any view that it is a fact that can only be correct or incorrect, in a positive economics sense, is of doubtful validity.

Scientifically based positive economics provides useful information about how the world works. However, economics is also interested in what we ought to do with that information.

For example, our study of the responsiveness of the demand for dental care to price might be used to determine what level of subsidy the government should provide to patients. Should it be reduced to deter excess demand, or increased to decrease unmet need? Such questions are typical of those that health economists are asked to investigate. Should we pay doctors on a fee-for-service basis or by salaries? Should the UK continue to fund health care through general taxation or should it adopt a French-style social insurance system? Should the government continue to subsidise primary health care fully or should GPs' patients be required to pay a fee? Should nurses be allowed full prescribing rights? Should Aricept™ be made available to people who have Alzheimer's disease?

In each case, scientifically based positive economics can be used to *describe* the outcomes, but a policy prescription ultimately relies on *value judgements* about their relative desirability. A value judgement is a weighing up of evidence based on the ethical and ideological values that a person or society holds. Analysis that relies at any point on value judgements is labelled *normative economics*. A normative statement can often be recognised by the inclusion of the word 'should'. For example, the NHS *should not* provide IVF because it provides small health benefits that are outweighed by its large costs. In summary, normative economics is concerned with the desirability of alternative economic outcomes; it is prescriptive in nature and rests on value judgements.

We noted above that an important implication of Arrow's observations about medical markets is that a reliance on private market interactions cannot be assumed to produce socially optimal outcomes. Although it does not make explicit recommendations, Arrow's paper is undertaken within a *normative* intellectual framework, observing, for example, that 'it is the general social consensus, clearly, that the *laissez-faire* solution for medicine is intolerable'. The appropriate balance between private markets and public involvement is a central theme of health economics, which we will return to throughout this book.

Finally, it is important to note that the distinction between positive and normative economics is not always as clear-cut as our definitions above might suggest. One extreme view is that *all* economics research is normatively driven, because people choose which questions form the focus of positive economic investigation. This reflects their view on the relative importance of the topics and variables selected for analysis (Katouzian, 1980). Moreover, the interpretation of theory and data can be selected to fit a particular set of values. For example, we could use the simple supply and demand model illustrated by Figures 1.2 and 1.3 to make two points supportive of publicly funded provision of health care. First, public funded systems do not create rationing of care. The price mechanism simply rations in a different way to mechanisms that are used in public services, such as waiting lists. Secondly, public funding exposes but does not create unmet need. Public and private systems may have an equal amount of unmet need, but it is manifest in public provision and hidden in private provision. However, we could equally use the model to make a normatively different point. Publicly provided health care is not related to the value that consumers attach to health care, as expressed by their willingness to pay, resulting in arbitrary shortages manifested as waiting lists. Given these ambiguities and complexities, a valuable skill for health economists to possess is the ability to scrutinise critically economic theory and empirical analysis – including the theory and analysis covered in this book! – so that its normative content, both explicit and implicit, can be identified.

1.9 Judging the use of health care resources

Economic analysis conventionally judges the use of resources using the criteria of *efficiency* and *equity*, which are dealt with in more detail in later chapters. These concepts arguably provide the main contribution of economics to decision making in health care. However, health economics inevitably has to deal with other criteria that may have analogies in other areas of economics but do not assume the same importance. The two most important are *effectiveness* and *ethics*.

Efficiency is one of the most important concepts in both positive and normative economics. Chapters 3 and 8 contain more precise and specific definitions, but for now a generic and non-technical definition is instructive. Knapp (1984) defined efficiency as 'the allocation of scarce resources that maximises the achievement of aims'.

The economic problem described earlier was that there are scarce resources and potentially unbounded uses for them. If our aim is to obtain the 'best' set of uses, defined in whatever way we like, then efficiency is simply the use of resources that maximises our achievement of it. For example, if our aim is to improve the health of the population given a fixed health care budget, an efficient allocation of resources will maximise the achievement of that aim.

In economic analysis more generally, efficiency issues largely concern the quantities provided of goods or services or the values attached to them. Whether or not the good or service actually 'works' is not usually a concern. However, health economics has to face this more fundamental issue: are health care services effective in improving health? Economic analyses often assume that it is not possible for health services to be efficient unless they are effective, but the nature of health and health care means that effectiveness is not a clear-cut issue. In particular, economic evaluation of health care, which is covered in Chapters 9–13, has to deal explicitly with the uncertainty surrounding health care effectiveness.

Efficiency is a relatively straightforward criterion compared with equity. It is far less clear how, for positive purposes, it should be measured and how, for normative purposes, it should be judged. It is far harder to give a general definition of equity, other than to distinguish it from efficiency and from other related concepts such as equality. Essentially, equity is a synonym for fairness. In this context, it means fairness in the distribution of health and health care between people. Equity is also relevant to assessments of the means by which health care is financed, principally the burden of finance, and whether the amount of money that people pay for health care is fair. Efficiency is largely concerned with the aim of maximising the value to society of health and health care, arising from production, consumption and distribution conditions, while equity is concerned with distribution itself. Equity, which means a fair distribution, is not synonymous with equality, which means an equal distribution. Under many circumstances equality may be fair, but not always; for example it may not be fair to devote equal amounts of health care to healthy and sick people.

Economic analysis of equity issues has both positive and normative aspects. Positive analysis focuses on measuring or describing distributional characteristics, such as how health, utilisation of health care or health care spending are spread over individual people or groups in society. Equity is not the same as equality, but positive analysis usually defines equity in terms of equality. For example, do people have equal access to health care given equal needs for it? Do people with equal use of health care services pay the same amount of money for that use irrespective of their ability to pay for it?

Normative analyses depend to a great extent on views about which equalities define fairness. We may come to different conclusions about equity if we define it as equal health outcomes for equal desert or as equal use of health services for equal willingness to pay for it. It should be said that there is far less agreement within economics about equity than about efficiency and that other disciplines such as philosophy have more to say about it. But it is always an important consideration in economics, and one of the special characteristics of health and health care is that people attach more importance to equity than for many other goods and services. Chapter 7 looks at these issues and their consequences in more detail.

As we have seen, normative economics requires us to acknowledge the role of values in making judgements. Usually these values are based on ideology, but in health and health care they are often based on ethics. In principle, ethical issues apply to the economic analysis of many goods and services, but in health and health care they are especially important. Health care professionals have developed normative criteria that, if implemented, impact on the way in which health care resources are used. For example, the Stanford University Medical Center Committee on Ethics (Ruark and Raffin, 1988) has promulgated a set of ethical principles: preserve life; alleviate suffering; do no harm; tell the truth; respect the patient's autonomy; and deal justly with patients. These principles are unexceptional when applied to individual patients but, taken literally, they may conflict with economic analysis when applied to society, where there are many patients. Given limited resources, preserving life for one person might have the opportunity cost of failing to alleviate suffering for another. A more sophisticated ethical code might resolve this conflict.

Ethical issues are also often raised about the way in which economic issues are addressed. A particularly widespread view is that it is ethically wrong for people to profit from others' ill-health. But what is meant by profit? Does this for example include the salaries of doctors and nurses? Does it include payments received for the use of land for hospitals and clinics? Or the income that firms obtain from selling medical supplies? Critics who take this view may really be referring to what economists call 'supernormal profits', an excess of revenue over costs, where the costs include a reasonable return on the person's human, physical or financial assets. Whatever the specifics of this view are, it does lead to a general discomfort with market-based solutions to health care issues. Box 1.2 provides an example of the discomfort generated by proposals to allow trade in human organs.

BOX 1.2   Why not allow a market in human organs?

The United Network for Organ Sharing (UNOS) reported in September 2011 that 72 500 USA citizens were waiting for organs, principally kidneys, for transplant operations that would dramatically improve their length and quality of life. UK Transplant reported in September 2011 that approximately 7 500 people are waiting for organs in the UK, but fewer than 4 000 transplants are performed each year. In nearly all countries there is a persistent shortfall between the number of organs available – the supply of organs – and the number of potential recipients – the demand for them. This results in a substantial loss of life and health. Human organs, tissues and blood products are clearly economic goods.

Why do these shortages persist? One reason is that medical technology has increased the success rate of transplantation, reducing the rate of rejection and increasing the number and type of operations that can be performed. It is alleged that another reason is that the supply of organs relies exclusively on voluntary donations: trade in organs is prohibited in the USA, as it is in all Western countries.

In 1999, the BBC reported that an eBay trader in Florida attempted to sell one 'fully functioning kidney'. Bidding started at $25 000 and reached nearly $6 million before eBay removed the offer from its web-based auction. In 2003 it also reported that a man had put a kidney for sale on eBay to pay for medical treatment for his daughter. The outrage surrounding these events suggests a widespread view that buying and selling human organs is abhorrent. In January 2011, *The Independent* newspaper reported that 'Leading surgeons are calling for the Government to consider the merits of a legalised market in organs for transplant. A public discussion on allowing people to sell their organs would, the doctors say, allow a better-informed decision on a matter of such moral and medical significance.' However, an 18-month enquiry by the Nuffield Council on Bioethics (2011), reporting later the same year, concluded that paying for organ donation should not be permitted because it might deter those who donate for free. It suggested that the NHS should test the idea of paying for the funerals of organ donors as an ethical way of encouraging more people to sign up as organ donors.

Economists have for many years debated the case for allowing markets in blood – for a famous example see Cooper and Culyer (1968) and Titmuss (1972) – and in organs. The main argument in favouring of legalising trade is that it would improve the supply of good-quality organs. Whether or not it will do so is a positive economics question. An economic evaluation could establish if the health benefits from the extra supply outweigh the health benefits that would be forgone by using scarce resources to collect organs commercially. If that were the case, then there is an ethical counter to the argument that trade in organs is abhorrent. The premature death and ill health resulting from an inadequate supply of donated organs is also abhorrent. Which is worse?

Sources:

Kidney sale on Web halted. BBC News, September 3 1999. www.bbc.co.uk/news

Father auctions kidney for daughter. BBC News, 4 December, 2003. www.bbc.co.uk/news

Doctors argue against changes on organ donation. The Independent, Wednesday, 5 January 2011. www.independent.co.uk/

United Network for Organ Sharing (UNOS). www.unos.org.

UK Transplant. www.uktransplant.org.uk/ekt/statistics.

Summary

1. Health economics is the application of economic theory, models and empirical techniques to the analysis of decision-making by people, health care providers and governments with respect to health and health care.

2. It is important because it offers a unique and systematic intellectual framework for analysing important issues in health care. This is useful because the health care sector consumes a great deal of resources, and because the organisation and delivery of health care are strongly influenced by the economic environment and economic constraints.

3. An economic good is any good or service that is scarce relative to our wants for it. Health care is an economic good.

4. A fundamental notion in economics is opportunity cost. The opportunity cost of committing resources to produce a good or service is the benefits forgone from those same resources not being used in their next best alternative. Consideration of opportunity cost means that the production and consumption of health care incurs real, human costs, as well as creating real, human benefits.

5. In order to understand the economics of health care it is important to understand the wants, needs and demand for health and health care by consumers, and the production of health and health care by producers.

6. Most health care systems are a complex mix of private and public sector activities. Government involvement in the finance and provision of health care is common. An important reason for this is the inherent uncertainty surrounding health and health care.

7. Economists often distinguish between positive and normative economics. Positive economics is concerned with investigating the relationship between economic variables. Normative economics is concerned with the desirability of alternative economic outcomes. Health economics has both positive and normative aspects.

8. In economics, it is conventional to judge the use of resources using the criteria of efficiency and equity. Efficiency can be simply defined as the allocation of scarce resources that maximises the achievement of aims. Equity is fairness in the distribution and finance of health and health care between people.

9. In health economics, we also have to take account of effectiveness and ethics. Effectiveness concerns whether or not health care 'works'; ethics essentially concerns strong value judgements widely held in health care.

CHAPTER 2

The demand for health care

2.1 Why study demand? Profits, policy and improving health

As we saw in Chapter 1, there are many different ways in which health systems may be funded and organised. But in every type of system, an understanding of the demand for health care is fundamentally important. In private health care markets, firms have a keen interest in knowing the determinants of demand for their products and services so that they can forecast responses to changes in prices and consumers' circumstances, and the consequences for their revenues and profits. In public systems, information on population and patient demands enables policy makers to predict health care use. They can then modify demand through measures such as charges or subsidies to meet health policy targets. Economic models of demand and of consumer choice theory are clearly of interest to providers and funders of health care. They also provide the fundamental basis for methods used to value health improvements and health services, as detailed in Chapters 9–13 of this book, which deal with the principles and methods of economic evaluation.

This chapter will familiarise you with economic theory of consumer choice applied to health and health care. It will show how that theory informs empirical analysis and the insights that research provides into consumers' behaviour. Throughout, we use the term 'good' to mean both services, such as consultations with a doctor, and more tangible physical products, such as hearing aids. We also use the term 'consumers' rather than 'patients'. This is both because this is consistent with the language of economic theory and also because not everyone who demands health care is a patient. Only those who become health professionals' customers are patients. We also use the term consumers for those who purchase health care services but who are not patients, principally those who act as agents on behalf of patients.

2.2 Consumer choice theory

2.2.1 Preferences and utility

Economists define the demand for any good, including health care, as the quantity that consumers are both willing and able to buy. Demand for a good therefore depends on both what consumers want and their ability to afford it. The law of demand evident in a downward-sloping demand curve, such as that shown in Figures 1.2 and 1.3 in Chapter 1, states that other things being equal, the higher the price, the lower the demand. Underlying this relationship between price and quantity demanded is a behavioural model of consumers' choices. Consumer choice theory explains *why* consumers behave or react in certain ways to changes in various factors. As we shall see, these models can provide rich insights into health-related choices and behaviours.

Consumer choice theory is based on the idea that people obtain *utility* by consuming goods. Utility describes the level of satisfaction that consumers obtain through having their desires met. Consumers' decisions are then driven by a single objective – the maximisation of utility. The relationship between the level of utility that they experience, U, and their consumption of different quantities of goods, X_i, can be represented as a *utility function*:

$$U = U(X_1, X_2, \ldots, X_n) \tag{2.1}$$

The *marginal utility* of a good is the additional utility obtained from one unit of it, which can be defined as

$$MU_{Xi} = \Delta U / \Delta X_i \tag{2.2}$$

If the good is infinitely divisible, so that the function in equation (2.1) is differentiable, marginal utility can be defined as a partial derivative, $\partial U / \partial X_i$.

Consumers are assumed to be *rational*, which essentially means that their behaviour is consistent with their aims. People behave as if they act in their own interest and make decisions with the aim of maximising their wellbeing. To do this, their utility function must obey certain conventions. A consumer must be able to compare any two 'bundles' – a term meaning a particular collection of different goods – and decide whether they either prefer one to the other or find them equally desirable. They must be capable of expressing such preferences for all possible bundles, which is known as a *complete preference ordering*. Preferences must also be logically consistent by being *transitive*. This means that if they judge one bundle a as better than another bundle b, and b as better than a third possible bundle c, then a should also be preferred to c. Finally, consumers' wants must be *non-satiable*. This means that increased consumption of any good will always increase their utility. Consumers always want more.

The effect of different bundles on utility can be represented as *indifference curves*, which are illustrated in Figure 2.1. An indifference curve shows all combinations of the consumption

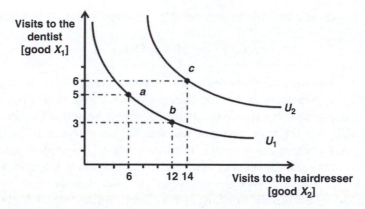

Figure 2.1 Indifference curves

of two goods that give a consumer the same level of satisfaction. In other words, the consumer is indifferent between these bundles of goods. For simplicity, imagine a world in which there are only two alternatives to choose between: visits to the dentist (good X_1), and visits to the hairdresser (good X_2). Points a and b in Figure 2.1 represent two quite different bundles of dentist and hairdresser services. However, each generates the same utility to the consumer, U_1. Indifference curves further from the origin generate higher levels of utility. For example, bundle c, which has more of both services compared to both a and b, generates a higher level of utility, U_2. Although only two indifference curves are drawn here, every conceivable combination of goods X_1 and X_2 can be placed on some indifference curve, giving an *indifference map*. Every possible bundle can therefore be compared with any other as giving either a higher, lower or the same level of utility.

Indifference curves have a negative slope, because if the person's wants are non-satiable, increases in consumption raise utility and decreases in consumption lower utility. It follows that an increase in the amount consumed of one good must be accompanied by a decrease in the amount consumed of the other good if utility is to remain the same. Any changes in the quantities of the two goods along an indifference curve must therefore have different signs, so the slope is negative. Different indifference curves also cannot cross.

The indifference curve also enables us to compare the utility that is gained from different goods. Using Figure 2.1, suppose that this person currently consumes bundle a, 5 visits to the dentist and 6 to the hairdresser. If the consumer changes to bundle b, they will gain utility from 6 extra hairdresser visits, but lose the utility from 2 fewer dentist visits. Since overall utility remains the same, these gains and losses must be equal. The change in utility for each good can be expressed in terms of their marginal utility by rearranging equation (2.2) to:

$$\Delta U = MU_{Xi}\Delta X_i \tag{2.3}$$

If overall utility remains the same, then ΔU must be equal for the two goods but with opposite signs. ΔU will be positive if ΔX_i is positive and negative if ΔX_i is negative, so that $MU_{X1}\Delta X_1 = MU_{X2}\Delta X_2$. Re-arranging this, it follows that the ratio of the change in the quantities of the goods is equal to the inverse ratio of their marginal utilities:

$$\Delta X_1 / \Delta X_2 = MU_{X2} / MU_{X1} \tag{2.4}$$

These ratios are known as the *marginal rate of substitution* (MRS) of good X_1 for good X_2, expressed as MRS_{X1X2}. The slope of the indifference curve between two points is also $\Delta X_1 / \Delta X_2$ although, as explained, because one of the ΔX_i must be negative, the slope must be negative. So the MRS has the same value as the slope of the curve, but the opposite sign.

In the example, to obtain the six extra hairdresser visits, the person must give up two dentist visits to retain the same level of utility. The MRS is therefore 2/6, and we can infer that the marginal utility of a dentist visit is 3 times that of a hairdresser visit.

Although those values apply to changes between bundles *a* and *b*, the MRS may be different for other changes. Indifference curves are usually depicted as convex to the origin, which means that the MRS_{X1X2} falls as we move along an indifference curve from left to right. Why? This assumed non-linearity in marginal utility means that as the amount of hairdresser visits increases, each additional visit confers a smaller increase in total utility than the previous visit. This assumption is known as *diminishing marginal utility of consumption*. In the same way, as consumption of dentist visits decreases, each additional visit given up generates a higher loss of utility.

The notions of utility, preferences and indifference in consumer choice theory are sometimes regarded as entirely abstract constructs. If you cannot measure utility, what practical purpose do such concepts serve? Box 2.1 shows how utility functions for health care can be estimated empirically by observing the choices that people make.

BOX 2.1   Using utility functions to understand patients' choice of hospital in the NHS

In 2002, the UK Department of Health (DH) set up an experiment to see how National Health Service (NHS) patients would respond if offered, for the first time, a choice of the NHS hospital in which they would receive their surgical procedure. The participants in the scheme had all been waiting for six or more months to receive elective surgery from their local hospital. The aim was to see how hospital demand patterns would change and what factors would affect patients' choices.

Burge *et al.* (2005) investigated these questions using a discrete choice experiment (Ryan and Farrar, 2000). This technique, discussed in more detail in Chapter 11, is based on random utility theory (Manski, 1977). It assumes that people choose between alternatives based on the alternatives' characteristics. By observing different choices when alternatives have different characteristics, the relative weight of those characteristics in the utility function can be estimated statistically.

The characteristics of hospitals that are important to patients were determined using focus groups and interviews with patients. These were: how long patients wait for surgery; the hospital's reputation; how far they travel to get treated; and where and how their post-surgical care is delivered. Patients were then asked to choose between two alternatives. One was their local hospital and the other was an alternative (hypothetical) hospital defined in terms of these characteristics – for example, the alternative might have a shorter or longer waiting time, be closer or more distant, and so on. Several such choices were offered, each with a different alternative that had varying levels of the characteristics.

The researchers found that patients like reduced waiting time, but other things matter to them as well. For every additional hour of travel time, patients require a two months' reduction in waiting time; to get treatment at a hospital with a better reputation, patients are prepared to wait an extra 3–6 months. Preferences and choices were affected by patients' own characteristics. For example, older and less educated patients were more likely to choose their local hospital, even if they could get quicker treatment elsewhere; and those on low incomes were less concerned than richer patients about hospitals' reputations. The results are being used to inform the introduction of hospital choice throughout the NHS.

2.2.2 Budget constraints and maximisation

The decisions that consumers make to maximise their utility are constrained by the budget that they have. The effective size of the budget constraint depends both on the income they have available to spend and the prices of the various goods between which they choose. The consumer receives an income (I) and faces a set of prices ($P_1, P_2, \ldots, P_n$) for each of the goods ($X_1, X_2, \ldots, X_n$). Consumers' behaviour can be modelled as a constrained maximisation problem. They maximise utility *subject to* their income and prevailing prices. In this simple example, we assume that consumers cannot borrow. Therefore the sum of the amounts that they spend on each good – the amount bought multiplied by the prevailing price – cannot exceed their total income.

$$\sum_{i=1}^{n} X_i P_i \leq I \tag{2.5}$$

Figure 2.2 illustrates the budget constraint where there are only two goods. A budget line shows the various bundles of goods X and Y that the consumer can purchase, given the constraints of their income and prevailing prices (P_X and P_Y). For example, suppose that a consumer allocates out of their total income a £500 yearly budget to hairdressing and dentistry. The price of dental visits is £100 and the price of hairdresser visits £25. The budget line's position is determined by the consumer's income and its slope is determined by the ratio of the goods' prices, P_X/P_Y. In Figure 2.2, the initial budget line, labelled P_{X1}/P_{Y1}, has the slope £25/£100 = 1/4. If the price of dental visits falls from £100 to £75 and there are no changes in other determinants of demand, the budget line will pivot upwards to P_{X1}/P_{Y2}, with a new slope £25/£75 = 1/3.

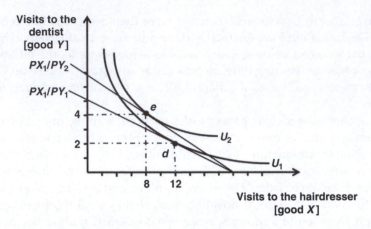

Figure 2.2 Maximising Utility

The consumer maximises utility (equation (2.1)) subject to their budget constraint (equation (2.5)). Utility is maximised when the consumer chooses a bundle of goods for which the ratio of the goods' prices (the budget line's slope) is equal to the ratio of the marginal utilities (the indifference curve's slope):

$$MRS_{XY} = -dY/dX = MU_X/MU_Y = P_X/P_Y \qquad (2.6)$$

In Figure 2.2, where prices are P_{X1}/P_{Y1}, the consumer's utility-maximising choice is point d, having 2 dentist visits and 12 hairdresser visits. When the price of hairdressing falls, the consumer's new utility-maximising choice will be at point e, having two more dentist visits and four fewer hairdresser visits. Another way of thinking about these points is that, in each case, given their preferences and prevailing prices, a utility-maximising consumer will divide their spending between the goods in such a way that $MU_X/P_X = MU_Y/P_Y$. In simple terms, the addition to utility per pound spent is equalised across all goods.

The assumptions of self-interest, rationality and utility maximisation that are central to economic models of consumer behaviour are frequently criticised on the grounds that they grossly oversimplify the factors that motivate human behaviour. For example, surely users of crack cocaine are not rational utility maximisers? Surprisingly, economic theory and evidence suggest this may not be so far fetched – see Box 2.2. Similarly, the assumptions appear to be incapable of explaining acts of charity and generosity to others, such as the donation of a kidney to strangers. Here too economic theory can cope. 'Caring' can be incorporated into economics models simply by making a person's utility function depend not just on their own consumption, but also on the consumption of others. And where one person's utility depends on the utility of others, redistribution or 'giving' can be modelled as utility-maximising behaviour (Hochman and Rodgers, 1969; Culyer, 1983). However, two important characteristics of consumer choice in health care are uncertainty and asymmetry of information between the consumer and the supplier. This has serious implications for the way health care markets might operate, which we discuss in Section 2.5 and in Chapter 5.

Nevertheless, it is worth emphasising that the purpose of economic models is to yield predictions that may be tested using data. The test of a good model is not whether its *assumptions* are realistic, but whether it is useful in explaining or predicting real-world behaviours (Friedman, 1953).

BOX 2.2 Rational addiction and price elasticity of demand

Consumer choice theory assumes consumers are rational utility maximisers. What about the consumption of heroin, cigarettes and other addictive products? Surely addicts cannot be described as rational or capable of making decisions in their own self-interest? A landmark paper on the economics of addiction, by Becker and Murphy (1988), suggests exactly that: addicted people maximise utility consistently over time.

Their basic model rests on the idea that a person's utility at any point in time (t) depends on the consumption of two goods, X and Y, where X is addictive and Y is not, and also on the past consumption of X (but not Y):

$$U(t) = U[Y(t), X(t), S(t)]$$

Past consumption of X affects current utility through a process of 'learning by doing', as summarised by the stock of consumption capital (S). The marginal utility of X depends on past values for X, as measured by S.

The definition of addiction is that a person is addicted to X if an increase in the current consumption of X leads to an increase in the future consumption of X. This is because past consumption of the good increases the marginal utility of present consumption. Assumptions are made that addicts attempt to maximise utility over their whole life, given a set of preferences and expectations about future prices.

Among the predictions of this theory is that price elasticity of demand will be lower in the short term than in the long term. This hypothesis has been tested and confirmed in a large number of empirical studies. The model itself has also been extended in various ways: for example, explicit modelling of withdrawal; incorporating uncertainty; and allowing the possibility of regret over past choices.

2.3 Demand functions

The demand curve shows the relationship between prices and the quantity of goods that consumers demand, but price is of course only one among many factors that affect demand. In economics more generally, prices are of great importance, which explains why the price/quantity relationship is at the centre of attention. However, in health care the role of prices is more subdued. In some cases, it is entirely missing, such as where the government fully subsidises a service or where it is fully covered by insurance. The demand curve is just one aspect of a more general concept labelled the *demand function*, which relates the level of consumer demand at a particular time and place to all of the factors that affect it. In this section, we will first look at what those factors are, then how we might in practice measure their effects, and finally what the evidence is of their effects on the demand for health care.

2.3.1 The determinants of demand

Health care includes a wide range of products and services, spanning health promotion, preventive interventions, diagnostic services, treatment, support services and palliation. Obviously, the nature of the relationship between demand and other factors will be quite different in each case, but the determinants of demand fall into some common categories. The most important of the factors affecting demand are generally held to be the price of the good, income, the prices of other goods, tastes and population size and composition.

Price

If the price of a good falls, we generally expect more to be demanded, other things being equal – a finding consistent with consumer choice theory and referred to as the *law of demand*. Recall that in Figure 2.2, when the price of a dental visit is £100, two are demanded. When the price falls to £75, four are demanded. Plotting these pairs of price and utility-maximising quantities on a diagram yields a downward-sloping demand curve. Such a demand curve relates to the demand by one consumer, but we can also define a market demand curve by calculating the sum of all of the individual consumers' demands at different prices, like those illustrated in Figures 1.2 and 1.3 of Chapter 1.

This law of demand is relevant for most goods. For example, we might observe a downward-sloping curve for a consumer's demand for food supplements. This relies on them buying more food supplements when the price falls. If all consumers responded to price changes in the same way, the market demand curve would also be downward sloping.

It is sometimes argued that for some sorts of health care this analysis makes no sense. For example, it might be argued that it is unlikely that anyone will purchase more cancer chemotherapy simply because its price has fallen. Chemotherapy is not in itself a desirable good, so people will only wish to consume it if they have to, and in as small quantities as possible, whatever the price. It might also be argued that some health care is life-saving, so even if its price rose the quantity that anyone would demand would not necessarily fall.

These issues about individual consumers' demand for some types of health care arise because this is often a unique event, particularly in the treatment of acute illnesses and conditions, so that only a single intervention is consumed. For example, a service such as corrective laser eye surgery is something which any given person will only demand once, so their demand curve is not downward sloping. At every price up to the maximum amount that they are willing to pay, demand is constant at one, and above that it is constant at zero.

However, because different consumers in the market are likely to have different willingness to pay, then the market demand curve will nevertheless be downward sloping with respect to price. This is because at lower prices there are more people who are consuming, rather than more consumption by individual consumers. Similarly, even for life-saving treatments such as chemotherapy there will be some observable response to price, both at the market and the individual patient level, as there are usually other treatments, in this case surgery or radiotherapy, that are substitutes.

When thinking about the price of a good, it is natural to think in terms of a payment made by a consumer to a provider. But this is often only part of the total costs that consumers must incur. As a simple example, if someone wishes to purchase a packet of aspirin, they may travel to a pharmacist, perhaps incurring transport costs, as well as paying for the drugs. In addition to these monetary outlays, there are also other costs such as the time spent travelling to and searching for the pharmacist, purchasing the drugs and returning home. Of course, this is the case for virtually all goods, but such costs are of particular importance in health care where there are subsidised user charges or even services free at the point of consumption. We can analyse the effects of such costs on consumer behaviour in the same way as prices.

Because the demand curve is of special importance in economics, it is also used to illustrate the effect on demand of factors other than price. There are some special terms used to distinguish changes in demand due to price changes from those due to changes in other factors. Figure 2.3 shows two demand curves, D_1 and D_2, that exist at different levels of the other factors. When the price of the good changes, there is a movement along the demand curve. For example, with the curve D_1, if price rises from P_1 to P_2 the quantity demanded falls from Q_1 to Q_2. When any of the other determinants of demand change, there is a shift in the demand curve. For example, if the size of the consumer population grows, the demand curve

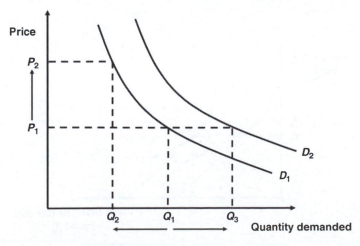

Figure 2.3 Movements along and shifts in the demand curve

will shift rightwards from D_1 to D_2, and at the price P_1 the quantity demanded will increase from Q_1 to Q_3.

Income

Demand is not simply the quantity of a good that consumers are willing to buy. They must also be able to afford it. So, there will be a relationship between a consumer's income and their demand. Again, this can be derived from consumer choice theory. Figure 2.4 shows what happens when income rises. Because prices have not changed, the budget line shifts outwards, retaining the same slope, and moves the utility-maximising point from d to e. In this case, the demand for good X rises as a result of the increase in income, but demand for good Y actually falls. The effect of income can be shown on a demand curve. For example, the shift in the demand curve shown in Figure 2.3 could be the result of an increase in income, assuming that the good is like good X. Another way to analyse this is to plot demand against income, other things held equal. This is known as an Engel curve.

Goods like good X are known as normal goods, because it is assumed that most goods are of this type. Goods like good Y are known as inferior. Examples include tooth extractions, the demand for which decreases as a consumer's income rises to be replaced by conservative treatments such as root canal surgery. A normal good is further categorised as being a necessity, such as toothpaste, if the increase in demand is proportionately smaller than the increase in income, or as a luxury, such as cosmetic surgery and dental veneers, if the increase in demand is proportionately larger. This terminology arises because it is assumed that at low levels of income people only buy necessities. As their income increases they buy the same amounts of these as before and spend additional income on luxuries.

There has been contrasting evidence about the impact of income on the demand for health care, including the thought-provoking assertion that health care in aggregate is a luxury good. This has led to controversies and conflicting policy conclusions about the provision of health care. We discuss this in more detail in Section 2.7.

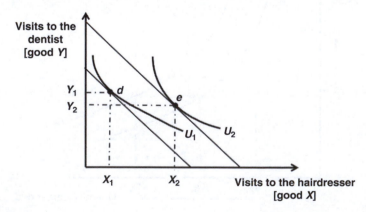

Figure 2.4 Changes in income

Prices of other goods

The demands for different goods are often interrelated since, as shown by the budget constraint, all goods compete for a consumer's limited income. In Figure 2.2, we saw that the demand for hairdresser visits changed simply because the price of dentist visits changed. Goods may be substitutes or complements. Other things held constant, if a fall in the price of one good causes a fall in the quantity demanded of another good then the goods are substitutes. An example of substitute goods is bariatric surgery and Anatrim^{TM} for the treatment of obesity. If a fall in the price of one good increases the demand for another good, then these goods are complements. An example of complements is general medical practitioner (GP) visits and prescription medicines. Prescription medicines can only be obtained if a registered physician prescribes them, so an increase in the price of attending a GP surgery will, holding everything else constant, lower the number of GP visits, and therefore lower the number of prescriptions.

Tastes and lifestyles

Even if two consumers have the same income and face the same prices, they may not demand exactly the same amount because their tastes for particular goods may differ. For foodstuffs, spreads made from yeast extract are an example of extreme divergence of tastes between different consumers. In health care, there are also differences in patients' tastes. An obvious example is the form in which oral drugs are taken, such as tablets, dispersible tablets, capsules, powders and syrups. Another is the taste for local anaesthesia for minor dental surgery, where some stoic patients prefer none to be used, where others always demand it.

Although tastes are personal, they are in part socially determined and may change over time, leading to changes in demand. If, for example, a good becomes more fashionable, demand for it will increase. A particularly important concept in examining demand for health and health care is the idea of a lifestyle, a set of attitudes adopted by groups of people that lead them to have similar behaviours, tastes and consumption demands. At least some health promotion activities are devoted towards understanding and modifying lifestyles, so that more people adopt health-promoting lifestyles, and fewer follow unhealthy lifestyles.

Changing tastes and lifestyles influence the demand for health care in different ways. First, lifestyle trends will affect overall population health, and ultimately the demands for health care. For example, in the 1950s smoking was seen as acceptable and desirable, with obvious consequences for long-term health and health care. Secondly, expectations and tastes regarding health itself also change over time, with consequences for the demand for health care. For example, in many countries in the 1940s, such as New Zealand and Scotland, it was viewed as normal to have all one's teeth extracted in early adulthood, whereas current generations expect to keep their adult teeth for life. The result is a fall in demand for dentures, and an increased demand for preventive and conservative dentistry. Thirdly, changes over time in tastes for specific types of health care might also affect their demand. Examples include termination of pregnancy and the rise in demand for a wide range of cosmetic surgical procedures, such as face-lifts, tummy-tucks and breast enlargements.

Box 2.3 outlines economic analyses of the rising prevalence of obesity. This is an example of a lifestyle trend that is having a major impact on population health and the use of health care services.

BOX 2.3   Why are people becoming more obese?

Rising obesity levels are a major problem in many countries. This is worrying because obesity is an important risk factor for a number of diseases, including coronary heart disease, type II diabetes, hypertension and stroke, as well as being a debilitating condition in its own right. Obesity has been shown to have a negative impact on life expectancy (Peeters *et al.*, 2003) and health related quality of life (Kinge and Morris, 2010).

Economic analyses have been used to explain the rise in obesity. A number of studies have investigated economic reasons for people to consume more calories or burn fewer calories or both. They tend to focus on the role of financial and time constraints on food consumption and physical activity. The studies show that reasons for the rise in obesity include:

- Technological innovation in food production and transportation that has reduced the cost of food preparation (Cutler *et al.*, 2003).
- Agricultural innovation and falling food prices that has led to an expansion in food supply (Lakdawalla and Philipson, 2005).
- A decline in physical activity, both at home and at work (Lakdawalla and Philipson, 2002).
- An increase in the number of fast-food outlets, resulting in changes to the relative prices of meals in fast food and other restaurants and meals prepared at home (Chou *et al.*, 2004).
- A reduction in the prevalence of smoking, which leads to increases in weight (Chou *et al.*, 2004).
- An increase in maternal employment, which can affect child nutrition and physical activity (Anderson *et al.*, 2003).

Obesity has substantial impact on the demand for health care. Müller-Riemenschneider *et al.* (2008) calculate that European countries spend 2–8% of health care spending on obesity, or 0.09–0.61% of national income.

Population size and composition

It seems obvious that as the size of the population increases, market demand is likely to rise. But the population's composition may also change, so that the relative size of different groups changes. The demand for goods consumed by this group will therefore increase relative to the demand for other goods. For example, if there are more women of childbearing age, the demand for obstetric services will grow more than proportionally.

Population size and composition are important determinants of the market demand for health care. Other things being equal, as the population size increases, the total amount of morbidity will increase and demand for health care will grow. It is also likely that the composition of the population will change over time. For example, advances in medical technology and improvements in living standards mean that life expectancy is increasing and people live longer. Older people will therefore form an increasingly large proportion of the population. We would therefore expect the demand for health care interventions typically consumed in the elderly population also to increase. However, the issue of how an ageing population will influence demand is not straightforward. Box 2.4 looks at this issue in more detail.

BOX 2.4   The effect of ageing on the demand for health care

A phenomenon that is widely blamed for rising health expenditures is an ageing population. The logic of this is obvious, and accounts for its popularity. Older people have more illnesses, are ill for longer and the treatments for their illnesses are more expensive. Seshamani and Gray (2002) estimated that NHS expenditure per person for people over 65 was 3.8 times that of younger adults. So, if there are more older people, the costs of providing health care must rise. But the evidence is that ageing is in reality a relatively small factor in rising health care costs.

The popular view is known as the 'expansion of morbidity' hypothesis. Gruenberg (1977) suggested that the decline in mortality that has led to an increase in the number of older people is because fewer people die from illnesses that they have, rather than because disease incidence and prevalence are lower. Lower mortality is therefore accompanied by greater morbidity and disability. However, Fries (1980) suggested an alternative hypothesis, 'compression of morbidity'. Lower mortality rates are due to better health amongst the population, so people not only live longer, they are in better health when old. Morbidity and disability are therefore at worst simply delayed until the last stages of life, suggesting that health care demands and costs will in the longer term not alter. More optimistically, the final stage may even be compressed into a shorter time, suggesting that costs will be lowered. Of course, it is possible that both of these hypotheses are true for different conditions, or that morbidity and disability will last longer but be less severe. In that case, the overall impact on demands and costs is difficult to predict.

Zweifel *et al.* (1999) examined the hypothesis that the main determinant of high health care costs amongst older people is not the time since they were born, but the time until they die. Their results, confirmed by many subsequent studies, is that proximity to death does indeed explain higher health care costs better than age *per se*. Seshamani and

Gray (2004) estimated that in the UK this is a factor up to 15 years before death, and annual costs increase tenfold during the last 5 years of life.

The consensus is that ageing per se contributes little to the continuing rise in health expenditures that all countries face. Much more important drivers are improved quality of care, access to care, and more expensive new technology. Of course, all of these may be largely devoted to older people, so that age may be associated with higher costs, but is not the causal factor.

2.3.2 Estimating demand functions

Although utility cannot be directly observed, the quantities of goods that consumers demand, such as visits to the dentist, generally can. If we can also obtain data on the prices charged to or paid by consumers, and on other relevant factors such as consumers' incomes, then the relationship between demand and each of these factors can be modelled using econometric techniques, and a demand function can be estimated. For example, we could hypothesise that the demand for dental care will depend upon the following set of variables:

$$D = D(P, I, N, P_C, P_S, T, S)$$

where P = price to the consumer, I = income, N = non-price access costs, P_C = prices of complements, P_S = price of substitutes, T = tastes and preferences and S = state of oral health. Estimating this equation would tell us which variables are or are not significant determinants of demand; what direction their influence has; the magnitude of their effect on demand; and what proportion of the variation in demand the model can explain.

Parkin and Yule (1988) estimated the demand for dental care in Scotland. Among other results, they reported the following function for the demand for dentures:

$$D_d = 157\,505 - 10\,960 \times P_d + 2\,141 \times P_o - 4\,432 \times I + 8\,867 \times A$$

where D_d = annual demand for dentures, P_d = price of dentures, P_o = price of other dental services, I = income, and A = availability. This suggests that the demand for dentures is negatively related to the price of denture services, and is positively related to the price of other dental care services. This is plausible, since other types of dental care, such as complex endodontic treatment, are probably substitutes for the extraction of teeth and the fitting of dentures. As a result, as the price of other dental care goes down, so will the demand for dentures. Income has a negative effect on demand. This suggests that as income increases, demand will fall, so that dentures may be regarded as an *inferior good*. This too is intuitively plausible. As consumers' incomes increase, we might expect fewer dentures to be demanded, as people instead choose other types of dental care. Finally, the authors included a variable for the number of dentists per 100 000 population, to capture possible effects on demand of the availability of dentists. This variable had a positive effect, suggesting that the greater the supply of dentists, the higher the demand for their services. The reasons why this might be are discussed in Section 2.5.

There is a considerable body of empirical evidence on the demand for health-related goods, in particular pharmaceuticals and health insurance. The demand for pharmaceuticals has been found to be reasonably price inelastic. (See Berndt *et al.* (1995) for an example of the antiulcer drug market in the USA.) Scherer (2000) suggests this is due to the role of health insurance (see Chapter 6) and the influence of prescribers (see Section 2.6).

There are some studies of the demand for health insurance in the UK, which are interesting because they explicitly address the possibility that the public and private health care sectors interact. Around 15% of the UK population has private medical insurance, despite access to comprehensive medical care services provided free at the point of demand through the NHS. Why would anyone buy private insurance? What are the determinants of demand for medical insurance policies? Besley *et al.* (1999) analysed data from a survey of insurance purchases and on local NHS services for 1986–1991. The greater the number of people waiting over one year for treatment, the higher the demand for private insurance. An increase of 1 person per 1000 waiting for more than a year was associated with a 2% increase in the probability of an average person purchasing insurance. The demand for insurance and the person's income, education level and age were strongly positively related. Propper *et al.* (2001) estimated a demand function for 1978 to 1996 and did not find a relationship between demand and NHS waiting lists, but this related to the total number waiting, which Besley *et al.* also found not to be significant, rather than the number waiting over a year. They also found complex links between the public and private sectors. For example, higher NHS spending lowers the demand for private insurance, with a lagged effect, and the availability of private sector facilities strongly increases the demand for insurance.

2.3.3 Price and income elasticity of demand

A useful way of summarising the relationships between price, income and other variables and the demand for health care is to express them as an *elasticity* measure. Elasticity measures the responsiveness of changes in one variable, for example quantities demanded or supplied, to changes in another variable, for example prices or income. The *price elasticity of demand* (PeD) is the percentage change in quantity demanded divided by the percentage change in price. If the price of an ophthalmology check-up in Singapore increased from $200 to $250, and the number of check-ups each week fell from 50 to 45, the percentage change in quantity is 10%, the percentage change in price is 25%, and the elasticity is 0.4. This elasticity is less than 1, indicating that, over the range of prices observed, demand is not particularly responsive to price. Price rose and demand fell, but it fell *less* than proportionately.

Elasticity is often measured over discrete ranges of price and quantity changes. A more precise measure is to calculate the elasticity at a given point on the demand curve, that is:

$$P\varepsilon D = (dQ/dP)(P/Q) \qquad (2.7)$$

where P/Q is a given price divided by the quantity demanded at that price and dQ/dP is the demand curve's slope at that point.

Elasticity provides a useful means of comparing the responsiveness of consumer demand to price and other variables between: different periods in time, in which the purchasing power of money may be different; different countries, where the currency is different; and different goods, where the units in which quantity is measured are different.

Further, the magnitude of price elasticity, that is whether it is <1, $= 1$ or >1, has direct implications for consumer spending and firms' revenues. For example, the Parkin and Yule (1988) study reported that the price elasticity of demand for dentures was 0.28. This suggests that an increase in the price charged by a dentist will reduce demand for dentures. But, because demand falls *less* than proportionately, both consumer spending and the dentist's revenue will increase. Consumers who continue to buy dentures will pay more and the extra revenue from them will outweigh the loss of revenue from those who no longer do so. Conversely, if the price elasticity were >1, an increase in price would reduce demand *more* than proportionately, and both quantity demanded and revenue will fall. In the special case where the price elasticity of demand equals 1, changes in price and quantity exactly balance each other and revenue does not change when prices change.

Income elasticity of demand is defined in a similar way, derived from the Engel curve. The point income elasticity is the percentage change in quantity demanded divided by the percentage change in income:

$$I\varepsilon D = (dQ/dI)(I/Q) \tag{2.8}$$

where I/Q is any given income divided by the quantity demanded at that income, other things (such as price) being held equal, and dQ/dI is the Engel curve's slope at that point.

The income elasticity is related to the change in the proportion of income spent on a good, and its size therefore determines whether the good can be labelled as inferior, necessity or luxury. Specifically, if $I\varepsilon D < 0$ the good is inferior, if $0 < I\varepsilon D < 1$ it is a necessity, and if $I\varepsilon D > 1$ it is a luxury.

Estimating elasticities for a good enables us to draw conclusions about the kind of good that it is – controversially, as we shall see in Section 2.7, in the case of health care.

The RAND Corporation's Health Insurance Experiment (Manning *et al.*, 1987) generated the most well-known and comprehensive findings on the demand for health care. Families from six areas of the USA were assigned to one of 14 types of health insurance plans. The study is unparalleled in health economics not just because of its sheer scale – the sample comprised over 5 800 people – but also because it is a rare example in economics of a controlled experiment. By assigning study participants to different health insurance plans, the effect of insurance cover, and thus prices to consumers, on the demand for health care could be observed, and other relevant factors controlled for. The study concluded that, overall, the price elasticity of demand for medical care was 0.22. Demand does respond to price, but is not particularly elastic.

Although there are important differences between types of medical care, the evidence on price elasticity of demand for health care, both in the RAND experiment and in other settings, generally estimates the price elasticity of demand to lie between 0.1 and 0.7. Thus, demand is responsive to price differences, but the elasticity is usually <1. A similar consensus is apparent on the effect of income: the income elasticity of demand tends to be positive but less than 1, suggesting that health care is a necessity. Non-price access costs, such as transport and time costs, are often also important determinants of demand, with an effect on demand as great as that of price.

Much of the evidence on the responsiveness of demand to price comes from observing consumers' demand under various insurance/co-insurance or subsidy/part-charge arrangements. Changes in these arrangements provide natural experiments in which subsequent changes in demand to changing out-of-pocket prices may be observed. The incentives to consumers arising from third-party health care financing are discussed in detail in Chapter 6.

2.4 Modelling choices about health

So far, this chapter's analysis has applied conventional consumer choice theory to health care. However, as Chapter 1 noted, health care is desired not for its own sake, but for its ability to improve health. Here we outline a theoretical framework for understanding choices about health and health care that was originally developed by Grossman (1972), based on Becker's theories of human capital (Becker, 1964) and household production (Becker, 1965). In Grossman's model, people both demand and produce health. They demand health because they derive utility from it. They produce health using different kinds of health-promoting inputs. They demand health care because it is one of those inputs, not because it provides them with utility directly. The demand for health care is therefore a *derived* demand.

Household production theory suggests that the true objects of human desire are 'basic commodities' such as nourishment, clothing, entertainment, transport and health. People create these using goods that they buy, called market goods, and their own time. They derive utility directly from basic commodities, but only indirectly from market goods. For example, in producing the basic commodity associated with nourishment, a household can have home-cooked, pre-prepared, restaurant or take-away meals. Each involves different combinations of time spent in activities such as purchasing, preparation and eating, and of market goods such as full meals or the ingredients for them plus energy for cooking. People divide their total available time between producing commodities and working for an income to buy market goods.

Grossman's model is founded on this view of health as a basic commodity. People produce health using their time and market good inputs, combined in packages such as diet, lifestyle choices and health care. The model goes beyond simply regarding health as a direct source of utility. Health is also demanded because it affects a person's ability to work, and therefore the total time available to produce an income. Essentially, poor health reduces both our happiness and our ability to earn.

This influence on the ability to work emphasises that health is a key component of *human capital*. This is the capacity that people have to produce goods that have economic value. In Grossman's model, health is treated not as a consumer good but as capital, with characteristics similar to more conventional capital goods. At any time, a person has a 'stock' of health. This depreciates over time with age and decreases when it is used in production and consumption of other commodities. It can be increased through investments of time, effort and knowledge in health-promoting activities. It is further linked to other human capital components, because a person's skills and knowledge affect how efficiently they produce health. The level of skills and knowledge in turn depends on how much has been invested through education.

Grossman's model is a powerful tool for analysing health and health care decisions, and we therefore outline it in some detail. Section 2.4.1 presents a simplified model based on an original geometric treatment by Wagstaff (1986a, 1986b). This is helpful in understanding the model's consumption features, but does not capture the human capital aspect. Section 2.4.2 presents the model more formally, with an emphasis on health care as an investment in health.

2.4.1 Understanding consumption of health and health care

In this simplified model, there are two basic commodities, health and other consumption, from which people derive utility. These are produced using just one market good each, health care and non health care inputs, respectively. There is a budget constraint that defines the amount of each market good that a person can buy at a given level of income. We are able to construct an indifference curve reflecting their preferences for the two basic commodities.

Figure 2.5 brings together these elements of production and demand. Graph 1 illustrates a budget constraint, like that illustrated in Figure 2.2. It shows every combination of health care

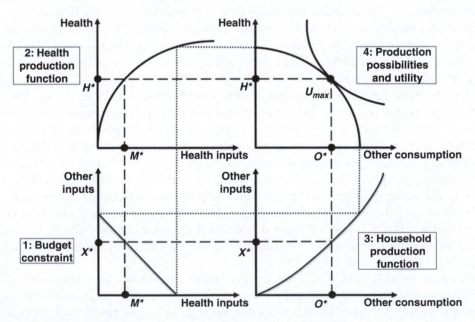

Figure 2.5 The demand for health

inputs (M) and non health care inputs (X) that a person can obtain, given their income and the prices of the inputs. Graph 2 shows the relationship between the amount of health care inputs and the amount of health that is produced (H). This is called a *production function*, which is analysed in more detail in Chapter 3. It describes how consumption of health care improves health and its shape incorporates assumptions about the effectiveness of health care. The shape in this graph assumes that more health care always improves health, but the size of the improvement is greater at lower levels of health than higher. This phenomenon, known as diminishing marginal productivity, will also be discussed in detail in Chapter 3. Graph 3 is another production function relating other consumption (O) to non health care inputs. It incorporates the same diminishing marginal productivity assumption. For ease of reference, we call this the household production function.

Graph 4 has two elements. The curve convex to the origin shows all combinations of health and other consumption that can be obtained from the budget in Graph 1. This is called a *production possibility curve* (PPC), which is also analysed further in Chapter 3. Any point on the budget line can be mapped to a specific point on the PPC by tracing two lines from the budget line point and marking their intersection in Graph 4. One line goes up to the health production function, then right. The other goes right to the household production function, then up. The dotted lines show how the PPC's boundaries derive from the budget constraint's boundaries. For example, the most health that can be produced is the result of spending the entire income on health care inputs. The dashed line shows one particular PPC point and how it is related to a budget line point. The PPC's convex shape is determined entirely by the assumed shape of the production functions.

The second element of Graph 4 is an indifference curve like that of Figure 2.1. Using exactly the same reasoning as in Section 2.2, the combination of health and consumption that maximises utility is where the indifference curve just touches the PPC. Any combination of health and consumption on the PPC could be chosen, but given the preferences represented by the indifference curves, utility will be maximised at the point marked U_{max}. H^* health and $O*$ consumption will be chosen, requiring the purchase of M^* health care inputs and X^* non health care inputs.

This simple model highlights that people choose a combination of health and other basic commodities that maximises their utility, and the demand for health care is derived from that choice. It will be a useful exercise for readers of this book to use this diagram to predict what effect changes in the different elements that make up the model will have on the combination of commodities chosen. For example, a change in income, which causes the budget line to shift, an improvement in health care technology, which causes the production function to change shape or position, and so on.

2.4.2 Understanding investment in health care

The geometric representation is a highly simplified version of the Grossman model that does not capture the important insight that health can be regarded as analogous to a capital good. In this section, a fuller treatment of the model is given, with an emphasis on this aspect of the theory.

The model starts with the same simplifying assumption as before, that people derive utility (U) from two goods: health (H) and a composite of all other basic commodities (O). The utility function of equation (2.1) therefore becomes:

$$U = U(H, O) \tag{2.9}$$

Both H and O are sums over time, weighted by the person's *time preference*, which is explained in more detail in Chapter 12. It reflects the fact that different people have different preferences for when they obtain benefits. Some are more impatient than others. H is the weighted number of healthy days that the person enjoys over their life. These derive from the person's *stock* of health (HS), so that the greater their health stock, the greater the number of healthy days they will have. Health stock at a particular time (HS_t) is determined by health stock in the previous period (HS_{t-1}) less any depreciation in health stock (d_t) that has taken place over that period plus any investment in health (I_t) that the person has undertaken:

$$HS_t = HS_{t-1} - d_t + I_t \tag{2.10}$$

Health, in this way of thinking, is analogous to other types of capital, such as a machine. For example, one's health can depreciate over time owing to excessive alcohol use or the effects of ageing. But this can be offset by investments – in terms of both time and money – that will maintain or improve health, such as regular exercise to reduce weight and improve heart function or medical care to repair damaged health. Both O and I are produced within the household, and we can define a production function for each of them. Production of O and I uses market goods, medical care (M) and all other market goods (X) respectively, and time spent either in production of health (T_H) or in producing other goods (T_O). A third input to both is human capital, usually characterised as the level of education (E). The production functions are therefore:

$$I_t = I(M_t, T_{Ht}, E_t) \tag{2.11}$$

$$O_t = O(X_t, T_{Ot}, E_t) \tag{2.12}$$

It is assumed that a person will attempt to maximise their utility, but there are two constraints upon this, a time budget and an expenditure budget. The time budget (T) is obviously fixed at 365.25 days each year on average; and as well as the time spent producing, the person must also spend time working (T_W) and suffer some time spent sick (T_S):

$$T_t = T_{Ht} + T_{Ot} + T_{Wt} + T_{St} \tag{2.13}$$

The constraint on the expenditure budget is income, which depends on how much time is spent working and the wage rate (W). How much is spent depends on the costs of market goods M and X and their prices (P_M and P_X respectively). It is assumed that all income is spent:

$$P_M M + P_X X = T_W W \tag{2.14}$$

Both sides of this equation should be regarded as *present values* (see Chapter 12), because they refer to a person's lifetime income and expenditure. They are therefore discounted at the interest rate r.

Maximisation of the utility function, subject to these constraints and taking into account the production functions, leads to an equilibrium condition which can be interpreted as a person making the marginal benefits of health capital equal to its marginal cost. Marginal benefit consists of two parts, one relating to the enjoyment of health resulting from the investment (MB_H) and the other relating to the monetary investment returns that it produces (MB_M). These are commonly known as 'consumption' and 'investment' benefits, although these terms are not entirely apt. An element that is common to them is the marginal product of health (MP_H), measured as the number of healthy days generated by one unit of health stock. The two elements of benefit are the product of these healthy days and the *value* of a healthy day in consumption and investment, which, because they are equated with costs, are expressed in money values.

The consumption benefit is therefore the MP_H multiplied by the value of a healthy day in consumption. This value is measured by the undiscounted ratio of the marginal utility of healthy days (MU_H) to the marginal utility of financial wealth (MU_W):

$$MB_{Ht} = (MP_{Ht})(1 + r)^t (MU_{HT}/MU_{Wt}) \qquad (2.15)$$

where $(1 + r)^t$ is a factor that ensures that the money value is not discounted. Healthy days can also be used for working to create income, so that the 'investment' benefit is the marginal product of health multiplied by the wage rate:

$$MB_{Mt} = MB_{Ht} W_t \qquad (2.16)$$

The marginal cost of health capital is the marginal cost of investment in health (MCI) multiplied by two factors: the real rate of interest, which represents the opportunity cost of investment, and the depreciation of health capital (d). The real rate of interest is the nominal rate (r) that could have been earned had the investment not been in health, less the change over the time period in the marginal cost of investment (ΔMCI), which can be interpreted as a capital gain, or a saving from investing now rather than in the future, assuming that marginal costs will increase over time. So, the equilibrium condition is

$$MB_{Mt} + MB_{Ht} = MCI_{t-1}((r - \Delta MCI_{t-1}) + d_t) \qquad (2.17)$$

This equation is the key result of the Grossman model. Although it derives from a complex model, it has an intuitively reasonable interpretation to it. The idea is that people invest in health up to the point where the marginal benefits from the investment, that is, the consumption benefit plus the investment benefit derived above, are equal to the marginal costs incurred by the investment. But as usual in economics it cannot be considered a good model until it is tested. We will therefore look at some of its predictions and their testing, and conclude with some criticisms that have been made of the Grossman approach.

2.4.3 Predictions of the Grossman model

Equation (2.17) is very important for empirical testing of the Grossman theory. Unfortunately, it is difficult to estimate as it stands owing to the complicated relationship between MB_H and MB_M. Testing has therefore worked mainly by looking at consumption benefits only, by setting $MB_M = 0$, or investment benefits only, by setting $MB_H = 0$. The model described earlier in effect assumes the first of these possibilities. To demonstrate some of the predictions of the model, we will look at the second of them, using the concept of the *marginal efficiency of capital* (MEC). This arises from an assumed relationship between the cost of capital, $(C = (r - \Delta MCI) + d)$, and the health stock, HS, which is illustrated in Figure 2.6. It is assumed that as the level of health stock increases it becomes more and more difficult to generate health by investing in it. In other words, investment is subject to *diminishing returns* (see Chapter 3), which explains the convex shape of the *MEC* curves.

This theory is useful because it provides a basis for hypotheses about the effect of important determinants of health on the demand for health and health care – propositions that can then be tested using data, which in turn enables more accurate predictions about health behaviour.

For example, the model yields hypotheses about age. Age is assumed to affect the depreciation of health capital; in particular it increases as people get older. Suppose that a person has the curve MEC_0 and an equilibrium at C_0, with health stock HS_0. In the next time period, they have a higher cost, C_1, owing to depreciation and therefore a lower preferred health stock, HS_1. However, the demand for investment in health – and therefore the demand for health care inputs – depends on what effect the depreciation had on the health stock. If it fell from HS_0 to HS_A, the actual stock would be higher than the new preferred stock, HS_1, so there would be no investment in health. However, if it fell to HS_B, investment would be necessary to raise it to HS_1.

Similarly, we can examine the effect of a change in wage rates (W). W affects both sides of equation (2.17). On the benefits side, an increase in W will raise the value of the production of

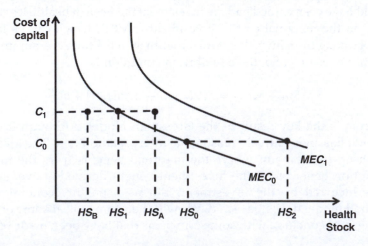

Figure 2.6 The marginal efficiency of health capital

healthy days, since working time is now more valuable. On the cost side, the opportunity cost of the person's time also increases, and because investment in health requires a time input, the opportunity cost of such investment also increases. But since there are other inputs to investment that do not increase, the proportional change will be greater for benefits than for costs, so the returns to health will increase at all levels of the health stock. In Figure 2.6, this is represented by a shift of the *MEC* curve from MEC_0 to MEC_1, accompanied by an increase in preferred health stock from HS_0 to HS_2. The demand for investment in health will therefore increase.

Much attention has been given to the relationship between health and education. An increase in education will increase the efficiency of non-market production, which increases the *MP* of health inputs. This would shift the *MEC* curve outwards, and raise the optimal health stock. Once again, however, the predicted effect on the demand for health care is ambiguous.

These propositions have been the subject of a considerable empirical literature. See, for example, Wagstaff (1986b, 1993). The model has been used to examine such diverse issues as socioeconomic inequalities in health (Muurinen and Le Grand, 1985), the impact on health of environmental quality, measured by the level of pollution (Erbsland *et al.*, 1995), and the demand for malaria treatments in a developing country (Masiye and Rehnberg, 2005). Empirical evidence about the model's assumptions has been mixed in terms of confirming or refuting them, but this should be seen as a contribution to its development and there is no doubt that this will be an increasingly important way in which economists examine health issues. A continuing interest has been in the use of the Grossman model to help understand inequalities in health between people and populations.

There are some problems with the way that the Grossman model is currently formulated, though these are the subject of a large ongoing research programme (Grossman, 2000). In the way that it is usually used, it rests on some rather strong assumptions. For example, it assumes that consumers have perfect information and perfect foresight about their health, the rate of depreciation of their health, and the effect of health care and other consumption on their health. Taken to the extreme, it suggests that people make well-informed and rational decisions about the date of their death! The model therefore does not take into account uncertainty – for example, about the timing of adverse health events – which, as we noted in Chapter 1, is a defining characteristic of health. This uncertainty extends to consumers' relative lack of information about the effect of health care on health. This has important consequences for the way consumers and providers of health care interact in the health care market, an issue we take up in Section 2.6 below.

2.5 Needs, wants and demands

The application of demand theory to health and health care gives valuable insights and one view could be that health is simply an interesting application of ordinary demand theory. But this is deceptive. In order to understand many aspects of health and health care it is necessary to look beyond straightforward economic concepts. In analysing the demand for health care, it is important to take account of the concept of *need*. This is true not only when considering the consumption of health care, it is also the case that a characteristic of health policy in most countries is that the concept of need, rather than demand, dominates views about the aims of health services.

If you ask people what determines their demand for health care, the most likely answer will be that 'people go to the doctor when they need it'. By contrast, the straightforward economics answer would be because they *want* to do so. That sounds peculiar, because unless they have a psychological disorder, such as Munchausen's syndrome, no-one wants health care for its own sake (Evans, 1984). On the face of it, Grossman's theory provides a reconciliation of these two views, because people *want* health improvements and *demand* care that will produce them. However, need is more complicated than that. Need implies an imperative to have health care, because it will deal with a health problem. By contrast, demand simply implies the willingness and ability to pay for health care. Moreover, people have limited knowledge about such needs, both the existence of health problems and the health care that will deal with them. By contrast, the usual assumption in economics is that in making demands people are the best judges of their own wants.

Economists prefer to define need as *capacity to benefit*, which means the capacity for a patient to benefit from health care. Even if someone is sick, they are not in need of health care unless they could benefit from it. This type of need must be distinguished from need that is related to a person's health state rather than health care, so that it is independent of whether that state can be improved through the provision of health care. Moreover, the generally preferred view of economists is that any definition of need relies on expert judgement of the likely benefits of treatment. Alternative definitions refer to each person's perception of their own needs, which depends on their knowledge of health care, their knowledge of health, and their expectations about what is 'normal' with respect to health. Of course, experts do not always agree and their judgements may change over time, so even this more rigorous definition of need is not at all straightforward to apply.

Needs and demands can thus be regarded as two very different ways of viewing matters, but taken together they give useful insights. Two extreme positions might exist. Sometimes there might be demand where there is no need. People might be pessimistically mistaken about their health state or optimistically mistaken about the possibilities for improving it. In practice, the more important case is that there might be need where there is no demand, and if health services simply respond only to demand, this implies that there will be *unmet need*. Some of this unmet need will be due to deficiencies in information, which will be looked at in more detail in the next section of this chapter. This kind of analysis views the other source of unmet need as *barriers* to the use of health care. From an economics viewpoint these can be categorised as supply factors, which are the availability of services to meet needs, and demand factors, such as prices and incomes, which affect people's ability to access services.

2.6 Asymmetry of information and imperfect agency

As we have emphasised, a characteristic of health care markets is uncertainty: about diagnosis, about available treatments, and about their effectiveness (Arrow, 1963). Some of this uncertainty is 'irreducible' (Pauly, 1978), meaning that neither the doctor nor the patient can know with certainty what the consequences of treatment will be. As suggested, this leads to the problem of unmet need. However, much of the uncertainty is one-sided. Consumers lack the medical training and knowledge to make truly informed choices.

Information is itself an economic good. Obtaining information, for example by engaging in consumer research to compare prices and qualities of alternative health care providers, or checking the relative cost and efficacy of alternative treatments, is worthwhile if the benefits exceed the costs. Where the costs of obtaining information are too high, if information is highly specialised or difficult to obtain, or the likely benefits too low, for example where it is for a one-off treatment, consumers may choose to remain 'rationally ignorant' and to delegate decision-making to the supplier. As McGuire (2001) puts it, 'In a patient's contact with the doctor, the doctor's position is not "Here is the price of my services, how many do you want?" It is more like "Here is what you should do".'

This relationship between doctor and patient is often presented as a principal–agent problem. The doctor is an *agent* acting on behalf of a *principal*, who is the patient, in making decisions about what health care to purchase. If doctors made these decisions in a manner fully consistent with patients' preferences, unaffected by the consequence for themselves, they would be acting as perfect agents – essentially, making the health care decisions that the patients themselves would do if they had access to the same information. Much of the economics literature has focused on the possibility that doctors either cannot or do not act as perfect agents. Specifically, the hypothesis of supplier-induced demand (SID) (Evans, 1974), sometimes referred to as physician- or provider-induced demand (PID), is that doctors 'engage in some persuasive activity to shift the patient's demand curve in or out according to the physician's self-interest' (McGuire, 2001).

There is an extensive theoretical and empirical literature on this subject. Early studies focused on testing whether or not greater availability of doctor services, measured by increases in doctor to patient ratios, increased the use of health care. Such evidence sounds convincing, but it may also be consistent with non-inducement models of how use is determined (Rice, 1998). The analysis that follows demonstrates why. It illustrates the power of a simple model to expose problems with seemingly straightforward evidence, but also shows the limitations of such models in generating predictions that can be tested in the real world. Much more sophisticated and realistic models have been used to analyse SID, though not necessarily with any greater success.

Recall from Figure 1.2 in Chapter 1 that a market may have an equilibrium price at which supply and demand are equal. This determines the level of usage. Suppose, as in Figure 2.7, that from an initial equilibrium price of P_1 and a usage level of Q_1, there is a change in supply conditions such that the supply curve shifts from S_1 to S_2. For example, a change in medical licensing regulations may result in an influx of doctors from overseas. The SID hypothesis suggests that each doctor will recommend more or more frequent treatment to their patients than before in order to increase demand. Suppose that they are successful in raising demand from D_1 to D_2. In the new equilibrium, quantity is higher ($Q_2 > Q_1$) and price is lower ($P_2 < P_1$). So, if we observed empirically that an increase in the supply of doctors coincided with increased numbers of doctor visits, does this prove that SID occurred? The answer is no, for three reasons.

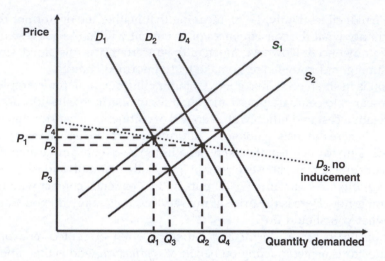

Figure 2.7 The problem of identifying supplier-induced demand

First, that observation is consistent with the predictions for any competitive market: if supply increases from S_1 to S_2, with *no* shift in the demand curve, we would get an equilibrium quantity of Q_3 which, like Q_2, is greater than Q_1, and price P_3, which, like P_2, is less than P_1.

Secondly, it is possible that the demand curve's shape is simply different to the way we thought. The equilibrium Q_2 and P_2, which we explained via an inducement effect, would be consistent with the equilibrium that would be observed if supply shifted from S_1 to S_2 and the demand curve was in fact D_3.

Thirdly, the increase in supply might result in a reduction in the costs of doctor visits such as searching for and waiting to see a doctor and travelling to the surgery, or might improve other aspects of quality, such as the length of each consultation. It may be these factors, which are themselves determinants of demand, that shift the demand curve from D_1 to D_2, rather than inducement. This third explanation could even explain cases where price actually *increases* following an increase in supply equilibrium, an empirical observation found by Fuchs (1978), for example a shift in the demand curve to D_4, resulting in a new equilibrium price of P_4, which is greater than P_1.

So, in general it seems that there is no way in which observed movements in prices and quantities can prove the existence of inducement. Of course, this also means that there is no way in which such data can disprove it.

A more general problem with this sort of approach is that it requires a *change* in supply in order to identify an inducement *response*. This does not tell us how much inducement was taking place before the change in supply conditions. If doctors can influence both prices and demand, how is equilibrium reached? A key point in understanding this is that economics assumes that people try to maximise their utility, not their income. Possible constraints upon SID include that medical ethics may act to constrain physician behaviour; that physicians' utility depends both on their income and the well-being, or utility, of their patients; and that physician behaviour is aimed at achieving a 'target income'. Ultimately, consumers also do act to constrain inducement. They may have less information, but the potential for consumer response restricts what even the most self-interested doctor can get away with. But a more fundamental problem with this way of analysing SID is that supply and demand models essentially assume that supply and demand are independent. They may simply not be a very good analytical tool if demand is partly determined by suppliers.

Some findings are clear: a comprehensive review of the evidence (McGuire, 2001) demonstrates that physicians do respond to financial incentives; they do appear to influence demand and to do so partly in response to self-interest. Box 2.5 gives an example of evidence that is available on this issue. However, notwithstanding the considerable body of research, a definitive understanding of SID remains elusive. To understand whether patients are being induced to demand more services than they really want, we would need to know how much they would have demanded if they were as well informed as the physician. No such study has been conducted (Mooney, 1994; Rice, 1998).

BOX 2.5   **Supplier-induced demand by Irish general practitioners**

Irish general practitioners (GPs) were the subject of one of the earliest studies of demand inducement (Tussing and Wojtowycz, 1986). GPs treat both public patients, paid for by the state, and private patients who pay for themselves, but at a higher rate. This gives them a financial incentive to treat more patients of all types, and private patients in particular. The authors surveyed 1 069 Irish households. They asked if, during a person's most recent GP consultation, the GP arranged a return visit. This was used as an indicator of whether or not the GP had stimulated the demand for their services. A regression model was used to explore variations in this according to patient variables such as gender, age, the distance from home to GP surgery and eligibility for free care, as well as local factors such as average income, the proportion of the population eligible for free care, and the number of GPs per person.

23.5% of all most recent GP visits led to the GP arranging a return visit. After controlling for other factors, GP-stimulated visits were positively correlated with the number of GPs per person and negatively correlated with the proportion eligible for free care and average income. The authors concluded that 'all three results . . . point to significant self-interested physician-induced demand by Irish GPs'.

Partly as a result of this study, the GP reimbursement system was changed in 1989. GPs are now paid by capitation for public patients. Madden, Nolan and Nolan (2005) compared visiting rates for public and private patients before and after this change. Eligibility for free care was associated with an increase in GP visits. However, the difference in visiting rates between eligible and other patients was the same after the change as before. If supplier-induced demand had been an important factor in the old system, this difference might have been expected to narrow.

2.7 Aggregate demand for health care: theory and evidence

Given the theory and evidence reviewed so far with respect to *individual consumers'* demand for health care, what factors would you expect to influence the demand of consumers *in aggregate* for health care, that is, the demand for health care by an entire country? Obvious answers might include the population age structure, levels of sickness and disease, the prevalence of smoking and obesity, and so on.

In fact, researchers have found that, using health care spending per person as a proxy measure for aggregate demand, most of the variation in health care demand between countries can be explained using just one variable: the country's income, generally measured as GDP per person. The strength of the relationship is evident even from a simple plot of GDP per person against health care spending per person such as Figure 2.8(a). This shows data for 184 countries in 2009, derived from data published by the World Bank. It is clear that the richer an economy, the more health care will be demanded.

An influential paper on this issue by Newhouse (1977), using a simple linear regression analysis on 13 countries, found that GDP per person of a country explains 92% of the variance in the level of spending between countries. Moreover, he calculated that the income elasticity of demand was greater than 1 at all levels of income, with an average value of 1.31. This led him to conclude that health care is, at a national level, a luxury good and that 'countries that spend more may well buy more caring, but little additional curing'. We can replicate his findings using the World Bank data. On close inspection, the data in Figure 2.8(a) suggest that the relationship is not a straight line, but is curvilinear. Figure 2.8(b) displays the data transformed into natural logarithms, and this looks much more like a straight-line relationship. The regression line on this is a good fit – in fact, it also explains 94% of the variation! The 95% confidence interval (CI) further shows that this is a phenomenon that applies universally to countries, as there are very few outliers. The income elasticity calculated from this regression line is 1.07, slightly less than Newhouse's value, but still significantly above 1.

Newhouse's original finding and conclusions were the catalyst for a vast literature re-examining the determinants of health care spending. Parkin *et al.* (1987) pointed out that Newhouse's use of exchange rates to make the currency conversions required to make between-country comparisons is not appropriate for goods, such as health care, which are not traded internationally. Re-estimating the income elasticity using purchasing power parity (PPP) conversions, they found income elasticity not to be statistically significantly different from 1, although subsequent empirical studies have not in general supported that finding.

More fundamentally, Parkin *et al.* (1987) and others have argued that the statistical relationship has a weak theoretical base, providing little guidance either to what explanatory variables should be included or to what the causal mechanisms are. Subsequent studies have explored more complex models, including variables to capture the population age structure, the extent of public sector provision of health care, urbanisation and number of doctors (Leu, 1986; Gerdtham *et al.*, 1998, 1992a, 1992b), tobacco and alcohol consumption, unemployment

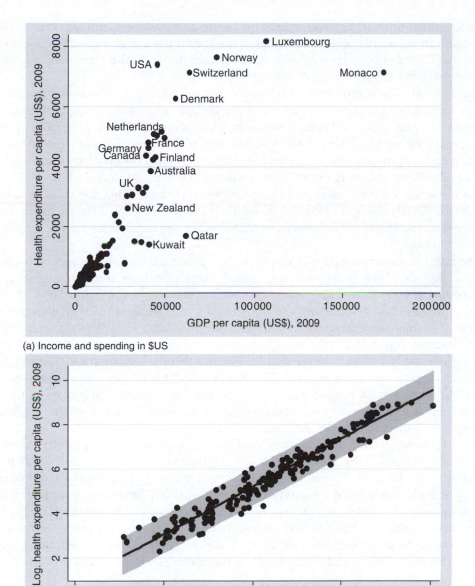

(a) Income and spending in $US

(b) Logarithms of income and spending in $US

Figure 2.8 The relationship between income per person and health care spending per person in 2009
Source: The World Bank website, www.data.worldbank.org

and various institutional characteristics of the health care system (Gerdtham *et al.*, 1998). The results from these studies, like our analysis of the World Bank data, nevertheless continue to suggest that GDP per person explains most of the variation in health care spending, although the estimate of the income elasticity varies.

More recently, contributions to this literature have focused on econometric issues arising from the time series and panel data properties of the data sets used, testing for unit roots and co-integration. McGuire *et al.* (1993) were the first to examine these characteristics of the data. Subsequently, Hansen and King (1996) looked at this in more detail and suggested that, given the time trends apparent in the data, previous estimates of income elasticity may be spurious. These results have variously either been confirmed (Blomqvist and Carter, 1997; Roberts, 1998) or contradicted (McCoskey and Selden, 1998). A review of this literature by Gerdtham and Jönsson (2001) suggests that the most likely reason for the differences in results is differences in methods. They conclude that further research is required to provide a definitive answer.

The original concern raised with respect to this issue remains. Is the observed relationship merely a statistical one or is there causation? Does the sheer strength of the apparent relationship between health care spending and income suggest an 'iron law'? If so, does this imply that the health sector will end up taking an ever larger share of GDP in the world's economies? Is this something we should be concerned about? Is it inefficient? Or is the unabated increase in health care spending an appropriate response to the preferences of increasingly wealthy economies? We should also note that the focus of these studies is on total and average health care spending and GDP per person. This may obscure important within-country differences both in *what* money is spent on, for example differences in the mix of inputs used in health care or the mix of outputs produced, and in the underlying *distribution* of health care and income between persons.

Finally, the suggestion that countries' additional spending is on caring rather than curing was probably intended by Newhouse to be deliberately provocative rather than a true deduction from the data. This is helpful in showing how the economist's technical term 'luxury good' does not always easily translate into ordinary language. In ordinary use, we might deduce that if extra health care is a luxury, that is because it has no effect on health, and only curative health care has an effect on health. In economics terms, however, there are no reasons why as incomes improve countries would not wish to buy, in increasing amounts, goods that improve their population's health or why caring services should not have a positive impact on health.

Summary

1. Economists define the demand for any good or service, including health care, as the quantity that consumers are both willing and able to buy.

2. The demand curve, which graphically is shown by a curve that is downward sloping from left to right, shows that – other things being equal – as prices rise, demand falls.

3. Consumer choice theory explains why consumers behave or react in certain ways to changes in various factors in order to maximise their utility. This theory underpins the demand for goods and services. Consumers are assumed to be rational, which means they have complete preferences, that their preferences are transitive, and that their wants are non-satiable.

4. The way in which the consumption of different bundles of goods and services affects utility can be illustrated using indifference curves. These show all the combinations of two goods that yield the consumer equal satisfaction.

5. The slope of an indifference curve is the marginal rate of substitution. This is the amount of one good that must be sacrificed if consumption of another good is increased in order for utility to remain unchanged.

6. The decisions that consumers make in the pursuit of utility maximisation are constrained both by their limited resources and by the prices of the various goods and services between which they choose. Hence, the consumption problem facing consumers is to maximise their utility subject to a budget constraint. Under these conditions, utility is maximised when the consumer chooses a bundle of goods for which the ratio of the goods' prices – the slope of the budget line – is equal to the ratio of the marginal utilities – the slope of the indifference curve.

7. There are various factors affecting the demand for goods and services, including the price of the good, income, the prices of other goods, tastes and trends for the good, and population size and composition. Changes in the price of the good result in movements along the demand curve. Changes in any of the other determinants of demand result in a shift in the demand curve.

8. Elasticity measures the responsiveness of changes in one variable, for example the quantity demanded, to changes in another variable, for example price. Evidence suggests that the demand for health care is price inelastic, that is, demand is not particularly responsive to changes in the price of health care.

9. A theoretical framework for understanding choices specifically relating to health and health care was developed by Grossman. In the model, people invest in health up to the point where the marginal benefits from the investment, which include a consumption benefit plus an investment benefit, are equal to the marginal costs incurred by the investment.

10. When analysing the demand for health care, it is important to take account of the concept of need. Economists commonly define need as the capacity for a patient to benefit from health care.

11. Health care is characterised by asymmetry of information. In particular, doctors are usually better informed about health and health care than are patients. For this reason, a principal–agent relationship usually develops in which the doctor (the agent) makes available their specialist knowledge to the patient (the principal).

12. If doctors acted as perfect agents they would maximise the utility of the principal. The hypothesis of supplier-induced demand is that doctors act as imperfect agents – failing to

maximise the patients' utility – in order to maximise their own utility. Unfortunately, supplier-induced demand is difficult to detect, since empirical findings may be consistent with a non-inducement hypothesis.

13. When considering the aggregate demand for health care (the demand for health care by an entire country), researchers have found that, using health care spending per person as a proxy measure for aggregate demand, most of the variation in health care demand between countries can be explained by the country's income.

CHAPTER 3

The production and costs of health care

3.1 Introduction

Applying economic theories of supply to health care requires us to consider its special characteristics as an economic good. Nevertheless, the same analytical framework can be applied to health care as to other goods and services. Supply theory analyses how 'firms' behave in the economic environment in which they operate. In health care, this can be applied equally to pharmaceutical companies selling in private markets and general medical practices serving the public sector. Supply of a good or service depends on its production: the amount that will be produced under different circumstances and the cost of production of different amounts. This chapter examines how economic analyses of production and costs are applied to health care. It is of interest in its own right, particularly in its analysis of efficiency. It also contributes to the theory of supply and market structure and behaviour, analysed in Chapter 4, to markets and market failure, discussed in Chapter 5, and to economic evaluation, the subject of Chapters 9–13.

To emphasise the fact that conventional economics tools are used, we will sometimes use generic descriptive terms that may seem unfamiliar when applied to health care. For example, health care comprises an extremely diverse range of goods and services, including surgical procedures, screening programmes, pharmaceuticals and counselling services. We refer to all of these as 'products'. There are also many different types of health care provider, including hospitals, GP practices, pharmaceutical companies and ambulance services. We refer to these as 'firms'. The quantity of health care 'product' produced by a health care 'firm' is referred to as its 'output'.

However, we must be careful in defining what health care output is, because an inappropriate definition may mislead. There are two opposing views about the nature of health care output. It is often argued that the ultimate aim of the health sector is to improve

① health outcome   ② amount of care

health. That implies that the output of health care facilities is changes in health. The other view is that only people can produce health, but they may use health care services to do so. In that case, the output of health care facilities is simply the amount of care provided and that can be regarded as an intermediate output that is used in the creation of the final output, which is health.

There are problems with each concept of output. Output that is measured as changes in health might not reflect the amount of health care provided, especially where there is uncertainty about whether or not treatments will be successful. Moreover, as discussed in Chapter 1, health is not a good that can be directly traded, so it is difficult to use this concept in analysing health care markets. However, viewing health care as output in its own right carries the danger of ignoring the main purpose of health care, which is to affect health. We might mistakenly judge one health care facility to be more productive than others when some of the health care that it provides does not affect health, or even is harmful.

Bearing these important issues in mind, we will regard both of these as valid measures of output. Our case studies include examples of output both as changes in health and as numbers of treatments provided.

The economic theory of production and costs is often presented using examples in which a firm produces a single product. However, an important aspect of health care production is that the more usual case is of a multi-product firm. Hospitals, for example, produce an enormous variety of health care products. We introduce each concept by looking at single product firms but then generalise it to cases that more nearly reflect what health care 'firms' do.

3.2 The theory of production

3.2.1 Production functions

Chapter 1 introduced the important concept of a production function. This is the relationship between the inputs to and outputs from a firm's productive process, as moderated by 'mediating factors' such as the environment in which the firm operates. The inputs are sometimes referred to as factors of production, factor inputs, or simply factors. They are commonly categorised into three broad types: labour; land or raw materials; and capital.

Consider the production of cataract removals in a surgical unit within an eye hospital. The inputs to production are labour resources such as the time of a surgeon, an anaesthetist and a nurse, and capital resources such as the use of an operating theatre and equipment plus materials such as drugs, dressings and disposables. There will also be inputs that are used in pre- and post-operative care of patients, including perhaps the use of hospital beds. The production function analyses how these various inputs combine to produce output, measured as the number of operations. For example, to what extent can different inputs, such as surgeons and nurses, be substituted for each other? If we employ more nurses, how many more operations will we be able to perform? How many more operations will we be able to perform if we use more of all of the inputs? How can we tell if production is being carried out efficiently?

For a firm producing a single output from n resource inputs, a production function may be expressed as

$$Q = Q(X_1, X_2, \ldots, X_n, s, e) \tag{3.1}$$

where Q is the output quantity, $X_1, \ldots, X_n$ are the input quantities, s represents *returns to scale*, which is described below, and e represents the managerial and organisational efficiency of the production process.

3.2.2 Marginal products

In analysing how output varies with the inputs employed, it is useful to consider how much extra output is produced when more of one of the inputs is used. In the example above, if we increase the number of nurses, but do not change the quantities of the other inputs, how many more cataract removals could the hospital carry out? An input's *marginal product* (*MP*) is the additional output obtained from one additional unit of it, other things remaining the same. For factor X_i, the marginal product can be expressed as

$$MP_{Xi} = \Delta Q / \Delta X_i \tag{3.2}$$

If the good is infinitely divisible, so that the function in equation (3.1) is differentiable, the marginal product can be defined as a partial derivative, $\partial Q / \partial X_i$.

The size of the marginal product may vary with the amount of inputs that are being used. If only a few nurses are employed, the extra output obtained by employing one more may be quite large. However, if there are very many, the output may be small. The *law of diminishing marginal returns* states that as the use of a particular input increases, the same increase will produce smaller and smaller increases in output. This law is observable in many production processes: Box 3.1 gives an unusual example in health care.

3.2.3 Technical efficiency and isoquants

The key issues in analysing production efficiency are demonstrated using a simple model in which there are only two inputs. Figure 3.1 shows, for each possible combination of these two inputs, the amount of output produced. This is analogous to how indifference curves (see Chapter 2) map the utility obtained from bundles of goods, but with an important difference. The indifference curve describes the utility that is actually gained from each bundle for a particular person. It would be possible similarly to describe what is actually produced from a particular combination of inputs. However, the curve shown, which is called an isoquant, maps the maximum output that the existing production technology can produce under ideal

BOX 3.1 ## Diminishing returns to health expenditure

All production functions relate inputs to outputs, but this need not be at the level of an individual type of health care or organisation. It is possible to look at different levels of aggregation. In the extreme, we can compare the total volume of inputs in a country with output indicators referring to the whole country. Since different countries have different levels of inputs and outputs, we can plot and estimate an aggregate world production function. Using World Bank data for 2009, total health expenditures per person can be plotted against life expectancy:

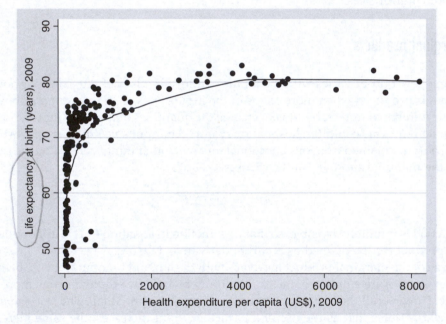

Health expenditures are a proxy for the quantity of inputs that a country devotes to health care and life expectancy is a proxy for health output. The relationship between them is consistent with the view that health expenditure has diminishing returns. It is positive up to an expenditure level of around $4 200 per person. Additional expenditure beyond this level has a negligible incremental effect on life expectancy.

Source: The World Bank website, www.data.worldbank.org.

conditions. Achieving this output is known as technical efficiency. Another way of viewing this is that if technical efficiency is achieved, it is not possible to produce more output without using more of at least one resource input. This definition is related to the concept of Pareto efficiency, which will be considered in more detail in Chapters 5 and 9.

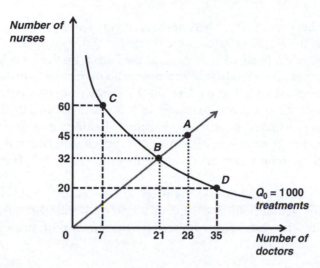

Figure 3.1 Production function and isoquant

There may be more than one technically efficient way to produce an amount of output. For example, the number of treatments that can be carried out in a hospital depends on the number of medical and nursing staff that the hospital has and on other inputs. To some extent, it is possible to substitute between medical and nursing staff, because either staff type could carry out some tasks. Ignoring for the present the other inputs, a hospital with a particular range of specialities might be able to produce a maximum of 1 000 treatments per year if it employs 60 nurses and 7 doctors, as at point C in Figure 3.1. However, it could produce the same amount in a technically efficient way with 20 nurses and 35 doctors, as at point D.

An isoquant shows every technically efficient combination of inputs that can be used to produce a specified output quantity in a defined time period. This isoquant, which includes points C and D, relates to 1 000 treatments but production functions generate a different isoquant for each output quantity.

Another way to view technically efficient production is that it uses the smallest possible amounts of inputs to produce a given output. It follows that it is not possible for a firm to use an input combination that lies below the isoquant. However, technically inefficient firms by definition have input combinations that lie above an isoquant. Point A on Figure 3.1 shows a technically inefficient hospital. It produces 1 000 treatments using 45 nurses and 28 doctors. If it were technically efficient it would employ either fewer doctors or fewer nurses or fewer of both. It could, for example, employ half the number of nurses or of doctors than it does.

Identifying inefficiency is useful, but it is even better to quantify the *amount* of inefficiency. However, there is a problem with that. Technically efficient firms may produce anywhere on the isoquant, so inefficiency cannot be expressed simply in terms of using too many of one type of input. Some technically efficient hospitals, such as those at points C and D, might actually employ either more doctors or more nurses than an inefficient hospital, but many fewer of the other type of staff. There are several ways to overcome this problem, but one of the most useful is the *Farrell radial measure* (Farrell, 1957). Essentially, the problem is that we are trying to compare a point with a line, and the Farrell method works by restricting the comparison to one point on the isoquant. It compares an inefficient firm with an efficient firm that uses the same proportions of inputs. The line $0A$ – a ray from the origin – shows all points that employ the same ratio of doctors to nurses as hospital A. One of them, point B, is on the isoquant and therefore technically efficient. Hospital A's degree of technical efficiency can therefore be measured by comparison with this point. Specifically, the ratio $0B/0A$ is an index of relative inefficiency, which can take values from just above 0 (very inefficient) to 1 (fully efficient).

With two inputs, the calculation is straightforward, because $0B/0A$ is identical to both the ratio of doctors employed at Point B compared to point A and also the equivalent ratio of nurses employed. In this example, comparing the number of doctors shows that the inefficiency index is $21/28 = 0.75$.

3.2.4 Substitutability between inputs

The slope of the isoquant is called the marginal rate of technical substitution (*MRTS*) of the inputs. It measures the degree to which different factors of production can be substituted for each other. The *MRTS* is given by:

$$MRTS_{XiXj} = \Delta X_j / \Delta X_i \tag{3.3}$$

As with the MRS of an indifference curve in Chapter 2, the *MRTS* is usually regarded as a positive number and is therefore strictly speaking the negative of the isoquant slope.

The *MRTS* at any particular point is equal to the ratio of the marginal products of the factors at that point. Using equation (3.2), the ratio of marginal products is

$$MP_{Xi} / MP_{Xj} = (\Delta Q / \Delta X_i) / (\Delta Q / \Delta X_j) \tag{3.4}$$

which rearranges to

$$MP_{Xi} / MP_{Xj} = \Delta X_j / \Delta X_i = MRTS_{XiXj} \tag{3.5}$$

Note that ΔQ disappears, which illustrates the point that output is the same everywhere on the isoquant. In Figure 3.1, for example, consider points C and B. If the number of nurses is decreased from 60 to 32, an increase is needed in the number of doctors from 7 to 21 to keep output at 1 000 treatments. But if the number of doctors is not increased, it will not be possible to undertake that number and output might, say, fall to 664 treatments, a decrease of 336. This implies that on average the marginal product of a nurse is $336/28 = 12$ treatments. Fourteen more doctors are needed to raise output from 664 back up to 1 000 treatments, implying that the marginal product of a doctor is on average $336/14 = 24$ treatments. The slope of the isoquant between points C and B is $-28/14$, which is the same as $-24/12$.

The isoquant is convex to the origin, so that as we move from left to right along the isoquant the *MRTS* decreases. For example, in Figure 3.1, the *MRTS* between C and $B = 28/14 = 2$, but between B and D it is $12/14 = 0.86$. In our example, this means that the fewer nurses we have, the more difficult it is to substitute nurses for doctors and attain the same number of treatments. What does this imply about the different inputs' *MP*s? A convex isoquant reflects an assumption that any factor's *MP* diminishes as the intensity of its use increases. In this case, the greater the ratio of nurses to doctors, the smaller the nurses' *MP* and the larger the doctors' *MP*. Strictly speaking, this is not the same assumption as the law of diminishing marginal returns, because that explicitly assumes that one factor is variable and all other factors are fixed. As we will demonstrate in Section 3.4, it is possible to have constant or even increasing marginal returns even with a non-convex isoquant. However, the rationales for these two assumptions are clearly very similar.

See Box 3.2 for an application of *MP* and *MRTS* to the production of live births in Thailand.

BOX 3.2   The production of live births in Thailand

Suraratdecha and Okunade (2006), using data from 1982 to 1997, constructed a production function for the health care system in Thailand, where 'the rapid growth in the use of limited resources and the escalating national health expenditure, raise the critical economic question of whether the use of health care resources [is] efficient'. The output measure was the number of live births per 1 000 population, which was related to three labour inputs (doctors, nurses and pharmacists) and one capital input (the number of hospital beds). The data also took into account regions within Thailand, time as an indicator of technical progress, and the number of hospitals and medical practices as an indicator of the effects of the scale of production.

It was found that the numbers of nurses and of beds had a positive influence on output, but that numbers of doctors and pharmacists had a negative effect. The calculated marginal products (*MP*s) for nurses and beds are therefore positive, but not only were the *MP*s of doctors and pharmacists negative, they were larger in absolute terms. However, the *MP*s varied widely across regions: for example, the nursing *MP* varied from 6.52 in Bangkok to 36.01 in the Northeast, with a national average of 16.48. This pattern was the same for all of the inputs; however, over time the regional *MP*s converged towards the Bangkok levels.

There was evidence of technical progress, with increasing use of physicians and to a lesser extent of pharmacists over time, but lower use of nurses and beds. The analysis suggested strong scale economies, with a 10% rise in health system capacity associated with a 26% rise in output, although this again varied by region. Estimates were made of the possibilities for substitution between inputs, which confirmed that the isoquants were of the theoretical shape, convex to the origin.

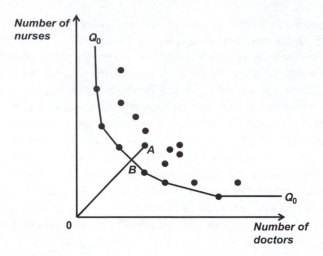

Figure 3.2 Production frontier

3.2.5 Production frontiers

Although the isoquant is a theoretical device, it can in principle be estimated from real data on inputs and output. However, it is important to remember that it assumes that production is technically efficient. In practice, firms will produce at different levels of efficiency relative to the theoretical maximum output. Indeed, there may be no observations of firms who are technically efficient relative to an absolute standard. A different view of the production process using real data is a *production frontier*, illustrated in Figure 3.2. The figure is based on a scatter diagram of observed input combinations that produce a given output Q_0. For example, each dot might represent an observed number of doctors and nurses for different health care providers producing a given number of operations. The frontier Q_0Q_0 is defined as a set of boundary points consisting of all firms that are technically efficient. All of the dots inside the boundary, such as point A, are technically inefficient. Again, the inefficiency level can be measured by the Farrell ratio $0B/0A$. Such a frontier is sometimes called a best practice frontier, because it does not compare firms to a theoretical standard but to the best observable performance within an industry.

3.3 Multi-product firms

Hospitals and other health care facilities do not usually produce only one generic output of, for example, 'operations'. Not only are there many different types of operation, hospitals also provide medical and other types of care as well as surgery. It would be possible to analyse production functions separately for each of the 'products' that a multi-product firm such as a

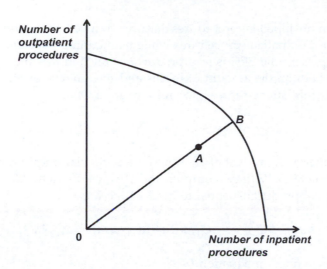

Figure 3.3 Production transformation curve

non-specialist hospital provides. However, this ignores three important economic issues. First, although there may be varying degrees of specialisation in the way in which different types of care are produced, there will be some input factors that could be used for many different types of care, for example basic nursing. The opportunity cost of using such inputs for one type of care is therefore that they cannot be used for another. Secondly, the hospital has to decide not only how many inputs to employ, but also which outputs should be produced, and how many of each. Thirdly, there may be some shared inputs, which are difficult to attribute to a single product. For example, a hospital normally needs only one Chief Executive, however many different types of care it provides.

A useful way to analyse the production of multi-product firms is therefore to look at how much of different types of product can be produced by a given amount of inputs. Figure 3.3 illustrates this for a simple case where a hospital has two products, inpatient procedures and outpatient procedures. The curve shown is a *production possibility curve* (PPC), which is also sometimes referred to as a production possibility frontier or boundary, or as a product transformation curve. It shows all the possible combinations of the two outputs that can be produced with a given amount of inputs. As with the isoquant, every point on the curve is assumed to be technically efficient.

The slope of this line is known as the *rate of product transformation* (RPT), which shows how substitutable the outputs are for each other. If there are two outputs, Q_1 and Q_2, and one input, X, the rate of product transformation of Q_1 for Q_2 is

$$RPT_{Q1Q2} = \Delta Q_2 / \Delta Q_1 \qquad (3.6)$$

The *RPT* is usually assumed to vary according to the mix of outputs that is chosen. Specifically, the larger the ratio of Q_1 to Q_2 is, the larger the *RPT* of Q_1 for Q_2 is. The shape of PPC shown in Figure 3.3 reflects this, because the further along the curve the output mix is, the lower the *RPT*. The more inpatient procedures that are produced, the more difficult it becomes to substitute them for outpatient procedures while maintaining the same input quantities.

One way to represent the PPC is as a production function in which production of one good is dependent both on the amount of inputs and the amount of other outputs. With n inputs and m goods this can be represented for any good Qi as

$$Q_i = Q_i(X_1, X_2, \ldots X_n, Q_1, Q_2, \ldots Q_{m-1}) \tag{3.7}$$

From this, the marginal product of an input for a particular output can be defined in the same way as equation (3.2). With two outputs, the *MP*s will be $\Delta Q_1/\Delta X_i$ and $\Delta Q_2/\Delta X_i$. The ratio of these marginal products is equal to the *RPT*, because

$$MP_{Q1}/MP_{Q2} = (\Delta Q_1/\Delta X_i)/(\Delta Q_1/\Delta X_i) = \Delta Q_2/\Delta Q_1 \tag{3.8}$$

which is the *RPT* as defined in equation (3.6).

This result is similar to the finding that the *MRTS* is equal to the ratio of two input *MP*s. Suppose that the *RPT* of inpatient (*IP*) for outpatient care (*OP*) is −10, meaning that the number of inputs used will be the same if we substitute one inpatient for ten outpatient procedures. Reducing the number of inpatient procedures by one would release $1/MP_{IP}$ units of the inputs; providing ten more outpatient procedures would use $10/MP_{OP}$ units. If the amount of inputs is to remain the same, these must be equal, so the ratio of MP_{OP}/MP_{IP} must be equal to −10, which is the $MRTS_{IPOP}$.

Again, it is possible to analyse this using the concept of frontiers and to measure efficiency using the Farrell measure. Figure 3.4 shows the equivalent production possibility frontier (PPF). The *RPT* does not decline smoothly. It is constant between frontier points and changes only at those points. In both Figure 3.3 and Figure 3.4, point *A* represents an

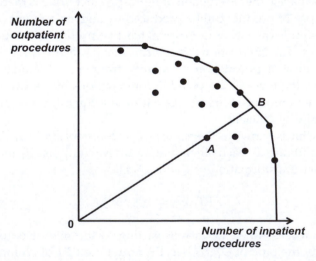

Figure 3.4 Production frontier: two outputs

inefficient hospital, as it lies within the *PPF*. An efficient hospital that produced the same ratio of outputs would produce at point *B*. The ratio $0A/0B$ measures the relative technical efficiency of hospital *A*. An example of this technique, applied to nursing home care, is shown in Box 3.3.

BOX 3.3   A multi-product production function for nursing-home care in the United States

Nyman and Bricker (1989), using data for one year, constructed a production frontier for nursing homes in Wisconsin, USA, noting that 'nursing homes, with expenditures nearing 1% of GNP, represent an important industry – one whose importance is expected to grow as the population ages'. They had five outputs; these were numbers of patients according to the kind of care they required: skilled nursing facility (SNF) intermediate nursing facility (INF), 'limited' care, 'personal' care and residential care. They included four inputs: these were hours of different types of labour: nurses, social workers, therapists and other staff.

Farrell technical efficiency scores were calculated for each nursing home. Those that defined the frontier had, of course, the highest possible efficiency score of 100%; the lowest score was 23% and the average was 89%. Factors that influenced these scores were analysed. For-profit homes had higher efficiency scores; for-profit nursing homes used 4.5% less labour per patient than did non-profit homes. Other factors that were associated with higher efficiency scores were a smaller proportion of SNF patients, lower wages and location in an urban area.

One problem with this kind of study is that it is important to make sure that the output measures used reflect important aspects of the service. In this case, the output is simply numbers of patients. Aspects of quality or what level of service patients received are not included. If, for example, staff in non-profit homes spent more time with patients, which led to an improvement in their well-being and satisfaction, the additional hours would in this kind of analysis simply be seen as inefficiency rather than a better service.

3.4 Returns to scale, additivity and fixed factors

A question that is often posed is how big health care facilities should be. For example, is it better for general practitioners to have separate facilities, or should they have a group practice? This question involves a number of different issues, concerned with demand as much as supply, but one of them is the extent to which merged practices can provide more health care than individual practices. This is the issue of *returns to scale*. It is closely related to *economies of scale*, which we consider in greater detail below.

The term 'scale' is a shortened version of 'scale of production'. Scale is defined by the quantity of output that is produced by an efficient firm. However, scale can be equivalently measured by looking at the quantity of inputs of all kinds that is required to produce a given amount of output. Returns to scale are then defined with respect to how the output quantity changes when the input quantities change, but with the mix of inputs remaining the same. If all inputs are multiplied by a number and output increases by the same multiple, there are *constant returns to scale*. For example, if there are 10 times the numbers of doctors and nurses and all other inputs, this will enable 10 times as many operations to be performed. If output increases by an amount greater than the input multiple, there are *increasing returns to scale*, and if by a smaller amount, *decreasing returns to scale*.

Figure 3.5 illustrates this using an isoquant map. It has two isoquants representing production of Q_0 and Q_1 operations, where $Q_1 > Q_0$. Point A represents 20 nurses and 17 doctors, and at that point the efficient amount of output produced is Q_0. Point B represents 40 nurses and 34 doctors, which is twice as many of each, and the efficient output is Q_1. If $Q_1 = 2Q_0$, then there are constant returns to scale. If Q_1 is more than double Q_0, there are increasing returns; if it is less than double, there are decreasing returns.

Increasing returns to scale have several sources. One is that large organisations can specialise, which applies to many inputs including the labour force, capital equipment and management. For example, a small hospital may have to employ general surgeons to deal with many areas of surgery, but a larger one may be able to employ specialist surgeons, who become proficient in performing specific types of surgery and can produce more output. A second is that there may be technical and managerial indivisibilities. Some inputs such as machinery are only efficient to use at a higher scale of production. They may have a fixed capacity, so that at lower levels of production there is spare capacity, and higher levels of

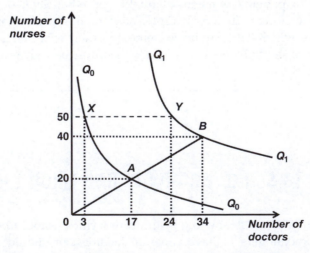

Figure 3.5 Isoquant map, returns to scale and returns to a fixed factor

production do not require an additional machine. For example, a body scanner in a rural area where there are only a few patients may not be used to its technically possible capacity. A third is that many aspects of a firm's overall activities may not increase proportionately as output increases, such as selling and promotion. For example, if a smoking cessation campaign is expanded to cover twice the number of people, that may not use twice the number of inputs. The initial work of devising the campaign and setting up a campaign structure does not need to be done again. Finally, where there is uncertainty in the required level of output, a larger scale takes advantage of the *law of large numbers*. This essentially means that predictions about the required level of output have greater precision. For example, a maternity hospital might wish to ensure that it has sufficient delivery rooms available on 99% of occasions. If it has an average of two deliveries per day, it might require four delivery suites to achieve this, with an average overcapacity of 100%. If it has an average of eight deliveries per day, it might require only ten suites, with an average overcapacity of 25%.

Whether *decreasing* returns to scale exist or not is disputed. They may arise from managerial inefficiencies, because at higher levels of production managers can be overworked making the decision-making process less efficient. An alternative view is that there are always increasing returns to scale in many areas of production, and those will always offset any managerial inefficiencies.

It is less easy to define returns to scale for multi-product firms. For example, it might still be the case that doubling the number of doctors and nurses in a hospital would enable twice the number of inpatient and outpatient procedures to be carried out. However, the mix of inpatient and outpatient procedures would be in the same proportions as before. There might be other efficient output mixes for the new level of inputs. For example, it might be equally efficient, given the doubled inputs, to have three times as many inpatient procedures and only 50% more outpatient procedures. If a firm does have a different output mix for different levels of inputs, scale economies are not unambiguously defined. Identifying and measuring returns to scale in real multi-product industries such as health care is therefore particularly difficult.

The sources of returns to scale are so-called 'long-run' factors, where all inputs are variable and can be flexibly assigned to different output combinations. Returns to scale for a hospital, for example, are relevant where all of the resources used by a hospital can be changed – buildings, equipment and consumables as well as staff numbers – to whatever amounts are required. The 'long run' is tautologically defined as the period of time that it would take to change the resource amounts to the desired level.

In the short run, which is simply a period of time shorter than the long run, the use of some resources will not be so flexible. For example, there may be temporary shortages of certain types of labour or equipment, or it may not be possible to expand the hospital site until new land is purchased and new buildings are constructed. In this case, we may be interested in what happens when some resource inputs are increased while others are fixed. Section 3.2.2 described the law of diminishing returns as the usual assumption about what happens when there are fixed inputs. The more of a variable input that is used, the smaller will be the increase in output from increasing the amount of the input used. Diminishing returns will definitely arise if the production function has constant or decreasing returns to scale. However, in theory this will not occur if there are very strongly increasing returns to scale. Figure 3.5 demonstrates this. If the number of nurses is fixed at 50 and there are constant returns to scale so that

$Q_1 = 2 \times Q_0$, the number of doctors would have to increase from 3 to 24, which is clearly more than double; hence there are diminishing returns. However, returns to increased numbers of doctors would actually increase if Q_1 were greater than Q_0 by a multiplication factor greater than $24/3 = 8$.

Because of the problem of defining output when there are many different products, it is difficult in practice to assess the extent of returns to scale and to fixed factors in health care. Many studies use a quantitative technique called Data Envelopment Analysis (Hollingsworth and Peacock, 2008) to overcome this problem, applying the Farrell measure described earlier. An example is a study of district hospitals in Namibia by Zere *et al.* (2006). However, evidence about scale, which as suggested is relevant to planning of health care facilities and mergers between them, comes mainly from studies of costs. The analysis of *returns* to scale is therefore best seen as providing one of the sources of *economies* of scale, which will be discussed below.

Returns to scale are not the only reason for expanding or merging health care facilities. Another reason is that this enables different *types* of health care to be brought together in the same facility, especially specialist health care services. This might be because of factors such as convenience to patients, but it might also be possible to produce more health care for a given set of inputs when it is produced in a shared facility than if it were produced separately. One reason would be if there were limited demands for each type of health care. Each type might use inputs that are indivisible, but can be used for a number of different types. If they are produced separately there will be spare capacity in those inputs. Having more products enables those inputs to be shared. There are many potentially shareable inputs in health care, such as inpatient beds, outpatient facilities, operating theatres, intensive therapy units and general nursing, medical, administrative and support staff.

This issue is known as *additivity*, which is closely related to *economies of scope*, discussed below. It is illustrated in Figure 3.6 using a production frontier. Suppose that a dentist can

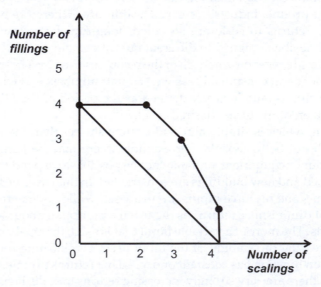

Figure 3.6 Additivity in production

provide one filling or one scaling in 15 minutes, including examination of the patient. If one hour of dentist's time is divided between practices that specialise in these different procedures, it is possible to provide four fillings only, three fillings and one scaling, two fillings and two scalings, three scalings or one filling, or four scalings only. The *RPT* is therefore one scaling for one filling, which is represented by the solid straight line. However, a general dental practitioner could, by combining examinations for the two procedures, provide more than this. The different combinations that the dentist can provide in one hour, for example three fillings and three scalings, are shown by a *joint production frontier*, the line connecting the dots. If, as in this case, output is greater with joint production than with separate production, there is *super-additivity*. It is also possible to have *sub-additivity*, where output is lower with joint production than with separate production.

If there is super-additivity, primary health care facilities that offer a number of services and general hospitals may be justified on efficiency grounds. Specialised facilities are justified if there are many highly specialised inputs that are not suitable for sharing, or where a high demand means that there is no spare capacity of shareable inputs. As with returns to scale, it is difficult to measure additivity in production directly. Relevant evidence comes from studies of costs, additivity in production being one of the sources of economies of scope.

3.5 Costs

So far, our analysis of how the output level is determined has regarded the inputs as resources that exist in a physical sense. However, a key aspect of economics is a concern with values. Economists measure the value of resources by their cost, in particular, the opportunity cost concept introduced in Chapter 1. Here, we investigate how costs vary as firms change the quantity of output produced. We are particularly interested in how firms can minimise costs, for two main reasons: first, it may be useful in explaining a firm's market behaviour; and secondly because this defines an important dimension of efficiency, different to technical efficiency.

3.5.1 Costs and production

The total cost of producing a particular amount of a good obviously depends on how much of each input is used and the cost of acquiring it. We will call the cost of one unit of an input its unit cost, although it is often called the input price. The total cost of each input is the unit cost multiplied by the number of units. The total cost of using a particular combination of inputs is the sum of the total costs of the inputs:

$$C = X_1 P_{x1} + X_2 P_{x2} + \cdots + X_n P_{xn} \tag{3.9}$$

where $X_1, \ldots, X_n$ are the input quantities and $P_{x1}, \ldots, P_{xn}$ are those inputs' unit costs.

This shows the cost of using a particular combination of inputs. However, this cost is not unique. There are many different combinations of inputs that would cost the same amount. For example, suppose the monthly costs of employing a nurse and a doctor are £3 000 and £6 000 respectively. The total cost would be £240 000 if, for example, 60 nurses and 10 doctors were employed or 40 nurses and 20 doctors or 20 nurses and 30 doctors. In Figure 3.7(a) this is plotted as a straight line, called an *isocost line*. It can also be viewed as a *budget constraint* similar to that introduced in Chapter 2, since it defines every input combination that can be afforded

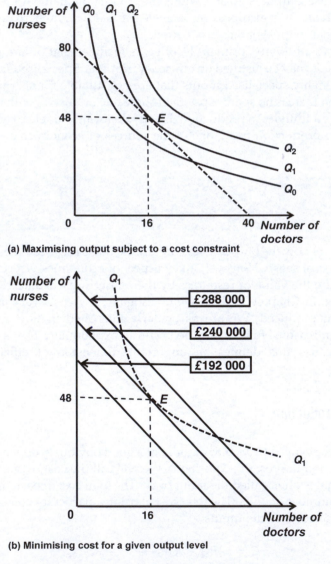

(a) Maximising output subject to a cost constraint

(b) Minimising cost for a given output level

Figure 3.7 Equivalence of maximising output and minimising cost

for a given budget. The limiting points are that 80 nurses could be employed if the entire budget was spent on them and similarly the maximum number of doctors that could be employed is 40. The slope of the isocost line is the ratio of the unit costs of the two inputs, P_{x1}/P_{x2}, which in this case is $3\,000/6\,000 = 0.5$.

Figure 3.7(b) shows three isocost lines representing different cost outlays. The input prices are the same for all of them, which is why they all have the same slope. The further they are from the origin, the greater the total cost.

The isocost line shows the relationship between cost and inputs. The production function shows the relationship between inputs and output. So, if these are linked, it is possible to analyse the relationship between cost and output. But, as with the analysis of isoquants, it is necessary to assume that production is undertaken efficiently. Isoquants are defined with respect to technical efficiency, achieving the maximum output from a given set of inputs. The cost-output relationship also requires technical efficiency, but in addition requires a separate type of efficiency. This has several different labels, including *economic efficiency*, *cost-effectiveness* and *allocative efficiency in production*. It means achieving either the lowest possible cost of producing a particular level of output or the greatest possible output for a particular budget. As we will show, these different definitions give identical results.

Figure 3.7(a) illustrates how output is maximised for a given cost. The greatest output that can be produced given the constraint on cost is Q_1, where the isocost line is at a tangent to the highest attainable isoquant. The optimal input combination is at point E, with 48 nurses and 16 doctors. Higher output levels such as Q_2 are not affordable and other points on the isocost line all lie on a lower isoquant such as Q_0.

Figure 3.7(b) illustrates how the cost of a given output is minimised. The isoquant denoting the desired level of output is Q_1. The lowest attainable isocost line that enables this to be produced is for £240 000 and production should be at their point of tangency, E. It is not possible to obtain the desired level of output at a cost such as £192 000 and other points on the isoquant all lie on a higher isocost line such as that for £288 000.

These solutions are identical. In both cases, at the point of tangency, the slope of the isoquant is equal to the slope of the isocost line. Using equation (3.5), this means that

$$MP_{X1}/MP_{X2} = P_{x1}/P_{x2} \tag{3.10}$$

which rearranges to $MP_{X1}/P_{x1} = MP_{X2}/P_{x2}$. More generally, the combination of inputs is efficient if

$$\frac{MP_{X1}}{P_{x1}} = \frac{MP_{x2}}{P_{x2}} = \frac{MP_{x3}}{P_{x3}} = \cdots = \frac{MP_{Xn}}{P_{xn}} \tag{3.11}$$

The numerator of this ratio is output measured in physical units, for example the number of operations. The denominator is a price measured in some currency, for example pounds. The ratio is therefore extra operations per pound spent. The condition in equation (3.11) means that when we have an efficient combination of inputs, the extra output per amount spent is the same for all inputs. If any input has a higher ratio than this, it is efficient to employ more of it, by substituting it for less productive inputs. Similarly, if any input has a lower ratio, it is efficient to employ less of it.

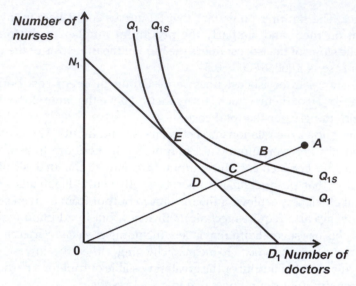

Figure 3.8 Technical, allocative and scale efficiency

There is another way of viewing the efficiency achieved by producing output at the lowest possible cost. For a given set of input prices, it is not possible to produce more of any good or service without incurring greater costs. As with technical efficiency, this is a definition related to Pareto efficiency (see Chapter 9). The terminology used in this context is *allocative efficiency in production*.

Figure 3.8 shows how allocative and technical efficiency can be quantified using a Farrell measure. Point A represents the input combination of an inefficient hospital producing Q_1. To be technically efficient, it should reduce its input use so that it was at Point C, as that is on the isoquant for Q_1. However, C is not the allocatively efficient point on that isoquant; that is point E. To be allocatively efficient the hospital should reduce its input use to point D, as that is on the isocost line N_1D_1. However, D is not the technically efficient point on that isocost line; again that is E. So we should really compare point A with point E. Unfortunately, we cannot do that directly. Instead, we have to decompose overall efficiency into separate allocative and technical elements.

As before, technical efficiency can be measured as $0C/0A$, the deviation of the hospital from the technically efficient output. Allocative efficiency can be measured as $0D/0C$, the deviation of the technically efficient point from the allocatively efficient point. Overall efficiency can be measured as $0D/0A$, which is simply the product of allocative and technical efficiency, since $0D/0C \times 0C/0A = 0D/0A$. This shows that technical efficiency is a *necessary* but not *sufficient* condition for allocative efficiency.

The final link in analysing the relationship between cost and output is to consider what will happen to the efficient input combination in response to changes in the desired output or to the budget. There is an efficient input combination for every possible isocost curve and isoquant curve. The way that efficient input combinations change as output increases is known as an *expansion path*, consisting of all of the tangency points.

3.5.2 Cost functions

Equation (3.1) relates quantities of outputs to quantities of inputs. Equation (3.9) relates quantities of inputs to cost. These can be combined to produce a cost function, which relates quantities of outputs to cost:

$$C = C(Q, P_{x1}, P_{x2}, \dots P_{xn}) \tag{3.12}$$

This is a general way of expressing the cost function, which emphasises that costs depend on both the quantity of inputs and input prices. However, for simplicity we will mainly use a shortened version of this, which assumes that input prices are fixed:

$$C = C(Q) \tag{3.13}$$

It is also possible to define a multi-product cost function:

$$C = C(Q_1, Q_2, \dots Q_m, P_{x1}, P_{x2}, \dots P_{xn}) \tag{3.14}$$

Two important measures derived from the cost function are *average cost* (*AC*) and *marginal cost* (*MC*). Average cost is simply total cost divided by quantity:

$$AC = C(Q)/Q \tag{3.15}$$

Marginal cost is the additional cost of an extra unit of output

$$MC = \Delta C(Q)/\Delta Q \tag{3.16}$$

or, for a differentiable function, $\partial C(Q)/\partial Q$.

The difference between *AC* and *MC* is very important in applied health economics. Very often data are available on the average cost of health care services but not on their marginal cost. However, using average costs as if they were marginal costs may mislead. For example, hospital costs will be reduced by schemes that allow some patients to be treated in the community rather than being admitted. Given data on total costs of inpatient stays, it is possible to calculate an average cost per patient. It is tempting to conclude that avoiding an admission will reduce costs by that amount. However, the average includes patients with different levels of illness severity, and the more severe the illness the more costly they will be to treat. Less severely ill patients are most likely to be suitable for treatment in the community, so *MC* will be lower than *AC*. Such schemes will therefore produce a lower cost reduction than the estimate of *AC* suggests.

A problem with multi-product cost functions is that it is not possible to define meaningfully what the *AC* of a particular product is. If different products share some inputs, the costs of those inputs cannot be solely attributed to any one of them. It is possible to define the *MC* of each product, because this is calculated holding the amount of all other products constant. In practice, when multi-product organisations such as hospitals calculate costs for particular products, they use accounting rules to share out the costs of all inputs and calculate average not marginal costs. See Box 3.4 for an example of a study estimating a multi-product cost function.

BOX 3.4   **Factors affecting the cost of hospital services in the USA**

Fournier and Mitchell (1992) estimated a multi-product cost function for 179 short-term general-care hospitals in Florida, USA from 1984 to 1986. The cost function included five different hospital outputs, hospital input prices and fixed inputs. They also studied the effect of hospital ownership and competition on the function.

Greater hospital output was associated with higher cost. The number of inpatient admissions, outpatient visits, emergency room visits and surgery minutes all had a statistically significant and positive effect on costs. Inpatient admissions had the largest impact. Input prices were highly significant predictors of cost, the salary of registered nurses being especially important. Capital stock also had a significant positive impact. This was interpreted as meaning that hospitals were employing too much fixed capital and equipment. The number of admitting physicians also had a significant positive effect. This was interpreted as evidence of either supplier-induced demand, or the positive effect of more physicians on quality, or both.

Investor-owned hospitals, and in particular those in a chain, had significantly lower costs than private non-profit hospitals and government-owned hospitals. Teaching hospitals had significantly higher costs.

The effect of competition depended on the type of health service. For maternity services, hospitals located in areas with a higher level of market concentration had higher costs. This implies that more competitive markets had lower costs. In contrast, higher concentrations of admissions, surgery, radiation therapy and diagnostic imaging procedures significantly lowered costs. This implies that greater competition raises cost. This may be because hospitals in more competitive markets engage in non-price competition, which adds to costs.

As with production functions, the cost function can be interpreted in two different ways depending on how relative efficiency is defined. As suggested above, the expansion path shows all technically and economically efficient input combinations at different levels of output. This enables a relationship between cost and output to be derived. However, the cost function can also be interpreted as an empirical relationship, in which efficiency relative to the theoretical minimum cost is not known or defined. In this case, the relationship between cost and output is best expressed in terms of a *cost frontier*. This has exactly the same relationship to a cost function as a production frontier has to a production function. It is again based on best practice from firms that achieve lower costs for the output produced. Efficiency is again defined in terms of performance relative to others, rather than to an absolute standard. Box 3.5 shows an example of the use of cost frontiers.

BOX 3.5   A cost frontier for hospitals in Finland

Linna (1998) analysed the efficiency of 43 acute-care hospitals in Finland in 1988–1994, using two different methods of estimating a cost frontier. He noted that 'economic recession and the Government's budget deficit have placed increasing pressure on hospitals in Finland to contain costs. The state subsidy reform of 1993 was expected to enhance productive efficiency by introducing competitive elements into health care.'

The data used were for four types of output (inpatient and outpatient treatment, teaching and research), two price variables (wage rates and general local health care prices), three other factors affecting cost (teaching status, readmission rate and year of observation) and an indicator of scale (number of beds).

Among the conclusions were that cost efficiency improved over time; teaching and research raise costs, but teaching hospitals were no more or less efficient than other hospitals; and technological change was also improving efficiency. There was a 3–5% annual average increase in productivity, due in equal measure to improvement in cost efficiency and to technological change.

It was estimated that improving efficiency, presumably to the level of the most efficient hospitals, would reduce hospital costs by 1.0–1.2 billion Finnish marks each year. Finally, the improvement in productivity occurred before and after 1993, so it appeared that the subsidy reform had no effect on efficiency.

3.5.3 Scale economies, long- and short-run cost functions and scope economies

As before, a distinction is drawn between the long run, where all inputs are variable, and the short run, where some of the inputs are fixed. Short-run and long-run cost functions therefore differ. We will consider long-run functions first.

As equations (3.13), (3.15) and (3.16) state, total costs, average costs and marginal costs all depend on the level of output. The relationships are illustrated in Figure 3.9 as cost curves, using the example of the cost of providing surgical care. The total cost (TC) curve in Figure 3.9(a) shows points of production at different levels of output, in this case the number of operations. The shape of the curve depends on *economies of scale*, how TC changes as the scale of operations changes. Scale economies arise from returns to scale, which define the relationship between scale and the amount of output, though they may also arise from other sources, which are discussed below. Constant returns to scale would produce a straight-line TC curve, meaning no scale economies, because both average and marginal costs would be constant.

Scale economies mean that there will be a less than proportionate increase in total cost due to an increase in output. It is usually assumed that these exist at low levels of output but that at some point there are no more to be gained. After that, there may even be diseconomies of scale. A long-run TC curve must start at the origin, because it is assumed that firms can close down and incur no costs by producing nothing. After this it follows an inverse S-shape, reflecting the

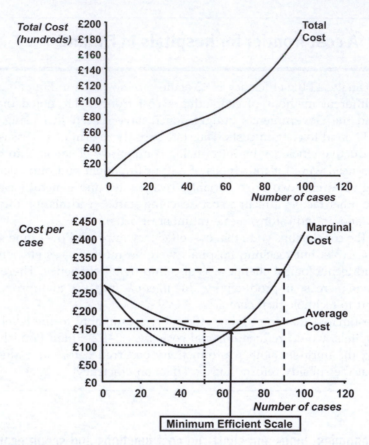

Figure 3.9 Total, average and marginal cost curves

U-shape of the average cost (*AC*) curve. At low levels of output, *AC* falls because of increasing returns to scale. However, returns to scale diminish, so *AC* falls more slowly until all scale economies are exploited. The point is then reached where there are constant returns to scale, shown by a constant *AC*. This point is known as the *minimum efficient scale*. In Figure 3.9, the minimum efficient scale is around 65 operations, at a cost of £145 per operation. In this figure, *AC* rises after this with more operations, implying decreasing returns to scale. However, as was discussed, this is a contentious concept. It is therefore often simply assumed that beyond the minimum efficient scale the *AC* curve is a horizontal straight line.

The marginal cost (*MC*) curve also reflects the pattern of economies of scale, and also has a U-shape. The *MC* curve is below the *AC* curve at lower levels of output but approaches it as output becomes greater and crosses it at the minimum point of the *AC* curve, which is the minimum efficient scale. As with any numbers, adding an item that is below the current average must cause the average to fall. So, if *MC* is less than *AC*, for example the dotted lines, where with 50 operations, *MC* = £105 and *AC* = £150, *AC* must be falling as output increases. Similarly, if extra units of output cost more to produce than the average, their production must increase average cost. So, if *MC* is greater than *AC*, for example the dashed line, where with 90 operations, $MC = £320$ and $AC = £170$, then AC must be rising. If AC is equal to MC, it is neither rising nor falling. This means that AC is both constant and at a minimum.

Scale economies that derive from returns to scale involve changes in the physical quantity of factor inputs required. However, some scale economies do not derive from increasing returns to scale. They result from paying lower prices for inputs because they are bought in large amounts; having lower costs of finance; and paying lower wages if the firm develops monopoly power in the labour market (see Chapter 8). Large hospitals, for example, are able to obtain large discounts by bulk buying not only of medical goods such as pharmaceuticals and disposables but also of goods used in their 'hotel' services.

Studies of economies of scale in the health sector do not give a consistent and general-isable picture. For example, a study by Weaver and Deolalikar (2004) examined cost functions for different types and locations of Vietnamese hospitals. They found that central general and specialty hospitals had approximately constant returns to scale, provincial general and specialty hospitals had large diseconomies of scale, district hospitals had moderate economies of scale and other hospitals had modest diseconomies of scale.

Long-run cost functions are useful in analysing the issue of the most efficient size for a firm. It assumes that all inputs are variable and can be obtained in exactly the amounts needed for a particular size. Short-run cost functions examine how costs vary with output when the firm is at a given size. This essentially means that some costs are fixed and some are variable. The short-run cost function can be expressed as

$$C = C(Q) + F \qquad (3.17)$$

where C is total cost, Q is output and F is fixed costs. Again, it is possible to define average and marginal costs, in the same way as in equations (3.15) and (3.16). Short-run TC, AC and MC curves have a similar shape to the long-run versions, but for rather different reasons.

In the short run, there are costs even if there is no output, because some costs are fixed. The short-run TC curve therefore does not start at zero but at the level of total fixed costs. It then follows an inverse S-shape, like the long-run curve, but for a different reason. With the long-run curve, this reflects the expansion path, the efficient level of costs at different levels of output. The short-run curve's shape reflects the law of diminishing returns. At low production levels the marginal productivity of variable inputs may increase, so the additional cost of producing extra units of output falls. TC therefore increases, but at a decreasing rate. As output increases further, eventually there are diminishing returns. The marginal productivity of the variable inputs falls, and extra units of output cost more to produce. TC therefore increases at an increasing rate. Using the example presented earlier of nurses employed on a ward, after diminishing returns have set in the marginal productivity of additional nurses falls. Therefore, the costs incurred employing each additional nurse achieve a lower return in terms of producing additional output. The marginal cost of producing additional output will rise as a result.

Short-run AC also follows a U-shape, for two reasons. First, AC initially falls as output rises simply because the fixed costs are spread over greater and greater output. Eventually, the fixed cost element may become so small that it is not a significant contributor to costs. Secondly, the pattern of increasing and diminishing returns causes AC first to fall and then to

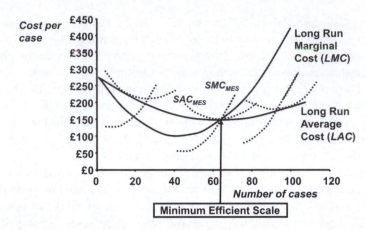

Figure 3.10 Short-run and long-run cost curves

rise. Short-run *MC* is of course unaffected by fixed costs, but it also has a U-shape, due to the changing returns to fixed factors. Again, it is equal to *AC* when *AC* is at a minimum.

What is the relationship between the long-run and short-run curves? There is only one long-run *AC* curve, but there are many short-run curves, one for each scale of output. The short-run *AC* curves, illustrated as dotted lines in Figure 3.10, should be interpreted as deviations from the long-run curve. A point on the long-run *AC* curve represents efficient production at a particular scale size. Short-run deviations from this cannot result in lower costs than the scale-efficient level of output. The short-run curves must therefore be higher than the long-run point at every level of output above or below this. They therefore lie at a tangent to the long-run curve. Note that the long-run curve is *not* composed of the minimum points of short-run curves.

At the minimum efficient scale, long-run average cost (*LAC*) is by definition at its lowest, and is therefore equal to long-run marginal cost (*LMC*). The short-run average cost (*SAC*) curve relevant to that scale (SAC_{MES}) touches the *LAC* curve at its own minimum point. This is therefore also equal to the short-run marginal cost (*SAC*) relevant to that scale (SMC_{MES}). So, if the firm's size is the minimum efficient scale and it is producing at the lowest possible *AC* for that scale, then *LAC*, *LMC*, *SAC* and *SMC* are all equal to each other.

Identifying this most efficient point is useful, because it enables us to examine the source of inefficiencies. It may be that a firm is inefficient because it is not producing the correct output for its size, or it may be that its size is wrong, or both. A Farrell measure can be used to quantify this. In Figure 3.8, the isoquant Q_{1s} represents efficient input combinations in the short run, while Q_1 represents the long-run or scale-efficient isoquant. Overall efficiency is measured, as before, by $0D/0A$. It can be decomposed into allocative efficiency, measured as before by $0D/0C$ and technical efficiency $0C/0A$. Technical efficiency can also be decomposed into pure technical efficiency, measured as $0B/0A$, which is the deviation from the short-run isoquant, and scale efficiency, measured by $0C/0B$, which is the deviation of the short-run from the scale-efficient isoquant. These measures are related by $0B/0A \times 0C/0B \times 0D/0C = 0D/0A$. As an example of this kind of analysis, the study of district hospitals in Namibia by Zere *et al.* (2006) found scale inefficiency to be as prevalent as pure technical inefficiency. They also found that the scale efficiency was mainly observed where there are increasing returns to scale, implying that the hospitals are too small, below the minimum efficient scale.

It was suggested earlier that a multi-product firm, such as a general hospital, might be more efficient than a single-product firm, such as a specialised hospital, because of the phenomenon of super-additivity. If so, we would expect this to result in lower costs for multi-product firms. This is called *economies of scope*. If there are scope economies, then, for example, a general medical practice and a general dental practice would have higher combined costs than a health centre that undertook both medicine and dentistry.

Scope economies may be defined using the concept of additivity in the cost function. An additive cost function means that the costs of joint production of outputs are the same as separate production of those outputs; in other words, there are no economies or diseconomies of scope. Similarly, a sub-additive cost function means that there are economies of scope and a super-additive cost function means that there are diseconomies of scope. It can be shown that the additivity properties of the cost function are equivalent to those of the production function. Sub-additivity of the cost function is equivalent to super-additivity of the production function and sub-additivity of the production function is equivalent to super-additivity of the cost function.

As with evidence on scale economies, studies of scope economies do not show any consistent and generalisable picture. For example, the study of Vietnamese hospitals by Weaver and Deolalikar (2004) referred to earlier found large scope economies for central and provincial general hospitals but small economies of scope for central specialty, district and other hospitals.

Summary

1. The inputs into a production process are commonly categorised into three broad types: labour; land or raw materials; and capital.
2. A production function summarises the relationship between the inputs to and outputs from a firm's productive process. It describes how the various inputs combine to produce output, and can be used to quantify how output will change as more of the inputs are employed, how the inputs can be substituted for one another to produce the same level of output, and how efficient a particular production process is. An isoquant is a graphical representation of a production function, showing all the combinations of inputs that will produce a particular output. The production function generates a different isoquant for each level of output, and a firm is technically efficient if it is producing at a point on the isoquant.
3. The marginal product of an input is the change in output resulting from a change in the quantity of the input used, other things held constant.
4. The slope of the isoquant is called the marginal rate of technical substitution of the inputs, which measures how substitutable the factors of production are.

5. Health care providers often produce more than one type of output. In economic terms they are multi-product firms. The production function for a multi-product firm can be shown graphically by the product transformation curve, the slope of which is the rate of product transformation. This defines the degree of substitutability of the outputs.

6. Returns to scale describe how output quantities change when input quantities change, but with the mix of inputs remaining the same. Increasing returns to scale in health care can explain why health care providers are often very large.

7. The concept of additivity can be used in health care to explain the merger of health care facilities. Super-additivity arises when it is possible to produce more health care for a given set of inputs when it is produced in a shared facility than if it were produced separately.

8. Costs of production depend on the quantity and combination of resource inputs that are employed, plus the unit costs of the inputs.

9. An isocost line defines all of the different combinations of the inputs that will cost a particular amount. The slope of the isocost line is the ratio of the unit costs of the two inputs.

10. Isocost lines can be combined with isoquants to determine the cost-minimising combination of inputs to produce a given level of output or the output-maximising combination of inputs for a given cost. These occur where the slope of the isoquant is equal to the slope of the isocost line, or where the marginal rate of technical substitution is equal to the ratio of the unit costs of the two inputs.

11. Cost functions relate the firm's costs to its level of output. Three useful ways of showing this relationship are total cost, average cost and marginal cost functions.

12. At low levels of output, average cost falls because of increasing returns to scale: there are economies of scale. However, returns to scale diminish, so average cost falls more slowly until all economies of scale are exploited; then there are constant returns to scale and average cost is constant. This point, which is the minimum point of the average cost function, is the minimum efficient scale. Beyond this point, average costs may start to rise, indicating decreasing returns to scale.

13. Economies of scope may be defined using the concept of additivity in the cost function. An additive cost function means that the costs of joint production of outputs are the same as separate production of those outputs; in other words, there are no economies or diseconomies of scope. Similarly, a sub-additive cost function means that there are economies of scope, and a super-additive cost function means that there are diseconomies of scope.

CHAPTER 4

The supply of health care

4.1 Firms, markets and industries in the health care sector of the economy

In earlier chapters we introduced a number of concepts that deserve further explanation. In Chapters 1 and 2, we referred to markets and introduced the analysis of health care markets as the interaction of the supply of and demand for health care. In Chapter 3, we analysed production of health care within firms and also referred to the health care industry. In this chapter, we analyse the supply side of the market and the role of firms and industries in markets. So it is useful to begin by defining what we mean by those terms.

A market is simply a place where those who wish to supply goods and those who demand them are brought together in order to effect an exchange. In economics, these suppliers and demanders are often called sellers and buyers, as the assumption is that the good will not be exchanged for free but for money or sometimes for other goods. A market need not be a single place. It would be hard to identify this for an internet pharmacy, for example. In health care, buyers include households, who buy health care services either directly out of their own pocket or indirectly via a third-party payer, and health care providers such as hospitals, who employ health care professionals via a labour market, and buy other inputs such as pharmaceuticals. Sellers include hospitals, which provide health care directly, and medical equipment and pharmaceutical companies, which provide inputs to the health care production process.

A firm is an economic unit that produces and sells goods, such as medical equipment, or services, such as dental care or health insurance. As suggested, it may sell directly to consumers of health care (people) or to other firms such as health care providers. An industry is a collection of economic units that sell similar products – for example the pharmaceutical, insurance or hospital industries. A stricter economics definition, which is important in analysing models of how markets work, is that the goods or services are close substitutes, as defined in Chapter 2.

The supply side of a market is the industry. In the same way as analysis of demand is based heavily on theories of how individual consumers behave, the analysis of supply is dependent on theories of how firms behave. Indeed, this topic is often called the *theory of the firm*. In this chapter we build on the analysis of production within firms dealt with in Chapter 3 and look in more detail at the operation of firms in the health care industry. The health care industry is large and heterogeneous, containing many different types of economic unit, which can be grouped into sectors depending on their area of specialisation. For example, health insurance companies cover the costs of health risks; pharmaceutical firms and suppliers of medical and capital equipment provide inputs into the provision of primary and hospital care; and general practitioners and hospitals provide outpatient and inpatient services. But it is important not to overlook other economic units that contribute to health overall, for example local authorities may run health promotion activities. Some of these economic units provide goods or services that are substitutes to those provided by the health care industry whilst others are complements.

Analysis of supply in economics is often dominated by theories of the firm that are based on an assumption that their overriding aim is to maximise profits. This can be viewed in two ways. First, such theories may indeed be reasonable descriptions of the aims of some firms and can therefore be used in a positive economics sense to generate predictions about the way that firms and markets operate. However, an important aspect of health care provision is that the

---

BOX 4.1   Profit maximisation in the health care industry

One area of the health care industry in which profit maximisation is commonly perceived to be an overriding aim is the pharmaceutical industry. The table below reports revenues and profits earned by the ten largest pharmaceutical companies in the USA in 2010. The figures indicate that a profit of US$0.25 was made on every US$1 of revenue.

Rank	Company	Revenue (US$ millions)	Profits (US$ millions)
1	Johnson & Johnson	61 897	12 266
2	Pfizer	50 009	8 635
3	Abbott Laboratories	30 765	5 746
4	Merck	27 428	12 901
5	Eli Lilly	21 836	4 329
6	Bristol-Myers Squibb	21 634	10 612
7	Amgen	14 642	4 605
8	Gilead Sciences	7 011	2 636
9	Mylan	5 093	233
10	Genzyme	4 516	422

Source: http://money.cnn.com/magazines/fortune/fortune500/2010/full_list/ Reproduced with permission from CNNMoney.com

more usual case is of firms that not only do not aim to maximise profits, but do not aim to earn any profits at all. The aim of most pharmaceutical companies and many insurance companies is to generate profits, and profit maximisation may be a reasonable assumption for them. Box 4.1 demonstrates how profitable health care can be. By contrast, most hospitals and nursing homes and some insurance companies do not aim to maximise profit. But theories based on profit maximisation have a second use, because they provide a useful set of performance benchmarks against which firms' actual performance can be compared. So, we will start by introducing theories based on profit maximisation, but stress that for much of health care other theories will be more appropriate.

4.2 Structure, conduct and performance in the health care industry

A useful framework within which to analyse supply is the structure–conduct–performance paradigm. The dominant features of market structure are how many firms are in the industry and how big each firm's market share is. There are other issues such as how similar the goods or services that the firms produce are and whether it is easy or difficult for new firms to enter the market. Conduct refers to how firms behave, which is in part determined by market structure. It mainly concerns whether firms compete or collude, covering issues such as their goals, pricing policies, investment and marketing strategies. Performance mainly relates to how efficient firms and industries are, either from a private or social point of view.

One of the key issues of structure is the degree of competition in markets, since that may have a large influence on the way in which firms have to operate. For example, hospitals operating in a highly competitive environment – the structure – may conduct their activities differently from those with few or no competitors. The more competitive the environment, the more aggressively the hospital may behave, in terms of pricing and the quality of care, in order to attract patients and raise revenue. This conduct will in turn influence performance, which may be measured in a variety of dimensions such as the number of patients treated, revenue earned, or profitability.

We can obtain an indication of how competitive a market is by observing the number of firms in the market. The greater the number of firms, the more competitive the market is likely to be. However, this is not an ideal measure because it does not account for the concentration of services within the firms in the market. For example, there may be many firms in the market, but if the largest provides 90% of total output the level of competition may not be as great as a market that has only two firms, each of which has 50% of the market.

A useful measure of market concentration, and therefore competition, is the Herfindahl–Hirschman Index (*HHI*), sometimes referred to as the Herfindahl Index or the Hirschman–Herfindahl Index. This is a measure of market concentration in areas served by providers, and is based on the market shares of all providers within a given market:

$$HHI = \sum_{i=1}^{n} s_i^2 \tag{4.1}$$

where s_i is the market share in percent of provider i and n is the number of providers in the market. *HHI* can take values ranging from close to zero (low concentration; much competition) to 10 000 (high concentration; no competition). If, for example, $n = 1$, there is a single provider in the market (a monopoly) with 100% of the market share. In this case $HHI = 10\ 000$. Conversely, if n is very large, indicating many different competing providers, and if each of these has a market share that is very close to 0%, then *HHI* will be very close to zero. Sometimes s is measured in proportions rather than percentages, in which case *HHI* can take values up to 1. Box 4.2 illustrates the use of the *HHI* to measure the degree of competition in the retail market for antimalarials in rural Tanzania.

BOX 4.2   **Market concentration in the retail market for antimalarial drugs in rural Tanzania**

Goodman *et al.* (2009) calculated the market concentration of private retail outlets of antimalarial drugs in three areas of rural Tanzania and looked at the impact this had on drug prices in those areas.

Markets were identified based on the geographical area over which most sales took place, which was the ward of residence, consisting of 2–8 villages. Data on treatment for malaria were obtained from a household survey. Data on drug sales and prices of antimalarial drugs were collected from a retail outlet survey and retail audits. The authors calculated market concentration, by both volume and value of sales, using the *HHI* in each market, with shares measured as proportions. The *HHI* based on volume of sales varied from 0.18 to 1 with a mean of 0.45. The *HHI* based on value of sales was slightly higher (range 0.24 to 1, mean 0.51). Regression analysis was used to assess the impact of market concentration on antimalarial drug prices. The authors found that on average a 0.1 unit increase in *HHI* led to a 9% increase in prices. The authors concluded that the anitmalarial drug market was highly concentrated, that prices were positively correlated with concentration, and that high prices were likely to be an important factor in the observed low uptake of treatment.

Other factors as well as market structure affect a firm's conduct and consequent performance. Ownership is important, because it may affect the firm's objectives. For example, state-owned hospitals may have very different aims and objectives, and conduct themselves very differently from privately owned hospitals, even those with objectives other than profit maximisation. There is a wide range of ownership arrangements in health care, probably greater than in any other sector of the economy. Examples are sole proprietors, such as single-handed GPs, dentists and pharmacists; partnerships, such as GP practice partnerships; privately owned or publicly quoted companies, such as those in the pharmaceutical and insurance industries; cooperatives, owned by consumers or workers; public sector ownership, the dominant form in many countries for hospitals; and medical charities.

The impact of ownership on a firm's objectives is moderated by another factor, which is that under many forms of ownership owners are not managers. So, in establishing what the goals of a firm might be, we must ask: whose objectives are we referring to? In Section 4.4, we will discuss some theories of the firm that explicitly recognise that owners and managers are two distinct groups with different aims and objectives. The answer to the question of whose objectives count is further complicated in the health care industry, where in addition to managers and owners there is a third group that can influence the objectives of the firm, namely health care professionals.

A further factor affecting the market structure is market definition. This is important because it determines the number of competitors and whether they supply differentiated or unique services. Market definition identifies which buyers and which sellers are included in a market. To define a health care market we need to determine its boundaries, which are defined by the geographical area covered by the market and the range of health care services included in it. For example, suppose a GP practice is located in a small village. If the market is defined as inhabitants of the village only, then the GP practice has no competitors and enjoys a monopoly. However, if the market is defined more widely and includes other villages in the surrounding area, each of which has their own GP practice, then the market is larger and more competitive.

We must also consider the range of products included in a market. For example, in the pharmaceutical industry, what are the product boundaries in the market for cholesterol-modifying drugs? Suppose a firm is considering developing a new drug within the class of drugs known as statins. The new drug may have an effect similar to but different from those of the other statins already available. How should the market be defined, and what competitors would the company have for its new product if it decided to develop it? One option might be to say that since the new product is different, even if only slightly, from current products, there are no competitors and the company will enjoy a monopoly. This would be unrealistic, however, and it might be more appropriate to define the market in terms of the other statins currently available (for example, simvastatin, pravastatin, rosu-vastatin, fluvastatin, atorvastatin). A further option would be to define the market even more broadly to include other cholesterol-modifying products, such as the bile acid sequestrants (colestipol, colestyramine, colesevelam), the fibrates (bezafibrate, ciprofibrate, fenofibrate and gemfibrozil), ezitimibe and nicotinic acid. Once it has decided who its competitors are, the company can then calculate the expected profits from the new drug and decide whether to invest.

In the next section we take a closer look at traditional economic theories of the firm based on profit maximisation. We then examine in more detail why this objective may not always be an appropriate assumption in health care and investigate theories based on alternative objectives.

4.3 Profit maximisation models

As suggested, traditional theories of the firm are based on the assumption that firms aim to maximise profits. Within this, there are different models depending on the market structure that is assumed. The following market characteristics are particularly important in defining market structure:

- the number of competitors;
- the freedom with which competitors can enter the market;
- whether the different firms in the market sell homogenous, differentiated or unique health care products.

Using these, we can distinguish four categories of market structure. Table 4.1 shows their key features and their applicability in health care. Three of them – perfect competition, monopoly and monopolistic competition – are specific models of market behaviour; the fourth – oligopoly – is actually a compendium term for many different models.

TABLE 4.1   Alternative market structures

Market structure	Number of firms in the market	Entry into market	Type of product	Control of provider over price	Examples
Perfect competition	Many	Unrestricted	Undifferentiated	None	Internet pharmacies
Monopolistic competition	Many	Unrestricted	Differentiated	Some	Medicines in the medium and long run
Oligopoly	Few	Restricted	Either undifferentiated or differentiated	Some	Hospital services, GP services, private health insurance
Monopoly	One	Restricted/ completely blocked	Unique	Considerable	Medicines in the short run, public health insurance

Before describing these models, we will discuss the mathematics of profit maximisation, since that is common to all of the models.

4.3.1 How firms maximise profits

The level of profit that firms make depends on the difference between the revenue that they receive from sales of their product and the cost of producing it. Revenue is dependent on price and the quantity sold at that price via the demand function analysed in Chapter 2; cost is dependent on the quantity of output via the cost function described in Chapter 3. From this information about demand and supply conditions, it is possible to determine the prices and quantities that will maximise the firm's profits and how much profit will be made at that level. To illustrate the key concepts, we will use the example of a profit-maximising fertility clinic that provides services in the form of assisted reproduction techniques (ARTs). It has a large enough share of the local market for ARTs to be aware that it faces a downward-sloping demand curve.

The total profit earned by the clinic (TP) is its *total revenue* (TR) minus its total costs of production (TC):

$$TP = TR - TC \qquad (4.2)$$

The total revenue earned by the clinic is its total earnings from the provision of a specific quantity of ARTs provided, Q:

$$TR = p_Q Q \qquad (4.3)$$

where p_Q is the price at which ARTs are sold. For example, if the clinic sells 500 ARTs per month at a price of £1 700 per ART, $TR = £850\,000$. *Average revenue* (AR) is the amount the clinic earns per ART, calculated as

$$AR = TR/Q \qquad (4.4)$$

Because we assume that the clinic sells each ART at the same price, AR is obviously equal to price. For example, if total revenue is £850 000 and the clinic provides 500 units of ART per month then its average revenue is £1 700. However, the same is not true of *marginal revenue* (MR), which is the additional revenue derived from providing an additional ART:

$$MR = \Delta TR/\Delta Q \qquad (4.5)$$

The reason that this is not necessarily equal to price is that there is a downward-sloping demand curve, and therefore the price is likely to change if the amount sold changes. For example, the clinic could employ an additional nurse and provide an additional 100 ARTs per month, giving a total of 600. However, suppose that to sell the additional 100 ARTs the price must be reduced to £1 600 each. The total revenue of the clinic is now £1 600 × 600 = £960 000, an increase of £110 000. So MR is £110 000/100 = £1 100. This is less than AR, because the increase in revenue due to increased numbers of ARTs sold is offset by a lower AR for every ART sold. In the extreme, MR can even become negative if the revenue increase is outweighed by the loss due to the fall in AR.

How does revenue vary with the number of ARTs provided by the clinic? We can define an AR curve relating AR to quantity. AR is equal to price, so the AR curve is the same as the demand curve, which is the curve relating price to quantity. The MR curve will also be downward sloping, but steeper than the AR curve, reflecting the fact that MR is less than AR at every quantity provided.

We can also define a TR curve which, with downward-sloping AR and MR curves, first rises and then falls. The turning point occurs at the point at which MR becomes negative.

The next stage is to combine this information with that on cost, which is also related to output. It is assumed in this that all output produced is sold. In Figure 4.1(a), we can see that TP, which is found by subtracting TC from TR, is maximised at the output where the distance between the TR and TC curves is greatest. In the data this occurs at around 625 ARTs per month. Notice that at this point the slopes of the TR and TC curves, which are, respectively, MR and MC, are equal. This equality is shown in Figure 4.1(b). Mathematically, it must be the case that the profit-maximising level of output, Q_{TP}, occurs where $MC = MR$.

The size of profit at this level of output can be demonstrated using the AR and AC curves, as in Figure 4.1(c). The profit per unit of output is the difference between AR and AC at the specified level of output. This is multiplied by the level of output to give total profits, shown as the shaded area. For example, at the profit maximising level of output the AR is £1 500 and AC is £1 100, so the total profit for the clinic is now £400 × 625 = £250 000.

The owners of the fertility clinic must earn a minimum amount of profit to prevent them from closing down their business and doing something else instead. This minimum profit can be thought of as a cost because, like other costs, it has to be recovered if the clinic is to continue to operate. It is an opportunity cost because it represents the profit that the owners could have earned in the next-best business alternative; if they can earn more than this running the fertility clinic, they will stay in business. This profit is referred to as *normal profit* and, because it is counted as a cost, it is included in the cost curves. Another type of profit is called supernormal profit. This is profit earned over and above normal profit. The profit shown by the shaded area in Figure 4.1(c) is supernormal profit.

4.3.2 Perfect competition

Of all market models based on profit maximisation, the perfect competition model is the most important, because of its strong conclusions, and also the most controversial, for the same reason. It is based on the following assumptions:

- a large number of sellers in the market;
- freedom of entry into and exit from the market;
- product homogeneity;
- perfect knowledge.

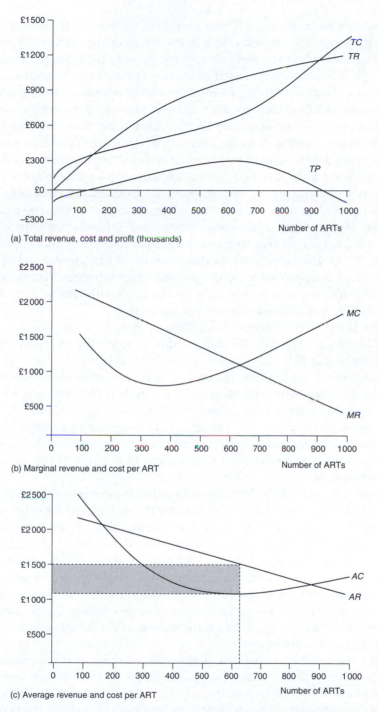

Figure 4.1 Revenue, cost and profit curves for a fertility clinic with some market power in setting prices

The first three assumptions imply that an individual firm in the market has no control over the price it charges for its goods. This is known as being a *price taker*.

In explaining these ideas and their consequences, we will discuss internet pharmacies as an example of a perfectly competitive market. In recent years there has been a massive increase in the number of companies selling products over the internet, including pharmaceuticals. Many of these companies sell their products directly to consumers, which is known as 'B2C' (business-to-consumers) e-commerce. For consumers, buying medicines from internet pharmacies can have many benefits, including access to drugs for the disabled or homebound, the convenience of being able to shop at any time of the day or night, privacy and anonymity for those who do not want to discuss their medical condition in a public place, and lower prices. However, internet pharmacies also create potential problems. Essentially, three types of internet pharmacy exist: pharmacies that only fill prescriptions written by a patient's doctor; pharmacies that charge for a 'cyber-consultation' and whose cyber-doctor then writes a prescription; and pharmacies that dispense prescription drugs without a physician's prescription (Rost, 2000). The latter two types of pharmacies can present significant problems, such as the sale of unapproved new drugs, sale of prescription drugs without a valid prescription, or marketing of products with fraudulent health claims, as well as bypassing the legitimate health care professional/patient interaction.

One of the benefits of internet pharmacies is that they are making the market for pharmaceuticals more competitive. We can see this by analysing the assumptions of perfect competition in more detail.

The market has a large number of firms so that each individual firm supplies only a small proportion of the total output provided in the market. The implication is that each firm is unable to affect the market price. There are also many buyers, who are also unable to influence the operation of the market. The growth of e-commerce generally has led to many firms selling pharmaceuticals starting up in business online. Since the reach of the internet is global, companies need to be aware of competitors in the rest of the world and not just regionally or nationally.

In the perfect competition model, there is a distinction between the *short run* and the *long run*, defined by how easy it is for new firms to enter the market and for existing firms to leave it. In the long run there are no barriers to entry or exit and new firms will be attracted into the industry if incumbent firms earn supernormal profits. In the short run freedom of entry and exit is restricted, but only because of the time it takes to start up or close down a firm. Internet companies have lower start-up costs than conventional rivals, because their premises can be smaller with no need for an expensive public 'shop-front', and marketing costs can be relatively low, especially with the use of internet search engines. Lower start-up costs also mean that internet firms have less to lose if the business fails. Therefore, the costs of entry to and exit from the market are lower.

A perfectly competitive industry is defined as a group of firms producing the same product, described as product homogeneity. The implication of this is that buyers cannot differentiate between the products sold by different firms in the market. While concerns exist surrounding the quality of products bought from internet pharmacies, the products supplied may be just the same as those purchased from other types of pharmacy.

All buyers and sellers in the market have complete knowledge of the conditions in the market. This means that firms are fully aware of market prices, the costs of production, and opportunities for making profits in other markets. Buyers are fully aware of the price, quality and availability of the products in the market. If you buy a product online it is possible to conduct an exhaustive search of suppliers and compare prices for the same product very quickly. This makes price competition more likely.

What happens in a perfectly competitive market?

The short-run equilibrium in the internet pharmacy market is shown in Figure 4.2. It occurs at price p^* and output Q^*, given by the intersection of the market demand and supply curves. An individual internet pharmacy, as a price taker, must sell its output at price p^*, which is set by the market. As a result, AR is equal to MR and the AR and MR curves are horizontal. At this price the profit-maximising level of pharmaceutical sales, Q_1, is determined by the intersection of the MR and short-run MC curves. The size of the profits earned at this level, which depends on the AR and short-run AC curves, is shown by the shaded area.

In the long run, if businesses in the sector are earning supernormal profits then market supply will increase as new internet pharmacies begin trading and existing businesses

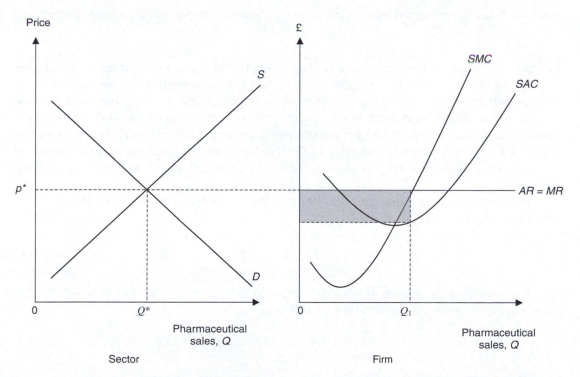

Figure 4.2 Short-run equilibrium in the internet pharmacy sector under perfect competition

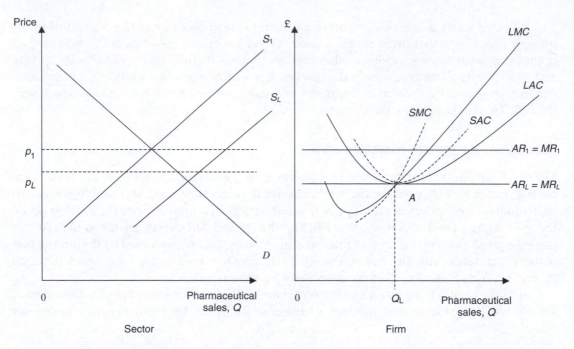

Figure 4.3 Long-run equilibrium in the internet pharmacy sector under perfect competition

increase the scale of their production. The overall effect will be an increase in market supply, as shown in Figure 4.3. At price p_1 firms earn supernormal profit. Therefore total supply in the market increases as the sector supply curve shifts to the right, leading to a fall in the equilibrium market price. Supply will continue to increase, and the price will continue to fall until firms no longer make a profit above the normal level. This is shown in Figure 4.3 at supply curve S_L and price p_L. On this basis, the long-run equilibrium output of the firm is Q_L. Note that no profits above normal are earned at this level of output, since $AR = LAC$.

The condition for the long-run equilibrium of the internet pharmacy market is that LMC is equal to price and LAC:

$$LMC = LAC = p \qquad (4.6)$$

The pharmacy adjusts its size so that it produces the level of output at which LAC is minimised. The long-run equilibrium condition is

$$SAC = SMC = LAC = LMC = p = AR = MR \qquad (4.7)$$

This equilibrium occurs at the bottom of the internet pharmacy's long-run average cost curve at point A. This means that given the current state of technology the firm will in the long run produce its output at the minimum feasible cost. Note also that consumers pay the minimum possible price for their medications, which just covers the marginal cost of production. Box 4.3 considers the marketing and pricing of drugs sold by online pharmacies.

BOX 4.3 Marketing and pricing of drugs sold by online pharmacies

The sale of drugs via online pharmacies might be one of the closest examples in the real world to the perfect competition model. For example, there are a large number of sellers in the market, who are free to enter and exit, and the product is homogeneous. One assumption that may not hold is perfect knowledge. While it is easier to surf the internet and access sellers, concerns have been raised about the quality and safety in what is a largely unregulated market where consumers may lack the information needed to make an informed choice. This raises questions about the need for tighter regulation, as exists elsewhere in the health care market.

Levaggi *et al.* (2009) looked at pricing and marketing practices of online pharmacies. They focused on four drugs that could normally only be purchased through prescription and were thought to have potentially high risks if used without appropriate medical supervision. Two of the drugs were antidepressant medications, and the others were sildenafil for erectile dysfunction and opioid painkillers. Risks were related to issues of dosage, interactions with other medications and adverse events affecting the nervous system. The authors analysed the marketing strategies used on the internet sites for these drugs and used regression analysis to look at variables important in price formulation.

They found that marketing and pricing strategies were sophisticated and varied according to whether the drug was branded or generic, the quality of the drug, the quantity demanded, and the target consumers. They found that online pharmacies provided drugs to consumers that other pharmacies cannot normally reach, such as those who would like to use the drug without consulting a physician or, would like to use it against the physician's advice. They also found that in cases like this, the online pharmacy usually charges a higher price, reassures consumers by minimising the significance of adverse events, and encourages them to buy in bulk.

We can conclude from this that online pharmacies may encourage the use of drugs when the marginal benefit to the consumer is less than the cost. In addition, rather than pricing at marginal cost they charge a higher price to consumers, especially to those normally denied treatment.

The authors concluded: 'This analysis suggests that the selling of drugs via the Internet can turn into a "public health risk", as has been pointed out by the US Food and Drug Administration'.

4.3.3 Monopoly

A monopoly is a market structure in which there is a single seller of a product. There are no close substitutes for the good sold by the firm, and there are significant barriers to entry for new firms. The main causes of these are:

- The size of the market. This may not be sufficient to support more than one firm. If a monopoly experiences substantial economies of scale, which may only be reaped at large scale levels of production, the industry may be able to support only a single firm. In this case the market creates what is called a natural monopoly.
- Lower costs for an established firm. Over and above the barriers caused by economies of scale, an established monopoly may have lower costs of production. This is because the existing firm is likely to have developed specialised production and marketing skills, to be aware of the most efficient production techniques, to have knowledge of the cheapest and most reliable suppliers of raw materials, and to have access to cheaper finance.
- Ownership of raw materials or exclusive knowledge of production techniques.
- Patent rights for a product or production process.
- Government licensing limiting the number of firms operating in a geographical area.
- Limit-pricing policy. This occurs when the existing firm adopts a pricing policy aimed at preventing new firms from entering the industry. This can be combined with other strategies to create barriers to new competition, including intense advertising and continuous product differentiation, all of which render entry for new firms unattractive.
- Brand loyalty. This might arise if the firm produces a unique product that consumers associate with the brand.

Patented drugs are an example of monopoly in health care. The justification for laws permitting such a monopoly is that developing new medicines is a lengthy and expensive process. Pharmaceutical company researchers in the USA have estimated that developing a new molecular entity from discovery to launch takes on average 13.5 years and costs $1.8 billion (Paul *et al.*, 2010). For these reasons, as soon as a promising new compound is found, the pharmaceutical company applies for a patent. This gives the company intellectual property rights over the compound for a period of 20 years. Effectively, the company is granted monopoly power in producing the compound, and other companies are legally prevented from producing it. This acts as a reward for the expenditure incurred in bringing the medicine to market, and to encourage future research and development.

What happens in a monopoly market?

We will use the example of a patent for a new type of drug that means there is a single pharmaceutical company in the market. As a result, the demand curve for the company is the demand curve for the whole market. Because the monopolist sells a unique product, it can raise its price and consumers have no alternative product to buy. They must either buy the product at the higher price or not buy it at all. Thus the firm is a *price maker*, and has the

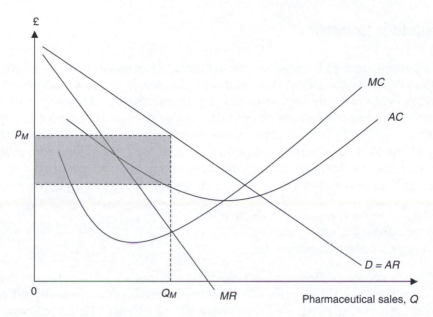

Figure 4.4 Monopoly equilibrium for a pharmaceutical company with a medicine under patent in the short run

downward-sloping *AR* and *MR* curves analysed in Section 4.3.1. Combining the cost and revenue curves produces the profit-maximising equilibrium shown in Figure 4.4.

The level of sales assuming profit maximisation is Q_M, which is the point at which $MC = MR$. The price of the medicine at this output is p_M and the level of profits earned by the monopolistic company at this price and output is given by the shaded area.

Since there are barriers to entry in the form of patent laws, the supernormal profit earned by the monopolist will not be eroded in the long run as with perfect competition, though it may be competed away once the patent expires. The only difference between short-run and long-run equilibrium under monopoly is that the long-run equilibrium occurs at the intersection of the *MR* and long-run marginal cost (*LMC*) curves. Thus, in contrast with long-run equilibrium under perfect competition, the firm does not operate at the minimum average cost, and price is greater than marginal cost.

A monopolist can also exploit their market power by selling their product at different prices in different markets. This is known as price discrimination. For example, a monopolist can increase their profit by setting a higher price in markets that are more price inelastic, as in the market for drugs in developed countries, and a lower price in markets that are more price elastic, like the demand for drugs in developing countries. In such an example, the monopolist will set the marginal revenue that is achieved in each market equal to the marginal cost of producing total output. Although it is possible for a country to legislate against price discrimination this sometimes has the unintended consequence of reducing the total quantity supplied. For example, if the market in developing countries is very small, legislation may result in the monopolist supplying only to developed countries where it can maximise its profits by charging a higher price.

4.3.4 Monopolistic competition

Perfect competition and monopoly are the extremes of possible models based on profit maximisation. While we have identified some examples, few health care markets can in reality be classified as being perfectly competitive or as pure monopolies. This is because providers of health care do compete with each other but also have some market power. Competition is therefore imperfect. Monopolistic competition is one type of imperfect competition. This model retains the idea from perfect competition that, at least in the long run, there may be many firms in the market, but relaxes the assumption that all products are identical, generating some monopoly power. It is based on the following assumptions:

- there are many firms competing in the market;
- there are no barriers to entry and exit;
- each firm sells a differentiated product.

The effect of product differentiation is that the firm has some discretion in the determination of price. The firm is not a price taker because its product is sufficiently different from its rivals to allow it to raise its price without losing all its customers. Each firm, however, faces competition from close substitutes in the market, and so this discretion in setting the price is limited. Product differentiation gives rise to a demand curve for the firm that is downward sloping with a corresponding downward-sloping MR curve.

What happens in a monopolistically competitive market?

Monopolistic competition has been applied to study the market behaviour of physicians (Pauly and Satterthwaite, 1981), psychologists (Klevorick and McGuire, 1987) and dentists (Grytten and Skau, 2009). In the short run the profit-maximising equilibrium of a firm under monopolistic competition is as shown in Figure 4.5. The profit maximising level of output is Q_{MC}, which is sold at price p_{MC}. The diagram is similar to the equilibrium for a monopolist except the demand curve is more price elastic due to the competition from close substitutes. The amount of supernormal profit earned by the firm is given by the shaded area. This depends on the degree of market power held by the firm, and hence on the slope and position of the demand curve.

In the long run new firms will enter the market and start to provide services. This will have two effects:

- The demand curve for the firm will shift to the left as the demand for its product contracts.
- The demand curve will also become more price elastic as the number of competitor products increases.

The demand curve will continue to shift leftwards and become flatter as long as supernormal profits are being earned. The long-run equilibrium is reached when the firm earns no supernormal profit. At this point there is no incentive for new firms to enter. This is shown in Figure 4.6. The demand curve shifts until it is tangential to the LAC curve. The equilibrium

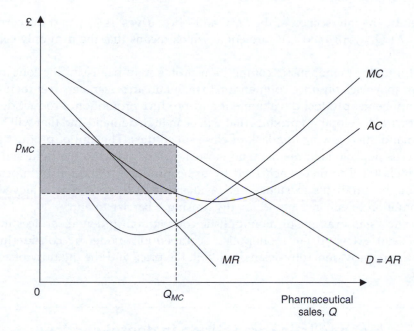

Figure 4.5 Monopolistic competition equilibrium in the short run

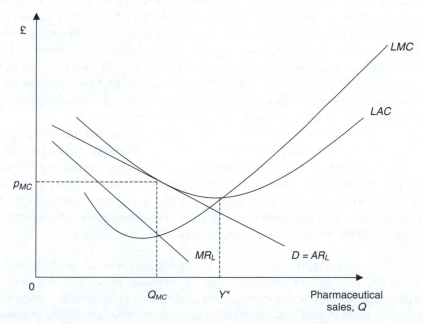

Figure 4.6 Monopolistic competition equilibrium in the long run

output, given by the intersection of the *LMC* and *MR*$_L$ curves, is Q_{MC} and the corresponding price is p_{MC}. At Q_{MC}, AR_L and *LAC* are equal which means that the firm only earns normal profit.

In reality, under monopolistic competition profits may persist in the long run. This is because firms may use non-price competition to maintain an advantage over their rivals. This has two components: product development and product promotion. Product development is concerned with developing a product that will be in high demand and that will have a price inelastic demand curve owing to a lack of close substitutes. The aim of product promotion, such as advertising, is to shift the demand curve for the product to the right and to make it more price inelastic. The first is achieved by using product promotion to inform potential consumers of the product's existence and availability. The second is achieved by using product promotion to enhance brand loyalty, raising a barrier to entry.

Box 4.4 shows an example of monopolistic competition in dental services in Norway.

Farley (1986) extended the monopolistic competition model by considering the case where health care providers (physicians) set both the price and the quantity of services that

---

BOX 4.4 **Monopolistic competition in dental services in Norway**

Grytten and Skau (2009) reviewed the competitiveness of dental services in Norway. These are divided into public and private sectors, and adults usually receive dental treatment from private general dental practitioners. In the adult dental market there are also oral specialists and private practitioners, some of whom compete for patients with general dental practitioners (prosthetists, periodontists and endodontists) and some of whom do not (orthodontists and oral surgeons). The fees of private sector general dental practitioners and specialists are determined by the market, and both groups are free to establish their practices in any location. Because the services provided by these groups are differentiated, the market resembles monopolistic competition.

Regression analysis of a representative set of data showed that net incomes per hour for orthodontists and oral surgeons (not in direct competition with general dental practitioners) were significantly higher than those for general dental practitioners and for the specialists that were in direct competition with general dental practitioners (prosthetists, periodontists, endodontists). They found that the net incomes per hour for prosthetists, periodontists and endodontists were not significantly different to those of general dental practitioners. The authors concluded:

> The results support our hypothesis that the specialists who have skills that give them exclusive possibilities to practice their profession have market power . . . [whilst] general dental practitioners give periodontists, endodontists and prosthetists so much competition that the market power of these specialists is limited.

their patients consume. She proposed that in this situation physicians would consider how best to maximise their own welfare, taking into consideration how this might impact upon the welfare of their patients. A physician's monopolistic power is limited by the ability of patients to go elsewhere for their treatment if their welfare from attending falls below that offered by other physicians.

In this model, the physician's profit function is given by:

$$TP_F = pqN - C \tag{4.8}$$

where q is the quantity of services provided per patient, N is the number of patients attending the physician and C is the cost function. N depends on the welfare of patients, which is affected by the physician's behaviour, and C depends among other things on N.

Patient welfare is measured in terms of the additional benefits they receive from consuming health care less the price paid, that is, the consumer surplus. The physician will set both the price and quantity of services consumed by patients, subject to patients receiving at least as much consumer surplus as they would from another provider. So, the equilibrium profit is given by

$$TP_F^* = CS_1 - CS_0 \tag{4.9}$$

where the consumer surplus for the current and alternative physician is CS_1 and CS_0, respectively. Farley shows that the equilibrium price is a markup over the marginal cost, where the amount of the markup depends on the consumer surplus received from another provider. The equilibrium output is the same as would be produced under monopolistic competition, but the price is higher and above the demand curve.

4.3.5 Oligopoly

Oligopoly is another type of imperfect competition in which, compared with monopolistic competition, there are fewer firms, and entry for new firms is restricted. Firms may sell either the same or differentiated products, and they have some control over price. This is the dominant market structure in many health care markets, for example for hospital services and for GP services, where there are more likely to be a few rather than many providers competing with one another, and where the providers have some market power. There are numerous models of oligopoly and we therefore give only a brief overview. The main features of an oligopolistic market are:

LTC

- There are barriers to entry for new firms. The main causes of these are the same as for a monopoly.
- Firms are mutually dependent. Each firm will be affected by the decisions made by its rivals. This interdependence arises because there are relatively few firms in the industry producing products that are close substitutes. Firms recognise that the other firms in the industry will

be affected by their pricing and output decisions and will react to them. Accordingly, they will attempt to predict the reactions and incorporate these predictions into the decision-making process.

These two characteristics lead to one of two behaviours by oligopolistic firms. Either firms will collude in order to limit competition among themselves or they will compete with each other in order to gain, for example, a larger share of the profits earned by the industry for themselves. The first is called a collusive oligopoly and the second a non-collusive oligopoly. Collusive oligopoly is more likely to arise when:

- There are only a small number of firms, who are well known to each other.
- There is no government intervention to prevent collusion.
- There is a dominant firm that the other firms will follow.
- Entry into the market by other firms is severely restricted, which makes it unlikely that new firms will enter the market and disrupt the collusion process.
- Firms are prepared to share information about their costs and production methods with each other.

Collusion between firms may be formal or informal (tacit). A formal collusive agreement is called a cartel. A cartel attempts to act like a monopoly, behaving as if it is a single firm. Informal or tacit collusion will usually take the form of price leadership, where firms follow the price set either by a dominant firm in the market (dominant firm price leadership), or by a firm considered to be a reliable gauge of market conditions (barometric firm price leadership).

In the case of a non-collusive oligopoly there is no agreement, formal or informal, between firms. With no collusion, price competition between firms is more likely to occur. Because each firm will be affected by its rivals' decisions – that is, the firms are interdependent – non-collusive oligopolists devise strategies that take into account the impact of their actions on the behaviour of their rivals. Therefore, the behaviour of a firm depends on how it believes its rivals will react to its policies.

Box 4.5 shows an example of the impact of oligopoly in the health insurance market in the USA.

4.3.6 Game theory

A key feature of oligopolistic markets is that the actions of one firm are dependent on and react to the decisions of other firms. This interdependence is a key feature of oligopoly. Game theory – mathematical models of decision-making that explicitly take into account interdependence – is therefore particularly useful in explaining firms' behaviour in this context. Game theory provides insights into a large number of economic phenomena, but we will here look at it only as an analysis of how firms behave in markets. Specifically, it is used to examine a firm's optimal pricing and output strategy, which depends on its views about how its rivals will behave in a non-collusive oligopoly. In game theory, oligopolistic or other firms are treated as

---

Oligopoly in health insurance markets in the USA

In the USA, where health insurance is provided predominantly by the private sector, the underlying assumption is that competition among health insurance providers produces efficient outcomes. There are conflicting views as to whether or not this is in fact the case. Dafny (2010) investigated the competitiveness of the group health insurance industry and the impact on premiums paid by employers on behalf of their employees as part of an employee benefit package. Using a national database of health insurance plans offered by a sample of large, multisite health insurance firms from 1998–2005 she tested whether or not health insurers charge higher premiums to more profitable employers. It was argued that price discrimination of this kind is feasible only if the market is imperfectly competitive.

The author investigated the size of the premiums for different group health insurance plans, where the plans were defined according to the employer, geographical market, insurance firm, plan type and year. She regressed health insurance premiums against employer profits plus a range of covariates and found that employers' profits were positively associated with the insurance premiums charged.

The author then considered the impact of the structure of the local health insurance market, and used interaction terms in a regression analysis to investigate if the impact of employer profits on the premiums paid depended on the number of insurance firms in the geographical market. The results showed that while more profitable employers paid more for their health insurance, the effect was statistically significant only in markets with 10 or fewer firms and was most pronounced in markets with six or fewer firms. In these markets, it was found that a profit increase of 10 percentage points was associated with an increase in health insurance premiums of 1.2%.

---

players in a game where for each action by one player another player may choose among several alternative reactions, either at the same time or in a subsequent time period. The actions of rivals are uncertain, yet it may be possible under certain circumstances to choose a strategy that will maximise the firm's expected gain after making due allowance for the effects of rivals' probable actions.

To illustrate how game theory might be used to devise an optimal pricing strategy in order to maximise profits, assume a local hospital market with two hospitals, A and B. The health care services provided by the hospitals are close substitutes, so that if their prices differ the hospital with the lower price will supply the larger share of the market. Suppose the hospitals charge one of two prices for each unit of health care they provide: £900 or £1 000. Each hospital has a different cost structure, and the total number of patients treated in the market is affected by the combined action of both hospitals. This means that the profit gains of one hospital will not necessarily be equal to the reduction in profit of the other hospital.

		Hospital A's pricing alternatives	
		Price = £1 000	Price = £900
Hospital B's pricing alternatives	Price = £1 000	Hospital A's profit = £10 million Hospital B's profit = £9 million	Hospital A's profit = £11 million Hospital B's profit = £5 million
	Price = £900	Hospital A's profit = £8 million Hospital B's profit = £7 million	Hospital A's profit = £9 million Hospital B's profit = £8 million

Figure 4.7 Profits under different scenarios in a non-collusive oligopoly

Figure 4.7 shows a payoff matrix for the two hospitals. Both decide what price to charge for their services, taking into account their rival's possible strategy. Let us assume that each hospital will choose its pricing strategy expecting its rival to take the worst possible action from the hospital's point of view. In this case if hospital A sets its price at £1 000 its minimum profit is £8 million, and if it sets it at £900 the minimum profit is £9 million. Among these two minima the hospital will rationally choose the largest, which results from the lower price. This is known as a maximin strategy, because it maximises the minimum outcome.

For hospital B, if it chooses a price of £1 000 the minimum profit it earns is £5 million. If it chooses a price of £900 its minimum profit is £7 million. The maximin strategy for hospital B is therefore also to charge the lower price. If both hospitals have a maximin strategy, then the outcome will be that both will charge the lower price.

Maximin is not the only possible strategy, however. The hospitals could, for example, adopt an optimistic approach that assumes its rival will act in the best possible way from the point of view of the hospital and again choose the pricing policy that will maximise its profits. This is called a maximax strategy. Under this strategy, hospital A will again charge £900 since its profits will be maximised at £11 million if hospital B acts favourably by setting a price of £1 000. Hospital A will in fact always adopt a low price strategy, since this will maximise its profits whatever price hospital B charges. This is called a dominant strategy. However, hospital B does not have a dominant strategy. Under maximax, it will charge a price of £1 000, hoping that hospital A will also charge £1 000, and thereby maximise its profits at £9 million.

In the next period, the hospitals will review their decisions. In the maximax case, hospital A has a dominant strategy, so it will conclude that it should maintain its price. Hospital B, however, will observe that if hospital A maintains its low price, hospital B will make greater profits if it also charges a low price. If it does change its policy, hospital B's profit will rise to £8 million and hospital A's profits will fall to £9 million. This produces the same pricing policies for the two hospitals as for the maximin case and therefore the same profit outcomes.

Given that both hospitals charge the low price, neither hospital has any incentive unilaterally to change its strategy, if it believes that the other hospital will not change its strategy. Hospital A's profits would fall from £9 million to £8 million if it increased its prices and B did not. Hospital B's profits would similarly fall from £8 million to £5 million if it increased its prices and hospital A did not. Unless there is some change in market conditions, the hospitals will continue with their pricing policies and the outcomes will remain the same in subsequent periods. This is known as a Nash equilibrium and is a key concept in game theory.

Note that in this case the equilibrium position puts both hospitals in a worse situation compared to a strategy where they both charge a high price, since they both earn a lower level of profit. Nevertheless, it is a stable position, and unless they collude it will persist. A special case of this is where both players have a dominant strategy that leads to an outcome that is worse for both of them than some other pair of strategies. This is called the prisoner's dilemma, after an example devised by the mathematician A. W. Tucker to popularise the work of its inventors, M. M. Flood and M. Dresher. In this example, two prisoners are interrogated separately about a crime. Both have an incentive to confess, because whatever their accomplice does, they will receive a lower sentence for giving evidence for the prosecution than if they do not. However, if neither confesses, both will receive a lower sentence than if they both confess.

Many other scenarios can be analysed using game theory, and the outcome need not necessarily be profit maximisation. It could be some other measure consistent with objectives other than profit maximisation such as number of patients treated, or number of staff employed. One advantage of the theory is that each player does not need to know the actual response its rivals will make to a particular strategy it adopts. However, it does need to know what the outcomes will be for each possible response to its actions.

4.4 Goals other than profit maximisation

Firms may not seek to maximise their profits. One possibility is that although a firm aims to make some profits, it does not aim to maximise them. Another is that the firm actually does not intend to make any profits at all, but to break even. Both of these occur in health care, but the second is particularly widespread.

One reason why for-profit health care firms may not aim to maximise profits is that the owners of the firm may not have complete managerial control. The owners of many health care provider units such as hospitals are not usually the managers who make pricing and output decisions on a day-to-day basis. The owners may want to maximise profit, but the managers may not necessarily share this view. Williamson (1963) argued that the separation of ownership and management in firms means that managers have some freedom in setting and achieving the goals within firms. As a consequence, managers will set goals that maximise their own utility. Factors likely to affect a manager's utility include their salary, power, prestige, job security and working conditions.

Therefore, while profit maximisation might be important, it is unlikely to be the only goal for managers. Firms may aim for a target level of profit rather than the maximum. They are therefore profit *satisficers* rather than profit maximisers. Managers ensure that they earn sufficient profits to satisfy the firm's owners, conditional on the other factors in the managerial utility function.

As mentioned earlier the separation of ownership and management in the health care industry is further complicated by the presence of a third group of influential decision-makers who have autonomy over patient care decisions: health care professionals. They are likely to set goals that maximise their patients' utility functions, assuming perfect agency, or their own utility function, assuming imperfect agency. Either way, it is unlikely that profit maximisation will be the most important goal. Some but not all of the arguments of the managerial utility function are also likely to feature in the utility functions of health care professionals, with an important addition – patients' utility. Hence, the likelihood of profit maximisation as a goal of the health care firm will diminish as the power of health care professionals becomes greater.

Many health care providers, particularly those that are publicly owned, are unlikely to be profit maximisers. This can stem from imperfect knowledge on the part of consumers, as discussed in Chapter 2, which results in an agency relationship between patients and health care professionals. Under these circumstances health care providers are instead more likely to favour goals such as utility maximisation, where utility is a function of the quality and quantity of health care services provided.

Even with the public provision of health care and health care professionals as key decision makers it is likely that some health care programmes will be perceived as being under-provided from the viewpoint of some sections of the population. These sections – special interest groups – might comprise patients, family and friends of patients, health care professionals or others who perceive that certain types of health care are under-provided both privately by the market and publicly by the government. These groups may themselves become involved in the provision of health care, and for reasons that are unrelated to profit. An example is the National Childbirth Trust in the UK, which is a registered charity launched in 1957 with the aim of providing information about pregnancy, childbirth and early parenthood to mothers and fathers. This is achieved via a number of routes including antenatal classes, breastfeeding counselling and mother-and-baby groups.

Taken together, the above factors suggest that goals other than profit maximisation are likely to be pursued by many firms in the health care sector. The consequences of this for hospital care in the USA are explored in Box 4.6.

4.4.1 Growth maximisation

Marris (1963) suggested that firms might have as their aim growth maximisation rather than profit maximisation. Firms aim to maximise their rate of growth, taking into account various indicators of size such as the demand for the firm's products, output, revenue and market share.

One justification for this goal is that although ownership and management might be separate, growth maximisation is consistent with the different goals of owners and managers. Growth may be correlated with profit, but also with factors such as managers' salaries,

| BOX 4.6 | The impact of hospital ownership in the USA |

Hospitals in the USA have three basic ownership types: public; private not-for-profit; and private for-profit. Public hospitals are owned by the government at the federal, state or local level to serve the military, rural residents, the poor, and/or the uninsured. Private not-for-profit hospitals are owned by a voluntary board of trustees to provide hospital care to paying patients and charitable services to the poor. Private for-profit hospitals are owned by private investors to make profits by serving patients in return for a fee. The key features of the three hospital types are:

	Ownership type		
	Public	**Private**	
Characteristic		**Not-for-profit**	**For-profit**
Owners	The public	Stakeholders	Shareholders
Key decision makers	Government officials	Volunteer Board of Trustees	Paid corporate officers
Goals	Multiple (for example equity, efficiency), often conflicting, frequently change with elections	Ambiguous	Profit maximisation
Sources of finance	Government, fees	Patient fees and charges, donations	Patient fees and charges
Market	Determined by government	Mission-driven, determined by clients	Determined by people's buying power
Number of hospitals in 2009	1 092 (21.8%)	2 918 (58.3%)	998 (19.9%)
Hospital beds per 1 000 population in 2009	0.4	1.8	0.2

Sources: Baker *et al.* (2000); www.statehealthfacts.org

The impact of hospital ownership type on a range of key outcomes is generally ambiguous, with different studies yielding conflicting results. Baker *et al.* (2000) reviewed 69 studies published between 1985 and 1999, analysing the impact of hospital ownership on hospital performance and outcomes. The main findings are:

- The degree of competition faced by the hospital is the major factor that influences the availability of services and pricing behaviour.
- Administrative costs are increasing in all three hospital types.
- For-profit hospitals are more profitable than private not-for-profit and public hospitals. Most of the research on profitability, revenue, and cost differences among hospitals is based on data gathered before 1990. Generally, these studies report that, although costs are similar, for-profit hospitals charge more for their services and are more profitable than private not-for-profit and public hospitals.
- The association between hospital ownership and patient outcomes is unclear. The evidence is mixed and inconclusive regarding the impact of hospital ownership on access to care, morbidity, mortality, and adverse events.
- Hospital ownership status has an impact on the type and degree of community benefits: public and private not-for-profit hospitals provide better access to care, a wider range of amount and type of health services, and greater involvement in professional education.

Horwitz and Nichols (2009) provided another example of an empirical study of the impact of hospital ownership. Consistent with the above, they find that not-for-profit hospitals' medical service provision systematically varies by market mix.

prestige and job security. Growth maximisation can result in the joint maximisation of both owners' and managers' utility.

Growth in a firm's size may be achieved either by internal expansion or by merger and acquisition. A merger is the result of a mutual agreement by two firms to come together. An acquisition arises when a firm succeeds in a takeover bid for another firm. Mergers and takeovers in the pharmaceutical industry are common. Two of the largest pharmaceutical companies are Pfizer and GlaxoSmithKline. Table 4.2 illustrates how these companies have grown in recent years as a result of mergers and takeovers.

4.4.2 Behavioural theories of the firm

Cyert and March (1963) developed a generalised behavioural theory of the firm which recognised that firms are complex organisational units with multiple goals and multiple decision-making units of different groups that are involved in the activities of the firm. These groups include managers, owners, workers and customers. Each group has its own demands on the firm, which may conflict with the demands of other groups. For example, managers want high salaries, power and prestige; owners want high profits; workers want high wages and good working conditions; customers want low prices and good-quality goods and services.

In this model the top management ultimately sets the goals of the firm through continuous bargaining with the different groups. The goals take the form of aspirations, or wishes, rather than strict maximising constraints.

Using this information the firm in a behavioural theory of the firm does not aim to maximise a single dimension of output, but instead seeks to attain a satisfactory

TABLE 4.2	**Some mergers and takeovers related to Pfizer and GlaxoSmithKline**

Company 1	Company 2	Date	New company name
Pfizer			
Parke-Davis	Warner-Lambert	1970s	Parke-Davis, Warner-Lambert
Pharmacia	Upjohn	1995	Pharmacia and Upjohn
Pfizer	Warner-Lambert	2000	Pfizer
Pharmacia and Upjohn	Monsanto	2000	Pharmacia Corp
Pfizer	Pharmacia Corp	2003	Pfizer
Pfizer	Wyeth	2009	Pfizer
GlaxoSmithKline			
Beecham Group	SmithKline Beckman Corporation	1989	Smithkline Beecham
Glaxo	Wellcome	1995	Glaxo Wellcome
Glaxo Wellcome	Smithkline Beecham	2000	GlaxoSmithKline

Sources: www.pfizer.com; www.gsk.com

performance in all relevant output dimensions in order to satisfy the wishes of the different groups. Hence the firm is a satisficing organisation rather than a maximising one, aiming to achieve satisfactory power, prestige and salaries for managers, a satisfactory level of profits for the owners, satisfactory wages and working conditions for workers, and satisfactory low prices and quality for consumers.

An example of this type of model in the hospital sector is given by Harris (1977). He argued that a hospital comprises two separate firms or divisions – the medical staff and the administration. Medical staff comprise the 'demand division', and are responsible for patient care decisions and ordering services from the administration – the 'supply division' – who are referred to as ancillary departments. These comprise laboratory, radiology, pharmacy and intensive care services, operating rooms, and the blood bank, plus other general services such as laundry and admissions services. The firms interact with each other in a complex way, and have their own managers, objectives, pricing strategies and constraints. The goals for the medical staff are related to patient outcomes, in their role as agents for patients, and their individual earnings. The administration is likely to be more concerned with maximising profit, maximising the utilisation of services and avoiding spare capacity.

4.4.3 Utility maximisation

Newhouse (1970) developed a model of utility maximisation applied to the hospital sector. The hospital aims to maximise both the quantity and quality of services provided subject to a financial constraint. Quality and quantity are each measured in a single dimension and together comprise the output of the hospital. The quantity of services Q may be measured in dimensions such as:

- the number of patients treated;
- the number of patient-days of care provided.

Quality k may be measured in dimensions such as:

- the expertise of the clinical staff;
- the status and prestige of the institution and its staff;
- the quality of care, as viewed by patients;
- the quality of care as measured using routinely collected statistics, for example readmission rates, length of stay, incidence of hospital-acquired infection;
- the non-health care characteristics of provision, for example the quality of the food and the décor.

The assumptions underpinning this model are:

- The demand for the hospital's services are a function of the quality of the care provided: $D = AR = f_1(k)$, where higher values of k denote higher quality. Other things held constant, k has a positive impact on demand.
- The average costs of production are also determined by the quality of services provided: $AC = f_2(k)$. Other things held constant, k has a positive impact on AC.
- The financial constraint faced by the hospital is that it breaks even. This occurs at the level of output Q at which $AR(k) = AC(k)$. If there is more than one point where this holds, the hospital will choose the one with the highest output.
- The utility of the hospital U is a function of the quality and quantity of services provided: $U = f_3(k, Q)$.

The outcome of the model is shown in Figure 4.8. Given quality level k_1 with corresponding cost and revenue curves $AC(k_1)$ and $D(k_1) = AR(k_1)$, the equilibrium (break even) level of output for the firm is Q_1. Depending on the relative movement of the cost and revenue curves as k changes the new equilibrium quantity might be higher or lower than Q_1. Figure 4.8 shows a situation in which, following an increase in quality from k_1 to k_2, the relative impact on the cost and revenue curves is such that Q_2 lies to the right of Q_1. Eventually, however, it is

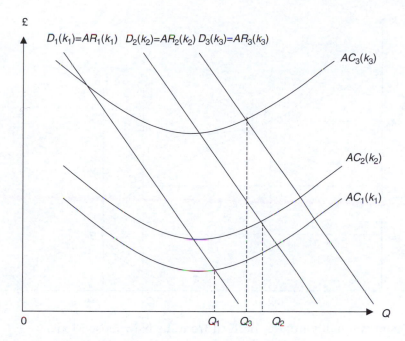

Figure 4.8 Quantity–quality trade-off in the Newhouse model

likely that increases in quality produce an increase in demand that is more than offset by the increase in costs. This is shown in the figure by an increase in quality from k_2 to k_3, which results in a new equilibrium output Q_3, which lies to the left of Q_2.

As k runs over its feasible range of values this will produce a locus of equilibrium of quality–quantity combinations. This yields the quality–quantity frontier as shown by FF in Figure 4.9, which at lower levels of quality, below k_B, shows a positive relationship between k and Q. Eventually, at higher levels of k, above k_B, the frontier bends back, demonstrating a quality–quantity trade-off.

The decision maker will choose a combination of quality and quantity on the frontier that maximises their utility. This will occur where the frontier is tangential to the highest attainable indifference curve. Assuming that $U = f(k, Q)$ and that there is a diminishing marginal rate of substitution between k and Q, then the indifference curves will have the usual shape, as shown for example by U_0. In this case the equilibrium quality and quantity combination is k_A and Q_X, which occurs at point A.

If the goal of the decision maker is quantity maximisation, subject to a break-even financial constraint, then $U = f(Q)$ and the decision maker's indifference curves will be vertical. The equilibrium of the firm is given by point B in Figure 4.9, which is on the highest attainable indifference curve U_1, with level of output Q_{MAX} at quality k_B.

Newhouse also discussed an alternative case where quality is a constraint on the decision maker's utility function, rather than component of it. The firm seeks to maximise output subject to a given level of quality and breaking even. Suppose the minimum acceptable quality

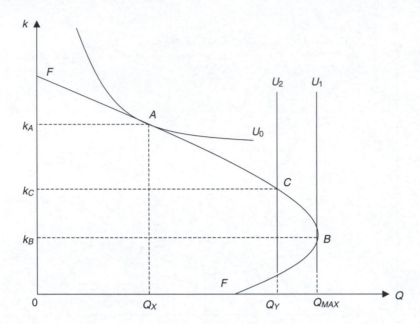

Figure 4.9 Quantity–quality frontier derived from the Newhouse Model

is k_C. In this case the equilibrium position is given by the intersection of the highest attainable indifference curve U_2 and FF, yielding an equilibrium quantity Q_Y.

4.4.4 Maximising net income per physician

Pauly and Redisch (1973) introduced a model of the hospital as a physicians' cooperative. Physicians control how the hospital operates and are able to appropriate any profits earned. They act as net-income-maximising agents who seek to maximise the sum of money incomes of all staff physicians. Net income per physician is given by:

$$\frac{TP}{M} = \frac{p_Q Q - p_x x}{M} = \frac{TR - TC}{M} \tag{4.10}$$

where TP is the total profit earned by the hospital, which is appropriated by the physician staff M. p_Q is the price of the output Q and p_x is the price of the non-physician inputs x. Figure 4.10 depicts the equilibrium of the hospital under these conditions. The physician supply curve S_0 is upward sloping. The net income per physician curve passes through the origin – net income per physician is zero with no physicians employed – and is an inverted U-shape. This is due to the relative shape of the cost and revenue curves assuming the hospital is a price taker, and is based on the shape of the TP curve in Figure 4.1.

If physicians can determine the number of physicians employed, the optimal physician staff size is M^*, where the net income per physician is $(TP/M)_{\text{MAX}}$. Alternatively, if any

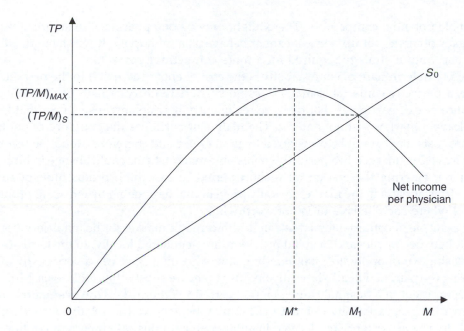

Figure 4.10 Maximising net income per physician

physician who chooses to do so can become a member of staff, the equilibrium number of physicians employed is M_1 with net income per physician given by $(TP/M)_S$. This arises from the intersection of the net income per physician curve and S_0.

4.5 Competition, contestability and industrial policy

A common feature of many models of supply is that they stress the importance of competition as a mechanism for regulating prices and quantities. The number of firms in the industry is the dominant feature that differentiates different market types, and this is a major determinant of the degree of competition. Under perfect competition, there are so many firms that none has any market power. Prices and costs are as low as possible and production is maximised. Monopolies have total market power. Not only do they have the highest possible price and cost and the lowest production outcomes, they are also able to indulge in cross-subsidisation and discriminatory pricing. Cases in between these extremes have corresponding intermediate outcomes.

Baumol *et al.* (1982) suggested that what is important in determining the degree of competitive pressure is how contestable the market is, not just how many contestants there are. A firm's behaviour is influenced as much by potential competitors as existing ones. Even if they have no actual competitors, firms may behave as if they face strong competition, if there are credible potential competitors. There might only be one pharmacy in an area, but if it is possible for others to set up there, it cannot behave as a monopoly. It will have to adopt the pricing and output strategy required for a more competitive market.

The key determinant of contestability is the cost of entry and exit into the market. At the extreme, a perfectly contestable market has no barriers to entry or exit. In this context, the importance of exit barriers is that they are really entry barriers, because a firm that thinks it cannot leave a market will not enter it. The main exit barrier is the existence of sunk costs, which are costs that cannot be transferred to another use and therefore cannot be recouped if the firm leaves the market. In a perfectly contestable market, firms could engage in hit-and-run competition, entering the market for a short period to earn high profits quickly and then exiting. Firms already in the market can only prevent that happening by reducing profitability to a level where such behaviour is not worthwhile.

An example of contestable markets in health care is a market for hospital services where contracts between payers and hospital providers are negotiated locally. In the local area there may be a single monopoly hospital. Building a new hospital is clearly a very costly exercise, and exiting the market will also be costly because there are substantial sunk costs. Much of the capital equipment in a hospital cannot be transferred to other uses. However, entry into any one particular geographically defined market may be achieved at relatively low cost for a hospital already in existence but located in another area. In this case there is an option for the local payer to contract with a non-local provider if necessary. The market is therefore contestable because there is a threat of competition from non-local providers.

Although contestability is the feature that provides the label for the theory, there are other elements that are equally as important. Contestability explains why the number of competitors may not determine market structure, but does not in itself explain what does determine it. That aspect is based on the concept of an efficient market structure, for example one that delivers the lowest prices to consumers for a given quality. Traditional theory identifies a single most efficient market structure, perfect competition. By contrast, it is asserted that each industry has a uniquely efficient market structure, which depends on the industry's production, cost and demand conditions. Perfect competition is the most efficient market structure only if all of the conditions assumed for it are met. However if, for example, economies of scale are very great, average costs may be so low that even a monopolist can deliver lower prices than a smaller number of competitive firms could achieve. That would then be the most efficient structure. A less extreme case, applicable to many hospital services, is that there may be a minimum efficient scale that implies there should be a few hospitals in a particular region, rather than many.

This is important because of the implications that it has for government policies about the regulation of industries, whether public or private. (Government intervention in health care is discussed more widely in the next chapter.) As a theory of how markets work contestability is different to older models, but it also suggests different government competition and regulation policies. Traditional competition theory assumes that the benefits of competition arise from having many competing, non-colluding sellers and assesses the degree of competition by the number of firms in the industry and their share of the market. If there are other market structures, such as monopoly, these should be broken up. If that is not possible, prices and profits should be directly regulated or firms nationalised.

Contestability theory suggests instead that the aim is to have efficient markets, which are maintained by firms experiencing the threat of competition. Policy analyses should be devoted to assessing efficient market structures rather than the level of concentration. If government intervention is required, it should be directed at lowering barriers to entry and exit. This might include support for initial financial investment, since this is the most important entry barrier. It might also include action to ensure that information about the market and technology in the industry is open and accessible. But lowering entry barriers in itself may not be sufficient to ensure that an efficient market structure is created and sustained. Other interventions may be required, for example to ensure that the market is not in practice affected by 'hit-and-run' operations and that existing firms do not create new entry barriers by branding, predatory pricing, maintaining over-capacity and other devices. Moreover, the efficient market structure for an industry may change over time, possibly requiring further intervention.

When applied to the public sector, the obvious implication is that promoting contestability might be an alternative to nationalisation as a means of dealing with issues such as natural monopoly. However, it also gives an alternative to privatisation as a means of promoting efficiency through competitive pressures, since privatisation might simply convert a public monopoly into a private one. The use of contestability to promote competition in the market for hospital services in the NHS in the UK was highlighted by Ham (1996), in an editorial in the *British Medical Journal*. He argued that:

> The middle way between planning and competition is a path called contestability. This recognises that health care requires cooperation between purchasers and providers and the capacity to plan developments on a long-term basis. At the same time, it is based on the premise that performance may stagnate unless there are sufficient incentives to bring about continuous improvement. [. . .]
>
> [T]here is the stimulus to improve performance which exists when providers know that purchasers have alternative options. [. . .] It is, however, a quite different approach than competitive tendering for clinical services, which would expose providers to the rigours of the market on a regular basis.
>
> The essence of contestability is that planning and competition should be used together, with contracts moving only when other means of improving performance have failed. Put another way, in a contestable health service it is the possibility that contracts may move that creates an incentive within the system, rather than the actual movement of contracts.

Subsequently, contestability became a key part of NHS policy. This obviously required removing legal restrictions on new providers, but other actions were also mainly directed towards reducing entry and exit barriers. This included improving cost and price information and offering favourable terms to new independent sector providers. The hope was that this would provide the alleged efficiency-creating benefits of competition. However, the policy, the way in which it should be implemented and the evidence about its effects all remain controversial.

Summary

1. A firm is an economic unit that produces and sells goods, such as medical equipment, or services, such as dental care or health insurance. An industry is a collection of firms that sell similar products, such as the pharmaceutical, insurance or hospital industries. An industry is the supply side of the market. To analyse the supply of health care we therefore need to develop a theory of the firm, which can be used to explain how health care firms behave.

2. A useful framework with which to analyse supply of health care is the structure–conduct–performance paradigm. Supply is strongly influenced by the market structure within which the health care firm operates. For example, a hospital operating in a highly competitive environment – the structure – may conduct its activities differently from a hospital with few or no competitors. The more competitive the environment the more aggressive the hospital may have to be to attract patients and revenue in terms of the price of services provided and the quality of care. This conduct will in turn influence the performance of the hospital, which may be measured in a variety of dimensions such as the number of patients treated, revenue earned or profitability.

3. Economists traditionally assume that firms aim to maximise their profits. The profit maximising level of output occurs where the marginal revenue received from sales of the product equals the marginal cost of producing it. There are different models of profit maximisation depending on the market structure that is assumed.

4. Market structure is commonly defined by the number of competitors in the market, the freedom with which competitors can enter the market, and whether the different firms in the market sell homogenous, differentiated or unique health care products. Common market structures are perfect competition, monopoly, monopolistic competition and oligopoly.

5. In perfect competition there are a large number of sellers in the market, there is freedom of entry and exit, firms sell undifferentiated products and there is perfect knowledge. Firms have no control over price: they are price takers. The implication of these assumptions is that in the long run firms will earn zero profits. An example of perfect competition in the health care industry is given by internet pharmacies.

6. A monopoly is a market structure in which there is a single seller of a product. There are no close substitutes for the goods sold by the firm, and there are significant barriers to entry. An example of monopoly in the health care industry is given by the market for medicines: pharmaceutical companies, having found a new molecule, are granted a patent which grants them monopoly power to produce the molecule. This acts as a reward for the expenditure incurred in bringing the medicine to market, and to encourage future research and development.

7. With monopolistic competition there are many firms competing in the market, there are no barriers to entry and exit and each firm sells a differentiated product from its competitors. An example of monopolistic competition in the health care industry is given by the market

for medicines when a product's patent may not have expired but there may be competitors producing a product in the same class of drugs; hence the firm will have some market power. In the long run after the patent has expired new firms will enter the market and start to provide generic copies of the medicine.

8. Oligopoly occurs where there are only a few firms in an industry, but more than one, and entry for new firms is restricted. An important characteristic of oligopolies is that firms are mutually dependent. Oligopolostic firms may collude in order to limit competition among themselves, and this collusion may be formal (in which case the oligopoly is called a cartel) or informal. In the case of a non-collusive oligopoly there is no agreement, formal or informal, between firms. With no collusion price competition between firms is more likely to occur. Due to the interdependence of oligopolistic firms, non-collusive oligopolists are required to devise strategies that take into account the impact of their actions on the behaviour of their rivals. An example of oligopoly in the health care industry is hospitals acting collusively in order to increase their revenue.

9. Game theory is an approach that can be used to examine the optimal strategy of the firm, depending on its views about how its rivals will behave, in a non-collusive oligopoly.

10. While the goal of profit maximisation may be applied to some sectors of the health care industry (for example, the pharmaceutical industry) goals other than profit maximisation also rise. This is due to the divorce of ownership and managerial control; autonomy of health care professionals; and, special interest groups.

11. Common alternatives to profit maximisation in the health care industry include: growth maximisation; behavioural theories, which recognise that health care firms are complex organisational units with multiple goals and multiple decision-making units; utility maximisation, where utility is a function of the quality and quantity of care provided; and, maximising net income per physician.

12. The theory of contestable markets says that what is crucial to the conduct of firms is not the actual degree of competition they face in the market, but the threat of competition. This is greater when the costs of entry and exit into the market are lower. At the extreme the cost of entry and exit might be zero. In this case the market is said to be perfectly contestable. Under these circumstances, even a monopoly provider is forced to adopt the same pricing and output strategy as it would if faced with a very large number of competitors.

CHAPTER 5

Markets, market failure and the role of government in health care

5.1 Introduction

Chapter 4 examined the way in which the characteristics of a market, such as the number of firms and barriers to entry, influence the way that firms decide about prices, output and profits. This chapter extends this by asking: Are private health care markets competitive? Do health care markets allocate resources efficiently? What might go wrong – and what should the government do about it?

We begin with a simple proof of an essential conclusion of conventional theoretical economics: perfectly competitive markets lead to an efficient allocation of resources. We then consider the relevance to real-world health care markets of the assumptions underpinning the perfectly competitive model and the characteristics of health care that lead to market failure. We conclude by examining the rationale for government involvement in health care markets to address their failures.

5.2 Using perfectly competitive markets to allocate resources

5.2.1 Equilibrium in competitive markets

Chapter 1 introduced a simple model of the demand for and supply of health care in private markets. Perfectly competitive markets are assumed to tend towards equilibrium. Market forces resolve mismatches between demand and supply. Shortages of goods and services drive prices up and unsold goods will result in falling prices. Prices result from interactions between buyers and sellers, and adjust to clear the market.

Chapter 1 noted that health care is an economic good, because it is scarce relative to our wants for it. Economic analysis deals with issues such as what health care to produce, how to produce it, and who should receive it. If health care were bought and sold in competitive markets, those issues would be resolved as follows:

- The market decides which types of health care and how much of each type is produced, by finding the price at which the quantity demanded equals the quantity supplied. The equilibrium quantity corresponding to this price defines how much of each health care programme is provided.
- Health care is supplied by providers who are willing to do so at the equilibrium price. They will produce it in an efficient way so that they can maximise profits.
- Health care is purchased by those consumers who are willing and able to pay the equilibrium price. Access to health care is based on ability to pay and not other factors such as need.

5.2.2 The efficiency of competitive markets

An important conclusion of economic theory is the First Fundamental Theorem of Welfare Economics. This states that a perfectly competitive market will generate an allocation of resources that is socially efficient. This idea is the basis for many economists' arguments in favour of free markets and minimal government interference.

What do we mean by social efficiency? In Chapter 3 we noted that definitions of technical and economic efficiency are based upon Pareto efficiency. Social efficiency is also based on this definition, using the concepts of Pareto improvements and Pareto optimality. These will be explained in more detail in Chapter 9. Briefly, if a change can be made to the health care system that benefits some people without making anyone else worse off, this is a Pareto improvement. When all Pareto improvements have been made, it is not possible to make anyone better off without making someone else worse off. The health care system would then be Pareto optimal, which is what economics conventionally defines as socially efficient.

Under certain assumptions, perfectly competitive health care markets, in the precise sense described in Chapter 4, can be shown to be Pareto optimal. In a perfectly competitive market, a rational consumer and provider will choose to purchase or provide health care if the gain from doing so exceeds the extra cost incurred. An activity is worth doing as long as the private marginal benefit to the decision-maker (PMB) exceeds the private marginal cost (PMC). So, if $PMB > PMC$, they should do more of the activity. If the gain is less than the extra cost ($PMB < PMC$), then they should do less of it. If the gain equals the extra costs ($PMB = PMC$), then they have achieved private efficiency and are acting efficiently in their own private interest. Pareto optimality is achieved when the gains to society (the social marginal benefit, SMB) equal the marginal cost to society (SMC). For a competitive market to be socially efficient, we must also assume that there are no costs or benefits to society over and above those experienced in the market by individual consumers and producers. These are known as spillovers or externalities, and are discussed in Section 5.3.1. If there are no externalities private marginal benefits exactly equal social marginal benefits ($PMB = SMB$), private marginal costs equal social marginal costs ($PMC = SMC$) and a competitive market will lead to Pareto optimality.

We will explain the efficiency of competitive health care markets using the example of an internet pharmacy market, first discussed in Chapter 4, as an example of perfect competition.

First, the privately efficient level of consumption of internet pharmaceuticals is achieved when $MU(= PMB) = p^C(= PMC)$. Under perfect competition, the marginal benefit to a consumer from consuming pharmaceuticals is their marginal utility (MU) from consumption. MU falls as consumption increases; that is, there is diminishing marginal utility of consumption. The marginal cost of consumption is the price the consumer has to pay, p^C, which is set by the market. A rational consumer will continue to consume pharmaceuticals up to the point where $MU = p^C$, or where the private marginal benefit from consumption equals the private marginal cost. This is shown by Q^* in Figure 5.1(a). Note that the MU curve tells us how much of the good is consumed at each price; it is therefore also the demand curve.

Secondly, the privately efficient level of production of internet pharmaceuticals is achieved when $p^P(= PMB) = MC(= PMC)$. The marginal benefit to the internet pharmacy from providing pharmaceuticals is its marginal revenue, which under perfect competition is equal to the price p^P. The internet pharmacy is a price taker and so price is set by the market. Under profit maximisation, the pharmacy will supply pharmaceuticals up to the point where $p^P(= MR) = MC$, or where the private marginal benefit from production equals the private marginal cost. This is shown by Q^* in Figure 5.1(b). Note that the MC curve tells us how much of the good is supplied at each price; it is therefore also the supply curve.

Thirdly, private efficiency is achieved when $MU = p = MC$. Under perfect competition, this is achieved because the same price is faced by both the consumers and producers in the internet pharmacy market. In other words, $p^C = p^P$ and the privately efficient levels of consumption and production are achieved simultaneously.

Fourthly, Pareto efficiency is achieved when $SMB = MU = P = MC = SMC$. With no externalities, private marginal benefits equal social marginal benefits ($PMB = SMB$) and

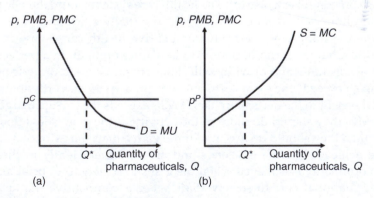

Figure 5.1 Private efficiency of the internet pharmacy market

private marginal costs will equal the social marginal costs ($PMC = SMC$). Therefore, the equilibrium prices and quantities yielded by a competitive market will also be Pareto optimal.

5.3 Market failure in health care

In the real world most health care markets rarely if ever achieve Pareto optimality. For example, the First Fundamental Theorem relies crucially on markets being perfectly competitive – and any breakdown in the underlying assumptions, such as freedom of market entry and perfect information, will lead to distortions in prices, quantities and social inefficiency. The term 'market failure' is used to cover all circumstances in which the market does not achieve Pareto optimality. The main causes of market failure in health care are discussed below.

5.3.1 Externalities

Externalities, or spillover effects, are costs and benefits incurred in the consumption or production of goods and services that are not borne by the consumer or producer involved. They may be positive or negative. Whenever other members of society are affected beneficially by externalities, there are said to be external benefits. Whenever other members of society are affected adversely there are external costs.

Health care markets will not lead to Pareto optimality if there are externalities. The full marginal cost to society from the production or consumption of health care (SMC) is equal to the private marginal cost (PMC) plus the marginal external cost (MEC), and the marginal benefit to society (SMB) is equal to the private marginal benefit (PMB) plus the marginal external benefit (MEB). If MEB or MEC or both are non-zero, then consumption and production decisions based on $PMC = PMB$ will not ensure that $SMC = SMB$. If there are external benefits, too little will be consumed or produced. If there are external costs too much will be consumed or produced. Table 5.1 illustrates the different types of externality.

Figure 5.2 illustrates consumption benefit externalities. The horizontal line shows price, which is assumed to be equal to both PMC and SMC. A person deciding on how much health care to consume will choose the amount at which $PMB = PMC$, resulting in Q^P being consumed. However, there are external benefits from the consumption of health care by this person, shown by the line MEB. The total marginal benefits to society are given by the line SMB, which lies above PMB. The socially efficient level of consumption is Q^S, where $SMB = SMC$, which is greater than Q^P.

An example of consumption benefit externalities is public health interventions such as vaccination. Each person's vaccination not only benefits them, by preventing them from catching the disease, but also benefits others, who might catch the disease from that person if they were not vaccinated. The greater the number of people who are immune to a communicable disease, the less likely it is that a susceptible person will come into contact with someone who has it. The externality that arises has been termed 'herd immunity'. This has interesting

TABLE 5.1	**Different types of externality arising from production and consumption**

Source and impact of externality	External costs	External benefits
Production externality that affects other production	MEC > 0 A pharmaceutical firm dumps its waste in a river and affects the production of a medical supplies firm downriver that uses the river's water	MEC < 0 A pharmaceutical firm's research benefits other pharmaceutical firms by improving scientific knowledge about a class of drugs
Production externality that affects consumption	MEB < 0 Smoke from a hospital's incinerator affects local people's enjoyment of their gardens	MEB > 0 A pharmaceutical firm's research enables people to be better informed about their health
Consumption externality that affects other consumption	MEB < 0 Consuming cigarettes and alcohol affects the wider society in the form of passive smoking and antisocial behaviour	MEB > 0 Vaccines directly benefit the health of others by reducing their chances of contracting the illness
Consumption externality that affects production	MEC > 0 The larger the market served, the greater the costs of reaching a more dispersed population	MEC < 0 Greater reliance on home care in a particular locality may reduce the travel time for home helps

economic implications, as the externality only exists if there are sufficient numbers of immune people.

Coase (1960) argued that the private market issues arising from externalities can in theory be resolved. This relies on the idea that it may be possible for people to be given ownership rights over externalities, so that they become part of private costs and benefits. With the further assumption that market transactions between private individual consumers and producers have no costs in themselves, markets will produce an efficient outcome irrespective of who is given ownership of any particular externality. In practice, of course, 'transaction costs' may be very large, especially where externalities are hard to define and 'property rights' may also be difficult or impossible to specify clearly.

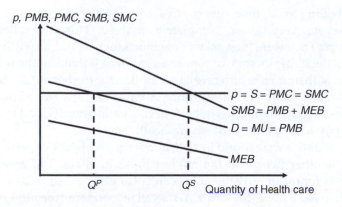

Figure 5.2 Pareto inefficiency with consumption benefit externalities

5.3.2 Caring externalities

The sorts of consumption externalities described above are sometimes referred to as 'selfish externalities', benefits that people value because they themselves receive them. However, people may also obtain an altruistic external benefit from other people's health care consumption, which is sometimes referred to as a 'caring externality'. The external benefit is gained by someone not from an improvement in their own health, but simply from knowing that someone else receives the health care that they need.

The existence of caring externalities in Sweden is discussed in Box 5.1.

BOX 5.1   Caring externalities in Sweden

Jacobsson *et al.* (2005) investigated the existence of caring externalities and examined whether the magnitude of the marginal external benefit of caring externalities is related to the severity of the illness being treated. They defined caring externalities using the utility function

$$U_i = U(C_i, H_1, H_2, \ldots H_n)$$

where U_i is the utility of person i, C is the consumption of goods and services, H is health (which is itself a function of health care received) and there are $i = 1, 2, \ldots, n$ people in society. The caring externality arises when the utility of person i is an increasing function of the health care received by other people in society.

The authors investigated how large the marginal external benefit due to caring is, by conducting a survey of 180 people in Sweden. Respondents were first asked how much they would be willing to pay for a cure from each of six ill-health states: slight, moderate, considerable, severe, very severe, completely disabled. This was called the 'internal preference group'. They were then asked how much they would be willing to pay for an improvement in the ill-health state of someone else, even if it meant the respondent must relinquish some of their own health care consumption for the benefit of the other person. This was called the 'caring externality group'. A ratio was constructed in which the sum of the willingness to pay for the two mildest health states was divided by the sum of the willingness to pay for the two most severe health states.

Caring externalities were found in all health states, with 52% of respondents willing to pay to cure another person in the mildest ill-health state. The mean value of the willingness to pay for the improvement in health of another person was smaller than that for the respondent in all ill-health states. Across all respondents the mild/severe ratio for the internal preference group was 0.30, while for the caring externality group it was 0.17. The authors suggest that this indicates 'a higher evaluation related to level of severity for caring externalities than for internal preferences'.

This study indicates the size of the marginal external benefit associated with caring. The authors conclude: 'Our results indicate that more attention and resources should be directed to severe health states, as compared to mild health states, than advocated by internal preferences in order to obtain more efficient resource allocation in the health care sector.'

5.3.3 Market power

Whenever there is a monopoly or imperfect competition, the market will fail to allocate goods and services in a Pareto efficient manner: the monopoly will provide less health care than is Pareto efficient. This is shown in Figure 5.3 in the case of a patented drug. As discussed in Chapter 4, a monopolist producing a patented drug is a price maker and has a downward sloping $D = AR$ curve. The MR curve is everywhere below the AR curve. A profit-maximising

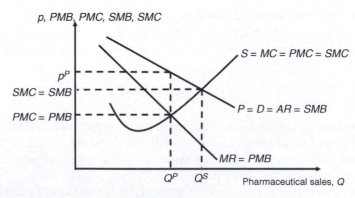

Figure 5.3 Pareto inefficiency with market power

monopolist will produce at the level of output where $MR = MC$, at output level Q^P in the figure. The Pareto efficient output is at the higher level Q^S, which occurs where $MSB = MSC$.

5.3.4 Public goods

Public goods are goods that are consumed *jointly* by all consumers. The strict economics definition of a public good is that they have two characteristics. The first is non-rivalry. This means that the consumption of a good or service by one person does not prevent anyone else from consuming it. Non-rival goods therefore have large marginal external benefits, which make them socially very desirable but privately unprofitable to provide. Examples of non-rival goods are street lighting and pavements.

The second is non-excludability. This means that it is not possible to provide a good or service to one person without letting others also consume it. In other words, if it is provided no-one can be excluded from consuming it. Anyone can obtain the benefits from consuming a non-excludable good without paying for it and therefore have no incentive to do so if someone else will pay for it. This may lead to a *free-rider problem*, in which people are unwilling to pay for goods and services that are of value to them. If everyone free-rides then the good or service will not be provided at all, which might lead to a loss to society. Examples of non-excludable goods are lighthouses and national defence.

When goods have these two features they will not be provided in a private market because there is no incentive for anyone to pay for them. The usual solution to this problem is for the government to provide them and compel people to finance this provision via taxation. Note the distinction between *public goods*, which are goods and services that are non-rival and non-excludable, and *publicly provided goods*, which are goods or services that are provided by the government for any reason.

Pareto efficiency requires that public goods should be provided at a level where $SMB = SMC$. The marginal social benefit is obtained by summing the private marginal benefits across all people. This is shown in Figure 5.4. Two people, Adam (*A*) and Zoë

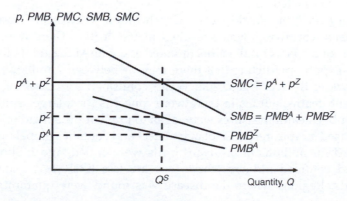

Figure 5.4 Pareto inefficiency with public goods

(Z), receive private marginal benefits from consumption given by PMB^A and PMB^Z, respectively. The social marginal benefit is the vertical sum of the private marginal benefits at each level of consumption, SMB. With a social marginal cost given by SMC the socially efficient level of provision is Q^S. At this level of provision, Adam would be prepared to pay price p^A and Zoë would be prepared to pay p^Z, which equates the private marginal cost with the private marginal benefits at the socially efficient level for each of them. Because both Adam and Zoë will free-ride, the good will be provided by the government and they will both be compelled to pay the price via taxation.

Most health care products and services are *not* public goods because they are both rival and excludable. For example, a hospital inpatient admission is rival because one person's use of a hospital bed prevents another from using it. It is also excludable, because the hospital can simply not admit someone. However, some health care, particularly public health programmes, does have public good properties. An example is measures aimed at preventing the spread of bird and swine flu – see Box 5.2.

BOX 5.2 **Public goods in health care: preventing a bird and swine flu pandemic**

Like humans, birds and pigs are susceptible to flu. Strains of animal flu have been found to pass into the human population, creating concerns of a flu pandemic with bird flu H5N1 in 2007 and swine flu H1N1 in 2009. Both strains can be fatal in humans. Bird flu spreads via migratory birds, which can then pass it on to domestic birds, and then on to humans. Humans catch the disease by being in close contact with live infected birds. The birds excrete the virus in their faeces, which then dry and become pulverised, and are then inhaled. However, the virus does not pass between humans. Swine flu spreads initially with close contact to infected herds and then spreads between humans. A similar flu strain to H1N1 was seen before 1957, offering some immunity to those who had previously contracted it.

By February 2007, the World Health Organization (WHO) confirmed 272 cases of H5N1 in humans worldwide, which resulted in 166 deaths. There were concerns of a larger epidemic of the H5N1 if the virus mutated and gained the ability to pass between humans, with experts predicting that there may be between 2 million and 50 million deaths worldwide. By April 2009, the WHO confirmed 257 cases of H1N1, which resulted in eight deaths, but again there were concerns for a larger epidemic.

Various public health measures were taken to prevent the spread of these diseases. The WHO devised a rapid-response plan to detect and contain a global flu pandemic. In the case of bird flu millions of farmyard birds were culled, and millions more were vaccinated and confined indoors where they are less likely to be contaminated by migratory birds. Regions where the disease was found were quarantined and some countries banned imports of live birds and poultry products. In the case of swine flu, the WHO advised against culling swine herds and instead countries were encouraged to selectively vaccinate high risk groups within the population.

These measures have public good aspects. With the imposition of controls to prevent the spread of bird flu and the use of vaccinations in the case of swine flu, the protection provided is non-rival in the sense that if one person is protected then others are also protected. It is also non-excludable in that it is not possible to exclude people in a region from being protected, and people who do not pay for the protection privately cannot be excluded from receiving it.

The measures seemed to have contained the spread of the disease. Worldwide bird flu has killed 303 people since 2003 and swine flu has killed over 18 000 people since April 2009. Though a higher death toll is reported for swine flu, this figure is in keeping with deaths from the seasonal flu.

5.3.5 Information imperfections

Imperfect information is another cause of market failure in health care, arising from uncertainty and imperfect knowledge.

Certainty in health care markets implies that buyers know exactly what they wish to consume, when they want to consume it, and how they can obtain it. Certainty is required for Pareto efficiency because consumers need to know the quantity of health care they would like to demand and providers need to know the quantity of health care to provide. If consumers have certainty, they are able to arrange their finances so that they can afford what they want to consume. With uncertainty, a market may be unable to function properly because consumers and producers do not know how much to demand and supply. They are therefore unable to equate the private marginal benefits of consumption with the private marginal costs.

Certainty is a reasonable assumption in the market for many goods and services. For instance, in the market for chocolate bars, people may know which items they would like to purchase. It may be possible for a person to predict when they would like to buy chocolate bars and how they can obtain them. However, the consumption of the majority of health care services cannot be planned in this way. This is because illness and deteriorations in health are often sudden and unexpected. Therefore, there is uncertainty in the market and the demand for health care cannot be predicted in advance.

The uncertainty surrounding the demand for health care seems to imply that markets may not allocate health care resources in a Pareto efficient manner. However, this problem can to some extent be addressed by insurance. Chapter 6 discusses health insurance and the various effects that it has on the demand and supply for health care services.

The problem of imperfect knowledge is that unless consumers and producers are well informed, they may take actions that are not in their best interests. They will be unable to equate private marginal benefits of consumption and production with the private marginal costs, and therefore both private and social efficiency are unlikely to be achieved.

Perfect knowledge on the part of consumers means that they are aware of their health status and of all the options open to them to maintain or improve their health. Although this may be the case for some illnesses, it is clearly not the case for the majority. Therefore, the market for health care is characterised by imperfect knowledge. Perfect knowledge is especially important in the market for health care since making the wrong decision may have much more serious consequences than choosing a chocolate bar that does not taste as nice as another does.

Imperfect knowledge in health care does not necessarily undermine health care markets. People are able to seek the help of suitably qualified and knowledgeable health care professionals whose job is to provide expert advice on health and health care so that people can formulate health care consumption decisions. However, health care providers who offer expert advice to consumers about health care may also supply health care and receive revenue from the services they provide. Therefore, the supplier of health care can influence the demand for health care. Contrary to the assumptions of competitive markets, supply and demand are not independent. Consumers of health care may be unable to act free of self-interested advice from health care providers, and the market may fail to provide an efficient level of health care. This is the problem of supplier-induced demand, whose existence and consequences are discussed in greater detail in Chapter 2.

5.4 Government intervention in health care

Governments intervene in the market for health care for two main reasons: because health care markets fail to achieve Pareto efficiency and because they are inequitable. A societal perspective might be that health care should be provided according to need and not ability to pay. The government might therefore become involved directly in the provision of health care in order to ensure greater access for certain population groups, for example low income groups and children, who might otherwise not receive the health care they need. We focus more fully on the issue of equity in health care in Chapter 7, but issues of equity are also relevant to the following discussion.

In the attempt to address these two issues there are many policy instruments affecting demand or supply that governments might use in the market for health care. Box 5.3 reviews policies that aim to reduce alcohol misuse whilst Box 5.4 reviews policies that aim to constrain pharmaceutical expenditure costs, particularly physician prescribing behaviour. A comparison of Boxes 5.3 and 5.4 shows that the reduction of alcohol misuse lends itself more to demand-side policies, whilst prescribing behaviour lends itself more to supply-side policies.

BOX 5.3   Policies to reduce alcohol misuse

Governments can use both demand- and supply-side policies to improve public health. Ludbrook and colleagues (Ludbrook *et al.*, 2001; Ludbrook, 2004) reviewed the cost effectiveness evidence of policies that could be used to reduce alcohol misuse.

Demand-side policies

Prevention. This includes mass media campaigns and school-based programmes to increase knowledge of the impact of alcohol dependence, aiming to change behaviour. School-based programmes tend to not teach facts, but skills to resist social and peer pressure.

Alcohol taxes. Taxation both raises revenue and reduces alcohol consumption.

Advertising controls. Legislation or voluntary agreements control the level and content of advertising, as well as the extent of promotional activities. Advertising controls are used to ban advertising that popularises alcohol related behaviours.

Screening and detection. Questionnaires have been developed to help GPs and other health care professionals detect patterns of harmful drinking or alcohol abuse. This enables them to intervene or give advice.

Brief interventions. This is counselling that aims to reduce alcohol consumption. The degree of alcohol dependence is assessed and reduced consumption goals are set through negotiation. Information is provided on ways to reduce consumption and further support is given in follow-up visits or telephone calls.

Detoxification. This mean abstention from alcohol for a time. Benzodiazepine can be used to alleviate withdrawal symptoms that arise.

Relapse prevention. This aims to maintain abstinence by psychosocial interventions to help the patient identify when relapse is most likely to occur, and medication taken to create an unpleasant reaction with alcohol or block its pleasant effects.

Supply-side policies

Legislation. This is used to control the opening hours of stores and bars selling alcohol, the types of outlets permitted to sell it, the number of outlets in an area and the legal age for purchase.

Enforcement. Successful legislation partly depends upon the action taken to enforce it. Enforcement of the drinking age includes age checks, media publicity and training schemes for alcohol outlets. Enforcement of drink driving laws includes random breath testing, suspending the licence of those failing tests and ignition interlock devices that require a breath sample to start the vehicle.

The authors found that taxation on alcohol reduced consumption overall but did not significantly affect the heaviest 10% of drinkers, who tended to substitute cheaper alcoholic drinks. The effects of other strategies are inconclusive. Some, like schools-based programmes, affect knowledge but not behaviour. They concluded that brief interventions, home and outpatient detoxification and relapse prevention were most cost-effective.

BOX 5.4   **Policies to control utilisation in the market for pharmaceuticals**

Bloor and Maynard (1993) discussed various policies to control utilisation in the pharmaceutical market.

Demand-side policies

   User (prescription) charges. These are used to raise revenue, reduce prescribing of unnecessary medicines and reduce the number of physician visits.

Supply-side policies

   Generic prescribing. Prescribing generic alternatives to brand-name drugs becomes possible when a drug goes out of patent. This also encourages price competition. There may be considerable savings to be made by prescribing cheaper generics, especially those produced by companies not involved in research and development. Some brand-name drugs may actually increase in price with the introduction of generics as the manufacturers attempt to indicate superior quality.

   Hospital formularies. These are preferred prescribing lists used in hospitals with the intention of providing guidelines for effective and cost-effective prescribing, without necessarily dictating which drug to use.

   Limited lists. These apply both to hospital formularies and drug reimbursement schemes. They limit the range of drugs that can be prescribed by doctors.

   Data on prescribing habits and cost. The dissemination of data on individual and mean prescribing patterns attempts to influence prescribing behaviour by increased awareness of costs.

   Indicative prescribing budgets. Upper-level targets for the volume of prescribing are set for prescribers based on factors such as existing prescribing costs, numbers and ages of patients and local social and epidemiological conditions.

5.4.1 Direct government involvement in the finance and provision of health care

The government might finance health care programmes directly, or provide public health insurance to enable people to obtain health care. It may do this for the whole population or for particular groups. It might provide all of the finance, so that it is free to consumers at the point of receipt, or subsidise it so that the costs to consumers are low. It might also provide some forms of health care directly, for example, publicly owned hospitals.

   Examples of these different types of involvement come from around the world. In some European countries hospital care is both financed and provided within a single government-based system. For example in the National Health Service (NHS) in the UK the government mainly controls both finance and provision of health care. In many countries self-employed general practitioners provide primary care, but they receive much of their funding from the government. There is therefore private provision with public funding. In other countries, private insurance companies might contract with hospitals of various ownership types, including publicly owned and privately owned not-for-profit and for-profit hospitals. There is therefore private funding but mixed public and private provision. We consider in more detail the role of the government in the finance and provision of health care in Chapter 6.

5.4.2 Taxes and subsidies

One consequence of market imperfections is that the level of output may not be socially efficient. It may be that the government can correct for some of these imperfections by introducing taxes or subsidies. Taxes are suitable for activities where the market level of provision is greater than the socially efficient level and subsidies where it is lower.

Where there are externalities, the government could impose a tax equal to the marginal external cost, or grant a subsidy equal to the marginal external benefit. One obvious area in which taxes might be used is to correct for external costs of consumption. For example, cigarette smokers pollute the air for other people but may take no account of this when deciding how much to smoke. There will be a 'passive smoking' consumption externality. The Pareto efficient level of cigarette consumption might be achieved via the introduction of a tax. This is illustrated in Figure 5.5. The privately efficient level of consumption is Q^P, where $PMB = $ price. SMC represents social marginal cost, which is the market price in the absence of any government intervention in the form of a tax. However, there is a negative MEB, so that SMB lies below PMB. The Pareto efficient level of cigarette consumption is Q^S, which is given by the intersection of the SMB and SMC curves. If a tax were levied on each unit of consumption of value equal to T, then the price and private marginal cost would rise to $p + T$ as shown in the figure. The correct level of T would ensure that the privately efficient level of consumption is also Q^S, the socially efficient level.

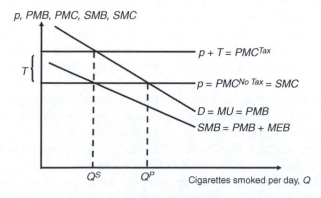

Figure 5.5 Imposing a tax to offset the external costs of consumption associated with cigarette smoking

5.4.3 Regulation

Governments influence the allocation of resources in the health market by establishing rules and regulations. At one extreme the government might prohibit certain activities entirely because of the adverse consequences they have on health. An example is the production and consumption of certain types of recreational drugs. At the other extreme the government might compel people to undertake certain activities, judging it is in their best interests to do so. An example is the mandatory wearing of seat belts in cars and helmets on bicycles. In addition, the government might regulate the market, determining the conditions under which goods and services are produced or consumed. For example, controlling the hours of operation for stores and bars selling alcohol, the types of outlets permitted to sell alcohol, the number of outlets licensed in defined areas and the age at which alcohol can be purchased. Regulation in health care can take many different forms, including price-setting, quantity-setting and quality controls.

The regulation of nurse migration into the UK is an example of the influence of regulation of both the source and destination country and is outlined in Box 5.5.

BOX 5.5   ## Regulation of nurse migration into the UK

All nurses working in the UK must be registered with the Nursing and Midwifery Council (*NMC*). Bach (2007) looked at the impact of regulations in both the source and the destination country and the impact this had upon the immigration of nurses.

In 2005 the NMC increased the educational requirements for registration of overseas nurses by introducing the 'Overseas Nursing Programme'. This programme required all overseas nurses to undergo a short additional training at a higher education institution to induct them into the NHS. The number of applications outstripped training places. Since 2005, 46 000 overseas nurses had applied for registration and were awaiting places, but only 8 000 places have been available each year. The training programme has therefore severely restricted the inflow of nurses into the UK.

But the regulation of the source country also has a large impact on those who apply, as shown in the case of the Philippines. The Philippines provides the largest source of nursing working overseas, and their nurses are especially popular in the USA and UK. This is partly due to their colonial past, giving proficiency in English and an education system close to the destination country. In addition, the Philippine government has for some time actively encouraged migration and eased regulation on the establishment of institutions offering nurse training to allow their expansion.

The UK government also uses 'soft regulation' in the form of a voluntary Code of Practice, to ensure that the NHS's international recruitment does not actively target developing countries, where nurses are in short demand already. In 2005 this Code was strengthened to require that recruitment agencies supplying nurses to the NHS must also adhere to it. A limitation of the Code is that it does not apply to nurses working in the independent sector, working in long-term care or social care. Despite this limitation, the Code has been successful in influencing the countries from which the UK draws its nurses, and is an acknowledgement of the impact of the UK's recruitment on the source countries. Moreover, other countries that also use international recruitment, like Canada and the USA, have yet to develop such Codes.

5.4.4 Provision of information

When market failure in health care arises due to imperfect knowledge, the government may help to correct the problem via the provision of information. An example is the provision of information for the general public on the benefits of certain types of health care. Box 5.6 considers an example of the provision of information by the government to reassure the population about the safety of the MMR vaccine.

BOX 5.6   The MMR vaccine

The MMR vaccine provides immunisation against measles, mumps and rubella. It is commonly given to children at around 1 year of age; a booster dose is usually administered at 3 to 5 years of age. The MMR vaccine is widely used around the world.

A controversy arose about the MMR vaccine when some parents and doctors alleged that it increases the risk of autism and other conditions. In February 1998, a paper published in the journal *The Lancet* suggested a link between the MMR vaccine and autism. As a result, uptake of the MMR vaccine fell sharply in the UK, leading to fears of a loss of herd immunity and a measles epidemic. The WHO has a target of 95% coverage amongst two-year-olds, but UK uptake fell from 92% in 1995 to 79% in 2003. In 2008, the number of measles cases in England and Wales exceeded 1 000 for the first time since 1995.

The research in the paper was severely criticised by scientists, and there was further controversy when it emerged that there had been an undisclosed conflict of interest, leading to a partial retraction of the paper by some of its authors. Further revelations of unethical behaviour and poor scientific practice led to it being completely withdrawn by *The Lancet*. The editor said "It was utterly clear, without any ambiguity at all, that the statements in the paper were utterly false." The editor of the *British Medical Journal* called it "deliberate fraud". The paper's main author has been disbarred from practising in the UK.

Because of this scare and its potential effect on uptake, the UK Department of Health, the NHS and others stressed that extensive research in numerous studies shows no link between MMR and autism. The Government's Chief Medical Officer, Professor Liam Donaldson, was very active in disseminating information to counter the effects of the scare. In a Department of Health press release on 12 January 2001 he said: 'Scare stories clearly worry parents but giving children separate vaccines unnecessarily exposes them to the risk of life-threatening infection. MMR remains the safest way to protect our children.' In February 2002, he promoted a TV campaign to persuade parents of the safety of the MMR and to immunise their children. By August 2008, it was necessary to set up an 'MMR Catch-up Programme'. He asked all Primary Care Trusts to offer the MMR to every unvaccinated child up to the age of 18 and to urge parents to have their children immunised. At the same time, the Department of Health made funds available for them to run a vaccination campaign.

In June 2011, the UK Health Protection Agency reported that coverage had for the first time since 1998 reached 90%.

Source: UK Health Protection Agency www.hpa.org.uk

The government may also provide information to patients and professional groups, for example, through such publicly funded bodies as the National Institute for Health and Clinical Excellence (NICE). NICE produces guidance in three areas: public health, health technologies and clinical practice. The guidance on health technologies and clinical practice is primarily for health professionals and patients. The audience of public health guidance is much broader than the NHS and includes those working in the fields of education, transport, environment, and criminal justice, in both public and private sectors. An important component of the advice is whether the intervention is cost-effective, a topic that we will return to in Chapters 9–13.

5.4.5 The theory of second best

If Pareto efficiency is achieved in the health care market, then we say that a first-best allocation of health care resources has been achieved. The failure to achieve a first-best allocation of resources may justify a role for government intervention. However, the question that then arises is how we can achieve a second-best allocation of resources, which is the best one that is feasible given the existence of market failures. The obvious solution would be to follow first-best rules, such as setting marginal cost equal to marginal benefit, whenever possible. Unfortunately, this is wrong. If we know that Pareto efficiency is not achieved in all parts of the health care market, then attempting to achieve Pareto efficiency by addressing market failures wherever possible may not be desirable. This is known as the *theory of second best*. It implies that the pursuit of perfect competition is not necessarily a desirable goal in health care if the first-best allocation of resources is not achievable.

To illustrate this, suppose that a pharmaceutical company enjoys a monopoly in the provision of a particular drug and that the drug's production process imposes an external cost of production on society in the form of pollution. Should the government intervene to reduce its monopoly power, that is, attempt to achieve the first-best rules of perfect competition without dealing with the first-best rule of no externalities? In this case the answer is no. Reducing the monopoly power enjoyed by the company and making the market more competitive will increase the production of this drug, with an increase in pollution and an even bigger negative production externality. Overall, society may be worse off than if the government had not reduced the monopoly power. To reach the first-best allocation would require further intervention, such as a pollution tax, to take account of the externality problem.

5.5 Government failure

gov't is too focused on election platform → to balance the desirable pareto efficiency.

We have examined a number of reasons why government intervention may be desirable in the market for health care. However, government intervention is not unambiguously a good thing. For example, for government intervention to be desirable it must be able to improve efficiency or equity or both. It may fail to do this because the government has imperfect knowledge about the marginal social benefit and marginal social cost of consumption and production of health care. In this case it is unlikely the government will be able to intervene to achieve Pareto efficiency and, more importantly, its interventions could result in an allocation of resources further from the optimum than a private market might achieve.

Public provision of goods may be inefficient compared to private provision. This might arise from excessive administration in government; a lack of market incentives such as the absence of significant competition, the lack of a threat of bankruptcy and difficulties in measuring performance; conflicting objectives in government arising from the interaction of different departments; and changes in government policy resulting from the political business cycle. Whatever the reason, if the problems created by government intervention are greater than the problems overcome by it, then there is *government failure* and a case for only limited government intervention.

The criticism made that the public sector is overly bureaucratic and inefficient is very widespread. The implication is that government intervention in health care leads to a waste of scarce health care resources. An alternative view is that administration costs are lower when there is one body, the government, dealing with health care finance and provision rather than a private market with many firms, each with their own bureaucratic procedures involving billing, consumer relations and cost and quality control. In Chapter 6, Box 6.1 compares health care administration costs in the USA (predominantly private market-based) and Canadian (predominantly government-based) health care systems, concluding that these costs are much lower in the government-based system.

Summary

1. If health care were bought and sold in a perfectly competitive market, this would determine what types of health care to produce, how to produce them and who receives them. The price system determines which types of health care and how much of each type

are produced, by finding the price at which the quantity demanded equals the quantity supplied. The equilibrium quantity corresponding to this price defines how much of each health care programme should be provided. Health care will be supplied by health care providers willing to supply health care at the equilibrium price. In an effort to maximise profits, health care will be produced in a manner that is technically efficient. Health care will be purchased by those consumers who are willing and able to pay the equilibrium price. Access to health care would be based on ability to pay and not other factors such as need.

2. Pareto, or social, efficiency occurs when it is not possible to make someone better off without making someone else worse off. The First Fundamental Theorem of Welfare Economics states that the allocation of resources in a perfectly competitive market will be Pareto efficient.

3. In the real world, health care markets rarely if ever achieve Pareto efficiency. The term market failure is used to cover all circumstances in which Pareto efficiency is not achieved by the market. Four causes of market failure that arise in health care are externalities, market power, public goods and information imperfections.

4. Externalities are costs and benefit incurred in the consumption or production of goods and services that are not borne by the consumer or producer involved. They may be positive or negative. Health care markets will not lead to Pareto efficiency if there are externalities. This is because private marginal costs and private marginal benefits deviate from the social marginal costs and social marginal benefits. An example of an externality in health care is the caring externality, which is an altruistic consumption benefit externality.

5. Whenever there is a monopoly or some form of imperfect competition, the market will fail to allocate goods and services in a Pareto efficient manner. For instance, a monopoly will provide less health care than is Pareto efficient.

6. Public goods are non-rival, non-excludable goods that are jointly consumed by everyone. Public goods will not be provided in a perfectly competitive market because there is no incentive for private consumers to pay for them; they will free-ride.

7. Information imperfections arise in health care because of uncertainty and imperfect knowledge. Uncertainty can be addressed via the introduction of health insurance. Imperfect knowledge can lead to physician-induced demand.

8. Governments intervene in the market for health care because markets fail to achieve Pareto efficiency and because markets can be inequitable. There are several policy instruments that governments might use to intervene in the market for health care: direct involvement in the finance and provision of health care; taxes and subsidies; regulation; and the provision of information.

9. The theory of second best states that if we accept that Pareto efficiency is not achieved in all parts of the health care market then attempting to achieve Pareto efficiency by addressing market failures wherever possible may not be desirable.

10. Government intervention in the market for health care is not unambiguously a good thing in the presence of market failure. There may be government failures which mean that intervention does not improve Pareto efficiency and equity. In addition, there may be inefficiencies in the public provision of goods compared to private provision.

CHAPTER 6

Health insurance and health care financing

6.1 Uncertainty and health care financing

Chapter 5 identified uncertainty as an important cause of market failure in health care. In this chapter we consider the implications of uncertainty, and some other related issues, for decisions about the way in which health care is funded.

It may be possible to predict future health states associated with chronic conditions and the magnitude of ill health for groups of people. This permits an assessment of the probability of future ill health for individual people. Generally, however, a person's future health state is uncertain. For health care that is not initiated by the onset of ill health, such as prevention or cosmetic surgery, it may be possible to predict demand. For most types of health care, demand is highly uncertain.

More specifically, health care is typically consumed under conditions of uncertainty with respect to the timing of health care expenditure (that is, when people become ill) and the amount of expenditure on health care that is required (what treatment is required and how much it will cost to become well again). People are at risk from unexpected ill health and of incurring possibly large unplanned expenditures for treatment. Health care expenditures may be 'catastrophic' if they require people to spend a significant proportion of their income at the same time that illness is reducing their ability to earn. As a result, they may be unable to afford the health care that they need.

The usual solution to such problems is insurance. This consists of an insurance contract between an insurance provider (the insurer) and a person who considers themself to be at risk of ill health (the insured). When someone buys health insurance he or she enters into an agreement with the insurer to pay an agreed price, called an insurance premium, in exchange for a payout to be made to the insured should they become ill.

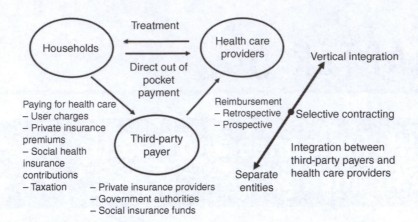

Figure 6.1 Health care financing relationships

Insurance works in the following way. Suppose that a group of 100 people each have a 1% chance in a year of becoming ill, which would require treatment costing £1 000. It is likely therefore that in a year one person out of the group will become ill, so the group's total expenditure would be £1 000. If each pays £10 into a fund, they will accumulate £1 000, which is exactly enough to meet their total expenditure. So, by *pooling risks* each of them converts an uncertain possible loss of £1 000 to a certain loss of £10.

The main model of health care markets used in Chapters 2–5 involves just two parties, and financing issues are very simple. Households demand health care and pay for it out of their own pocket. Health care providers supply health care in return for payments made by households. Most health care markets do not work that way. More commonly, a 'third party' is involved in financing, which may be an insurance organisation or the government or both. Financing is complicated, as shown in Figure 6.1.

The third-party payer can be one of three broad types: private insurance companies; the government; or social insurance funds. Private insurance companies operate in the same way as any private firm, with the making of profits as their main goal, although in health care insurance there are many companies that are not-for-profit.

In tax-based systems, the third-party payer is the government, local, regional or national. In effect it acts as both a provider of insurance and a purchaser of health care. The government therefore has considerable market power in setting payments for health care providers for the services it purchases. Any lower payment rates achieved may be passed on to households. Additionally, with a dominant large insurance provider administration costs may be lower than in a system with many individual private health insurance providers, each with different payment systems and their own bureaucracy.

In social health insurance systems, the third-party payer is effectively the social insurance fund, which is usually independent of direct government control. There might be numerous individual funds or a single national fund with market powers equivalent to those of government authorities.

We explore models of health insurance and examine the main features of the market for health insurance. We outline various reasons why the health insurance market might fail to provide appropriate protection from catastrophic expenditure. In the last section we explore the various ways in which health care is financed, and summarise the main mechanisms that are used to correct for market failures. We begin by looking at attitudes towards risk and investigating why people will pay to reduce uncertainty via insurance.

6.2 Risk and the demand for health insurance

The role of health insurance in addressing uncertainty in the demand for health care depends on attitudes to risk. Risk and uncertainty are different. Uncertainty exists when any one of a number of states of the world may occur and we do not know which one will arise. Risk exists when the probability of each possible state of the world occurring can be estimated.

Attitudes to risk can be analysed using the concept of a *fair gamble*. Suppose someone plays a game that offers a 50% chance of winning £10 and a 50% chance of losing £10. On average they would expect to make no money because the expected value of the gamble is zero: $(+10 \times 0.5) + (-10 \times 0.5) = 0$. This is called a fair gamble.

Now suppose that this person plays a game that offers a 25% chance of winning £20 and a 75% chance of losing £10. This is an unfavourable gamble. The expected value is negative and they will lose £2.50 on average. If the chances of winning and losing are reversed, this is a favourable gamble because on average the gamble will be profitable. The expected value is positive and the average gain is £2.50.

We can use these ideas to classify attitudes to risk. A risk-averse person will refuse a fair gamble. This does not mean that they will never undertake risky behaviour, only that the gamble needs to be sufficiently favourable to overcome their dislike of risk. The more risk-averse the person, the more favourable the gamble must be. A risk-neutral person is indifferent between accepting and not accepting a fair gamble. They will only accept a favourable gamble and will refuse an unfavourable gamble. A risk-loving person will accept a fair gamble, and may even accept an unfavourable gamble. The more risk-loving a person, the more unfavourable the gamble must be before they will not accept it.

Risk attitudes arise from two sources. One is whether someone likes or dislikes taking risks. Risk aversion may be due to a specific disutility from taking chances, and risk loving to utility from gambling. However, as the next section demonstrates, there is another explanation – essentially that a fair gamble in money terms may not be a fair gamble in utility terms.

6.2.1 Risk attitudes and the diminishing marginal utility of income

Friedman and Savage (1948) explained individual attitudes towards risk and insurance by looking at how people maximise utility and observing that people may have a diminishing marginal utility of income. The concept of diminishing marginal utility was used in Chapter 2 to explain the shape of indifference curves.

In Figure 6.2, $U(Y)$ shows the total utility attained by the person at each level of income. The slope of the $U(Y)$ curve gives the marginal utility of income. As income Y rises, the $U(Y)$

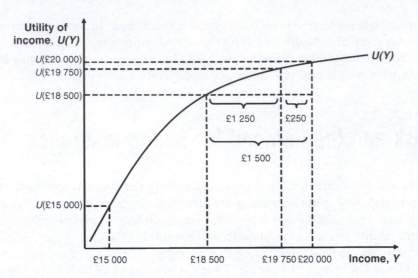

Figure 6.2 Insurance and the diminishing marginal utility of income

curve becomes flatter and the marginal utility of income diminishes. This is known as a concave total utility function.

Suppose that Figure 6.2 represents the total utility function for Adam, a 55-year-old man. He has hypertension and is considering whether or not to buy health insurance to cover himself for the risk that he will have coronary heart disease (CHD) over the next year. He has an initial level of income $Y_2 = £20\ 000$. He would have to pay £3 000 in treatment costs if he develops CHD and lose £2 000 in wages. If he is uninsured, his real income would therefore fall to £15 000. He faces a risk of two possible outcomes $Y_2 = £20\ 000$ and $Y_1 = £15\ 000$, associated with the utilities $U(Y_2)$ and $U(Y_1)$ respectively. If he has a probability of developing CHD of $p = 0.05$ then the probability of remaining well is $(1 - p) = 0.95$.

In deciding whether or not to purchase insurance Adam must weigh up the benefits and costs of insurance. Without insurance, he has an expected income $E(Y)$ of (£20 000 × 0.95) + (£15 000 × 0.05) = £19 750, an expected loss of £250. An insurance premium, which essentially is a certain loss incurred to remove an uncertain loss, will be a *fair premium* if, in this case, it is set at £250. However, economic theory suggests that people base their demand decisions on utility. Adam will assess the expected utility from his income, rather than the income itself, that is $(U(Y_2) \times 0.95) + (U(Y_1) \times 0.05)$. If he has a diminishing marginal utility of income any loss of income will lead to a proportionally higher loss of utility. The utility loss will therefore be greater than the utility that would be lost by a certain income reduction of £250.

Adam will therefore be risk-averse and willing to pay more for an insurance policy that removes risk. If, for example, his level of risk aversion results in an expected utility without insurance equal to $U(Y_3)$, where $Y_3 = £18\ 500$, the maximum premium he will be prepared to pay for insurance is £1 500. The risk premium is then £1 250. If he has to pay more than £1 500, the utility he gets from insurance will be lower than that without insurance, so he will not buy it.

Analysing the utility of income rather than its absolute value provides a plausible 'natural' explanation of risk aversion, which is a very common characteristic of people. However, it suggests that those who experience a diminishing marginal utility of income will always be risk averse. But an equally common observation is that many people both insure and gamble. This might be explained by gambling having a utility of its own, but Friedman and Savage (1948) explained this observation using a utility function that is concave below a person's initial income level, and convex above it.

6.2.2 The demand for insurance and indifference

Another way to view this is using indifference curves (Rothschild and Stiglitz, 1976; Rees, 1989). Figure 6.3 illustrates the insurance decision facing Adam. The horizontal axis shows his income when he is well, Y_W, and the vertical axis shows his income when ill, Y_I. Every point on the diagram represents a pair of incomes. The line $Y_I = Y_W$ is an equal income line (EIL), where Adam's income is the same in both states of the world, well or ill.

Point A shows Adam's actual income when well (Y_{W1}) and ill (Y_{I1}). The expected value of this, given the probability of being ill, is

$$E(Y) = \overline{Y} = (1 - p)(Y_{W1}) + p(Y_{I1}) \tag{6.1}$$

Point A is not, however, the only income pair that would have this expected value given those probabilities. The line DE is an *expected value line* (EVL), which shows for a particular probability of being ill all income pairs that give the same expected income as point A. The EVL is similar to the budget line of conventional indifference curve analysis, introduced in Chapter 2. Its slope is determined by the relative size of the probabilities of being well and ill. If these probabilities change, the line will pivot around the point A, becoming flatter if the probability of being ill is higher and steeper if the probability is lower.

Point B is of special interest, because it also lies on the EIL. Adam's income when well is Y_{W2} and when ill Y_{I2}, with $Y_{W2} = Y_{I2}$. His expected loss if he is ill, which is $(Y_{W1} - Y_{I1})$, is

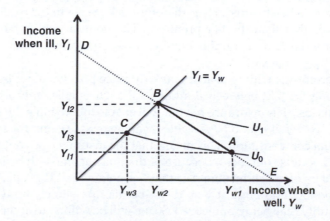

Figure 6.3 Indifference curve approach to the demand for insurance

therefore fully covered. The difference between his uninsured and insured incomes when well is the premium that he pays. $(Y_{W1} - Y_{W2})$ is the fair premium.

It is very unlikely that Adam would choose an insurance policy that lies on the EVL below point A. Points between A and E mean that Adam would accept a lower income when ill in exchange for a higher income when well. Similarly, it is unlikely that he choose a policy that lies on the EVL above point B. Points between B and D mean that Adam would accept a higher income when ill than when well. We therefore ignore those points, indicated by drawing BD and AE as dotted lines, leaving only points on AB as feasible.

Adam's utility level depends on his expected income, which means that it is determined both by the incomes that he will obtain when well and ill and also on the probability of being ill. We assume that his utility function is:

$$U(Y_1, Y_2, p) = (1 - p)\ln Y_2 + p\ln Y_1 \qquad (6.2)$$

An important point about this is that, other things being equal, Adam's expected utility will be maximised if his income when well is equal to his income when ill. The reason for this is the diminishing marginal utility of income. For example, point B is an equal income point. Any other point on AB has the same expected income, but a lower expected utility. The utility gained by having a higher income when well will be smaller than the utility lost by having a lower income when ill. The EIL therefore not only shows points where well and ill incomes are equal, it also shows all points of maximum expected utility.

Another way to view this is that if Adam is to obtain the same utility as given by an equal income point, he will require a greater expected income. As a result, indifference curves, representing equal levels of utility, have a slope that diminishes as income when well increases. This is shown in the diagram by, for example, indifference curves U_o and U_1, with $U_1 > U_0$.

Adam's utility when uninsured, at point A, is therefore U_o. If he were able to obtain insurance at the fair premium, he would be at point B, with a higher utility, U_1. He would willingly pay a fair premium of $(Y_{W1} - Y_{W2})$ to cover his expected loss of $(Y_{W1} - Y_{I1})$, which maximises his utility. However, he would be willing to pay a larger premium than this, as long as his utility is greater when insured. He is therefore risk averse to the extent that he is willing to pay a premium higher than the fair premium. The point at which he will be indifferent between being insured and uninsured is point C, where the premium is $(Y_{W1} - Y_{W3})$, with a risk premium of $(Y_{W2} - Y_{W3})$.

Adam will therefore be willing to accept an insurance policy that will give him an income pair anywhere along the EIL between B and C. All such policies mean that Adam is fully compensated for his loss. His insurance payout will enable him to have the same income when ill as when well. However, it would be possible for an insurance company to offer a policy that provides only partial compensation. This means that the insurance payout will not fully cover the loss that he has because of illness. Because of that, his income will be lower when ill than when well. The policy offers an income pair that lies below the EIL. Will Adam be willing to purchase such a policy? Although it would not be his first choice, he would, as long as it provides greater utility than being uninsured. So, he will be willing to accept any policy whose income pairs lie within the area ABC.

6.3 The market for health insurance and market failure

In this section we analyse the market for health insurance, starting with some issues related to the supply of insurance and finishing with an analysis of possible market failures. The key issues in market failure are *adverse selection* and *moral hazard*, though there are other characteristics of insurance that can cause insurance markets to fail.

6.3.1 The supply of health insurance

We have shown that health insurance enables people to swap uncertain for certain outcomes. It can remove the uncertainty that people face with respect to the timing and magnitude of health care expenditure. Insurance passes the uncertainty from the insured to the insurer. So, why do insurers take on the risks that their customers are prepared to pay to avoid? The answer is that the insurance provider is able to pool its risks. It can do this using the law of large numbers, which we first came across in Chapter 3 in the context of increasing returns to scale. Essentially, this suggests that predictions based on larger samples have smaller confidence intervals. Put another way, the larger the number of events of a particular type the more precise predictions of the average outcome will be. Using the law of large numbers, people may face uncertainty but insurance providers, who insure a large number of people, may face approximate certainty. Using the example of CHD risk, our 55-year-old man with hypertension does not know whether or not he will get CHD in the next year, but the CHD rate in the population for 55-year-old men with hypertension is known. It is the relative certainty of the average outcome resulting from the law of large numbers that allows insurance providers to provide insurance profitably.

Given this, what determines the price that insurance providers charge for health insurance? We saw previously that the expected loss for an uninsured person is given by $p(Y_2 - Y_1)$. Using the example earlier, the insurance provider knows that Adam has a probability of 5% of developing CHD, and that if he does develop CHD he will lose £5 000 in treatment costs and wages. It therefore calculates that the expected loss – the average payout it expects to make to him – is $(£5\ 000 \times 0.05) = £250$.

This is the average payout that the insurance provider would expect to make to people like Adam that it insures. The total premium charged by the insurance provider, q, is defined as

$$q = p(Y_2 - Y_1) + F \tag{6.3}$$

where F is called the loading factor. This covers the insurance provider's administration costs and the normal profit – which we discussed in Chapter 4 – that it needs to earn for each insured person to remain in the market. This is the price at which health insurance will be supplied in a competitive insurance market.

Suppose that the average cost of administering the insurance contract held with each insured person is £25 per year, and the additional administration and other costs of dealing with a claim are £600. The expected costs of dealing with a claim are (£600 × 0.05) = £30. The insurance provider also needs to earn a certain level of profit if it is to remain in the market, achieved by a mark-up of £150 on every contract. F is therefore £25 + £30 + £150 = £205, and the price that Adam is charged for insurance to cover his expected loss of £5 000 is £250 + £205 = £455. He will be willing to pay this, because it is lower than the maximum premium that he is willing to pay, which in our example is £1 500.

The size of the administrative burden of health insurance is important because of its impact on the affordability of insurance. Box 6.1 compares administrative costs in the USA and Canada, which have quite different arrangements for insurance.

BOX 6.1   Health care administration costs in the USA and Canada

In assessing the administrative costs of health systems, it is useful to compare the USA, with a large private insurance sector, with Canada, whose third-party payers are predominantly government authorities. Woolhandler *et al.* (2003) studied this issue using data from 1999, and Pozen and Cutler (2010) published a similar comparison for 2002.

Woolhandler *et al.* obtained data on insurance overheads, employers' costs to manage health care benefits, hospital administration, practitioners' administrative costs, nursing home administration and administrative costs of home care agencies. These were from published sources, surveys, employment data, and cost. Pozen and Cutler classified health care costs as arising from provider incomes, additional procedures for hospitalised patients and administrative costs. Administrative costs included hospital administration and administrative costs of practitioners but excluded insurance overheads, employers' costs to manage health care benefits, long-term care and nursing hours devoted to administrative tasks reports filed by hospitals, nursing homes and home care agencies.

In both studies, the costs were summed and those for Canada were converted to US dollars using gross domestic product purchasing power parities.

Woolhandler *et al.* found that administration accounted for 31.0% of total health care expenditures in the USA compared with 16.7% in Canada. Administrative costs in the USA were US$294.3 billion, or US$1 059 per person. In Canada, they were US$9.4 billion, or US$307 per person. This is a difference of US$752 per person. Applying this to the 1999 US population suggests that the total excess administrative cost is US$209 billion.

Pozen and Cutler estimated that the difference between the two countries in hospital and physician costs per person was $1 589. Health care administration accounted for 39% of this, provider incomes for 31% and additional procedures for 14%.

Pozen and Cutler also compared the staff numbers in the USA health system with those in other countries. Adjusting for population size, the USA had more administrative personnel, but approximately the same number of clinical staff: 25% more administrative staff than the UK, 165% more than the Netherlands and 215% more than

Germany. They offered two explanations for these higher administrative costs. First, there is a public goods problem, because insurers lack incentives to coordinate billing, as the costs of different rules are spread across all insurers. Secondly, insurers would tolerate a complex administrative system if it lowered overall payments.

The conclusions of both studies suggest that large savings in costs might be made in the USA if they had a Canadian-style government-based health insurance system. Woolhandler *et al.* end their paper with the question: 'Is $294.3 billion annually for US health care administration money well spent?'

6.3.2 Adverse selection

Adverse selection exists when exactly the wrong people, from the point of view of the insurance provider, choose to buy insurance: those with high risks. For example, suppose that everyone is charged the same premium as Adam (£455), based on an average probability of illness. Unless they are more risk averse than Adam, people whose probability of illness is lower than this may choose not to buy insurance at this price. Those who are most likely to buy health insurance are those who have a relatively high probability of becoming ill and maybe also incur greater costs than the average when they are ill. If such high-risk people are the only ones who take out insurance, the insurance provider will make a loss.

An obvious solution is to raise the insurance premium, to reflect the true average expected costs of those insured. However, this will simply deter those whose expected costs were above the old average, but are below the new average. This has two implications: the average person is deprived of insurance and premiums continually increase until insurance is not attractive to anyone. The costs of insuring those with the highest risks of illness approach pre-payment rather than insurance, and such people may not be able to afford that, especially because they may also have relatively low incomes. This has been referred to as the 'adverse selection death spiral' (see for example Buchmueller and DiNardo, 2002).

Adverse selection arises because of the asymmetry of information between insured and insurer. People who wish to buy insurance often have a good idea of their own risk status. The insurance provider does not know the risk for a specific person but does know the *average* risk in the population. Insurance providers base their assessment of risk, and therefore insurance premiums, on the average experience of the whole population, which includes both high-risk and low-risk people. This is known as *community rating*. Anyone who feels that their probability of illness is greater than the community rate will have an added incentive to insure, and those with a lower than average probability may choose not to insure unless they are sufficiently risk averse.

Suppose that the numbers of high-risk, medium-risk and low-risk people in the population are N^H, N^M and N^L, respectively. The probability of illness in each group is p^H, p^M and p^L, respectively, where $p^L < p^M < p^H$, and the insurance premiums that people in each group are prepared to pay are q^H, q^M and q^L, respectively, where $q^i = p^i(Y_2 - Y_1) + F$ for $i = L, M, H$ and $q^L < q^M < q^H$. The insurance company knows N^H, N^M and N^L, but does not know to which group any individual person who wishes to buy insurance belongs. They set a community rate q^{C1} payable by everyone, equal to the average of the amounts each group is prepared to pay, weighted by the proportion of the population in each group:

$$q^{C1} = \left[\frac{p^L N^L + p^M N^M + p^H N^H}{N^L + N^M + N^H}\right](Y_2 - Y_1) + F \tag{6.4}$$

Suppose that $q^L < q^{C1} < q^M < q^H$. The community rate will be unacceptable to the low-risk group because it is more than they are prepared to pay. They will therefore drop out of the health insurance market and will be uninsured.

The insurance provider will then make a loss, because only the high- and medium-risk groups remain in the market. It will therefore set a revised community rate q^{C2} based on the weighted average premium the remaining two groups will pay:

$$q^{C2} = \left[\frac{p^M N^M + p^H N^H}{N^M + N^H}\right](Y_2 - Y_1) + F \tag{6.5}$$

Since $q^M < q^{C2} < q^H$, the new community rate is more than the medium-risk group is prepared to pay; they too will drop out. The insurance provider will again make a loss, because only the high-risk group still wish to buy insurance, so it will set a rate given by

$$q^{C3} = p^H(Y_2 - Y_1) + F \tag{6.6}$$

In this case $q^{C3} = q^H$, and only those with the highest risk of illness will buy health insurance. However, if p^H is close to 1, then insurance is no longer feasible and the insurance market will collapse. An example of this phenomenon in the USA is given in Box 6.2.

BOX 6.2   Adverse selection in health insurance in practice

One way to examine adverse selection is to look at how people move between different insurance plans over time. Cutler *et al.* (2010) analysed claims data from 1994–2004 for 225 000 employees and family members employed by the state of Massachusetts who bought insurance from the state's Group Insurance Commission. They analysed the movements between a more generous fee-for-service indemnity plan (FFS), and a Health Maintenance Organisation (HMO). The generous plan offers more freedom of choice of providers, but costs more. The authors refined the concept of adverse selection, defining adverse *selection* as less healthy people moving to more generous plans and adverse *retention* as less healthy people staying in their current plans.

The authors' theoretical model assumed that someone will stay in a plan if the utility obtained from doing so is higher than if they switch to a different plan. The data were analysed using logistic regression analysis, in which the probability that people will switch plans from one period to another is related to variables that impact on their utility. These were demographic variables that might affect their propensity to switch, the level of copayment, the number of visits made, the number of claims, expected future claims, and the expected differences in premiums between FFS and HMO.

They predicted that a higher copayment would encourage people to switch, so this variable's coefficient would be negative. For FFS patients, if there is adverse selection or retention, higher current or expected claims and a greater number of visits will encourage people to stay, so those variables will have a positive coefficient. Adverse selection and retention work in the same way, so they cannot be separated. However, that is not the case for HMO patients. For them, adverse selection implies that the claims and visit variables will have positive coefficients and adverse retention implies negative coefficients.

The authors found clear evidence of adverse selection in the fact that an increased number of claims was associated with a greater number of switches from an HMO to FFS, but a lower number of switches from FFS to HMO. The logistic regression analysis found strong effects of demographic variables, in particular households containing older people were less likely to switch. Copayments had a negative effect, as expected, though this was small. Crucially, households having high claims and expecting high claims in the future are less likely to switch from the FFS plan, but more likely to switch from the HMO. This suggests that there is adverse selection rather than adverse retention.

Because the government heavily subsidises premiums, few people change plans, despite the fact that adverse selection occurs. The authors simulated long-run enrolment to look at the impact that different government subsidies have upon adverse selection. If the government contributes 85% of the premium, as it did in 2004, 37% of the sample will enrol in a FFS plan. This falls to 18% if the government pays 50%, and 11% if the subsidy is discontinued altogether. The people that remain in the FFS as the subsidy is phased out are those with high costs, so the FFS plan is forced to increase its premiums. The authors concluded that an adverse selection 'death spiral' is likely to occur if the government significantly reduces its subsidies.

Two approaches are adopted to prevent adverse selection. The first is experience rating, where the insurance provider sets a different insurance premium for different risk groups. Those who apply for health insurance might be asked to undergo a medical examination and to disclose any relevant facts concerning their risk status. For example, they might be asked to declare if they have been tested for the gene mutation that carries Huntington's disease. There are two problems with this approach. First, the cost of acquiring the appropriate information may be high. The cost will be passed on to insured people in their insurance premiums via the loading factor, which may mean that health insurance is no longer affordable or attractive. Secondly, it might encourage insurance providers to 'cherry pick' people, only choosing to provide insurance to the low risk. This may mean that high-risk people are unable to obtain health insurance at all. Box 6.3 discusses the UK's moratorium on the use of genetic tests for insurance purposes.

BOX 6.3 **Should insurance companies have access to genetic test results?**

Genetic testing is increasingly widespread, and its accuracy continues to improve. Genetic tests offer the potential for people to be more informed about their future risks than insurance companies. This asymmetry in information may lead to adverse selection, since people with high and low risks of certain genetically related diseases are being offered the same insurance contracts.

In the UK there is a moratorium on the use of genetic test results in insurance until 2014. Huntington's disease is the only exception to this. The test for Huntington's disease predicts its occurrence quite accurately. Currently there is no cure.

Those in favour of allowing these test results to be used in insurance argue that the insurance companies can already use family history to determine the susceptibility to some diseases. Those in favour of the moratorium argue that mandatory disclosure of test results may discourage people from been tested, and therefore reduce early identification of risks and uptake of treatment. For example, early testing and diagnosis of bowel cancer can significantly improve the chances for successful treatment. There is also a concern that the tests may lead to prohibitively high premiums for those found to have the disease, leading to a 'genetic underclass' who cannot get insurance.

The evidence from the UK for Huntington's disease seems to confirm that people will choose not to take a test if there is little to be gained from the test and it adversely affects their insurance premiums. In 2010, *The Guardian* reported that Professor Sarah Tabrizi, who leads research into this, said that about 20% of those at risk of Huntington's disease take a test to establish whether or not they will develop the disease.

In 2001, *The Economist* observed that the USA insurance market has not lobbied hard for the use of genetic information. The view seems to be that the medical benefits of early identification outweigh the benefits that would arise from reducing adverse selection.

Sources:

Fear of insurance penalties keeps Huntington's sufferers in the shadows. *The Guardian*, Wednesday 30 June 2010. http://www.guardian.co.uk

Special report on genetics and insurance. *The Economist*, 2001. http://www.economist.com/

The second approach is to make health insurance compulsory. The problem of adverse selection arises because low-risk people drop out of the market. By making health insurance compulsory this is prohibited and adverse selection will not arise. This approach is typically used with publicly provided health insurance, which is discussed below. The problem with this is that low-risk people effectively subsidise the health insurance payments of those with higher risks, which may be regarded by some as inequitable.

6.3.3 Moral hazard

Health insurance changes the economic incentives facing both the consumers and the providers of health care. One manifestation of these changes is the existence of *moral hazard*. This is a phenomenon common to all forms of insurance. The suggestion is that when people are insured against risks and their consequences, they are less careful about minimising them. If someone has vehicle insurance, they may be less careful to ensure that they do not damage their own or others' vehicles. Moreover, they may be more likely to claim for more trivial damage to their vehicles and to receive and accept higher estimates for repair from repairers. The problem with this is that the increased costs will be passed on to those insured in the form of higher premiums. As with adverse selection, this may affect the viability of insurance and its accessibility to those on lower incomes.

Moral hazard arises when it is possible to alter the probability of the insured event, p (that is, the probability of claiming), or the size of the insured loss, $Y_2 - Y_1$ (that is, the payout required by the insurance provider). Moral hazard can be avoided as long as insured people cannot influence p and $Y_2 - Y_1$. If they can, p and $Y_2 - Y_1$ are said to be endogenous; if they are free from influence then p and $Y_2 - Y_1$ are exogenous.

With endogenous p, people can influence the probability of the insured event. This is probably not a large factor in health insurance. Being ill and receiving treatment are intrinsically unpleasant, so there is a non-monetary disincentive for people to put themselves at a greater risk of illness just because treatment would be paid for. One example where this might arise in health care is planned pregnancy, which is influenced by individual action. The probability of making a claim for normal maternity care is not exogenous and it is usual for this to be excluded from private health insurance plans. Complications of pregnancy are often covered, however, because they are exogenous.

In the case of endogenous $Y_2 - Y_1$, people can influence the size of the payout that the insurance provider is obliged to make. This may take the form of an increased number of claims or a higher cost for each claim. Consumers and providers of health care may both be a source of this payout inflation. Consumer moral hazard arises because they have an incentive to gain additional benefits for themselves at the expense of the insurance provider. This is simply normal economic behaviour, consumer demand increasing in response to a lower price, as discussed in Chapter 2. The extent of the problem depends on the price elasticity of demand, as shown in Figure 6.4. Suppose that the market equilibrium price is p^*. With health insurance, the price facing the insured is zero, shown by p^0. If demand is perfectly inelastic, as in Figure 6.4(a), then Q^* is demanded whether or not the consumers are insured. If demand is price elastic, as in Figure 6.4(b), then the introduction of health insurance causes the demand for health care to rise from Q^* to Q^0.

Provider moral hazard arises from the fact that health care providers can also influence the size of the payout that the insurance provider is obliged to make. One way to view this is that in their role as the patient's agent health care providers will demand more health care for their patients when they are insured. If the provider is acting as a perfect agent, this is similar to the analysis of consumer moral hazard. However, it may also be more accurately described as supplier-induced demand, which was discussed in Chapter 2.

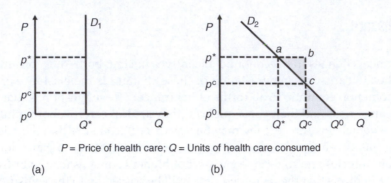

P = Price of health care; Q = Units of health care consumed

(a)   (b)

Figure 6.4 Moral hazard, price elasticity, co-insurance and deductibles

Three main mechanisms can be used to reduce moral hazard. The first is *co-insurance*. Many insurance policies require that when an event occurs the insured shares the insured loss $Y_2 - Y_1$ with the insurer. The *co-insurance rate* is the percentage of the insured loss that is paid by the insured. The *co-payment* is the amount that they pay. For example, with a co-insurance rate of 10% on an insured loss of £2 500 the insured would be required to make a co-payment of £250 and the insurer would pay the remaining £2 250. Co-insurance simply acts as a price attached to health care. For example, p^c in Figure 6.4(b) represents a co-payment that the insured is required to pay to their insurer if they make a claim. Assuming health care is price elastic, demand will then fall from Q^0 to Q^c.

The second is deductibles. A deductible is an amount of money the insured pays when a claim is made irrespective of co-insurance. The insurer will not pay the insured loss unless the deductible is paid by the insured. For example, a deductible of £100 would mean that the insured would pay the first £100 of all insured losses claimed for. This is also sometimes referred to as an *excess*. This is also illustrated in Figure 6.4(b). The insurance company must pay p^* for every unit of health care that the insured consumes, incurring a total cost of $p^* \times Q$. By setting a deductible, it in effect sets a number of units of health care that the insured must pay for before getting any additional units for free. Suppose that it sets a deductible such that the number of units that it will pay for is Q^c; the deductible will be $p^* \times Q^c$. This is more than the insured would pay if they were not insured; that would be $p^* \times Q^*$. However, the insured will not simply compare these two amounts, because if they are insured they will receive more health care, which is valuable to them. For some of the additional units, from Q^* to Q^c, they pay more than they would be willing to pay for them. The total 'overpayment' is the triangle *abc*. For the remaining units, from Q^c to Q^0, they pay less than they would be willing to. The total 'underpayment' is the triangle cQ^cQ^0. In the example given in Figure 6.4(b), the gain is greater than the loss, so the insured person will make a claim and pay the deductible. This deductible therefore does not deter excess consumption, but does raise revenue for the insurer.

The third is no-claims bonuses. These are payments made by insurers to discourage claims. They usually take the form of reduced insurance premiums in the next period. Suppose someone currently pays an insurance premium q^1. If they make no claim on an insured loss in the current period, then in the following period they receive a no-claims bonus equal to $q^1 - q^2$. The premium they are charged by the insurer will be q^2, where $q^1 > q^2$.

Suppose that the insured requires treatment that costs $Y_2 - Y_1$. If $(Y_2 - Y_1) > (q^1 - q^2)$, then treatment costs more than the no-claims bonus and it makes sense for the insured to claim a payout to cover the insured loss from the insurer and forgo the no-claims bonus. If, on the other hand, $(q^1 - q^2) > (Y_2 - Y_1)$, it makes financial sense for the insured not to claim from the insurer, to pay the cost of treatment $Y_2 - Y_1$ out of their own pocket, and obtain the no-claims bonus in the next period. No-claims bonuses typically discourage insurance claims where the payout by the insurer is small.

6.3.4 Non-price competition

Insurance can have a perverse effect on the efficiency of health care providers. Because price is no longer important to patients, there is a smaller incentive for health care providers to make their services affordable by minimising costs.

If patients have a choice of provider, price will be an important part of any choice decisions by those who have to pay out of pocket. Insured patients will not be price sensitive, and are more likely to choose a provider on the basis of non-price factors such as comfort, facilities and perceived quality. The costs of making improvements in these will be passed on to the insurer. So, health care costs will rise as providers compete for patients on these factors. Contrary to the normal conclusions of economic theory, a greater level of competition leads to higher costs and prices.

Because such cost escalation raises the total bill faced by third-party payers, there is an incentive for them to introduce cost-containment measures. Many such measures in effect attempt to replace the market power that patients do not wield with the market power of insurance providers. The most powerful of these is the ability to restrict patients' choice of health care provider.

6.3.5 Incomplete coverage

Another problem that arises in health insurance markets is incomplete coverage. Even if adverse selection does not occur, some population groups might find it difficult to buy health insurance. Low-income groups may not be able to afford health insurance, even if it is charged at a fair premium and there may be incomplete coverage for high-risk groups. Box 6.4 discusses the problem of uninsured people in the USA.

There will be incomplete coverage when the probability of illness tends towards 1. In that case, payout by the insurance provider is a near-certainty and insurance becomes more like pre-payment. Recall from equation (6.3) that the total premium charged by the insurance provider, q, is equal to $p(Y_2 - Y_1) + F$. As $p \to 1$, then $p(Y_2 - Y_1) \to (Y_2 - Y_1)$ and the premium charged by the insurance provider exceeds the insured loss $[q > (Y_2 - Y_1)]$ owing to the loading factor. Using again the example of Adam, if his probability of illness was in fact equal to 1 he would have to pay a premium of £5 205 to cover treatment costs of £5 000. Private health insurance will not be offered because there is no demand for it. In health care this problem can arise for people with chronic or congenital illnesses, such as cancer, if they attempt to buy health insurance after the condition has been diagnosed. Typically, private health insurance providers exclude treatment for pre-existing conditions, precisely because the probability of requiring treatment is too high to insure. The likelihood of incomplete coverage is compounded in low-income, high-risk groups, for example, older people.

Incomplete coverage might be remedied using cost-containment policies, which will cause treatment costs to fall. If the insurer passes this reduction to the insured, then premiums may become more affordable. Another solution would be to make health insurance compulsory and calculate individual insurance premiums not on the basis of individual risk but on ability to pay. This would mean that low-income and high-risk groups would be more likely to be able to afford health insurance. Addressing the problem of incomplete coverage in this way provides an important justification for tax-based health systems and those based on social health insurance.

BOX 6.4   Mind the gap: 50 million uninsured Americans

Data released by the US Census Bureau (2010) showed that the number of Americans without health insurance cover (either public or private) in 2010 was 49.9 million, or 16.3% of the total population. This represents an increase of 900 000 people from the previous year, of nearly 10 million compared with 2000, and of nearly 20 million since 1987. The proportion with no health insurance was not distributed uniformly across the population. For example, people with low incomes were more likely to be uninsured. 26.9% of people whose annual income was less than $25 000 were uninsured, compared with 8.0% of those whose income exceeded $75 000. Overall, 9.8% of children under age 18 had no health insurance but for children in poverty it was 15.4%. Blacks (20.8%) and Hispanics (30.7%) were much more likely to be uninsured than white non-Hispanics (10.7%). Because these people are required to pay for their health care directly, that is out of their own pocket, they are at risk from potentially catastrophic health expenditure.

Figure 2.8(a) shows that the USA has one of the highest levels of spending per person on health care in the world. The difference between the magnitude of US health care expenditure and the number of Americans who are uninsured has been famously described as 'a paradox of excess and deprivation' (Enthoven and Kronick, 1989).

6.4 Reimbursement

The method of reimbursement relates to the way in which health care providers are paid for the services they provide. It is useful to distinguish between reimbursement methods, because they can affect the quantity and quality of health care. We focus on methods for reimbursing hospitals, though the principles could apply to other providers.

6.4.1 Retrospective reimbursement

Retrospective reimbursement at full cost means that hospitals receive payment in full for all health care expenditures incurred in some pre-specified period of time. Reimbursement is retrospective in the sense that not only are hospitals paid after they have provided treatment, but also in that the size of the payment is determined after treatment is provided. Total reimbursement R is given either by $R = W \times AC$ or by $R = W \times S \times I$, where $W =$ workload (for example, number of cases treated), $AC =$ average cost of services provided per case, $S =$ number of services provided per case, and $I =$ fee per item of service. Which model is used depends on whether hospitals are reimbursed for actual costs incurred, or on a *fee-for-service* (FFS) basis.

The main features of retrospective reimbursement are that in the actual costs model hospital income depends on workload and the actual costs incurred. In the FFS model reimbursement depends on workload and the services provided. The fee, I may be set by competition or by the third-party payer. Since hospital income depends on the actual costs incurred (actual costs model) or on the volume of services provided (FFS model) there are few incentives to minimise costs. For example, hospitals might encourage excessively long lengths of stay or may over-order diagnostic tests.

6.4.2 Prospective reimbursement

Prospective reimbursement implies that payments are agreed in advance and are not directly related to the actual costs incurred. This does not mean that the hospital receives the payment in advance, only that the size of the payment is determined in advance. Since payment is not directly related to the actual costs incurred, incentives to reduce costs are greater, but payers may need to monitor the quality of care provided and access to services. If the hospital receives the same income regardless of quality, there is a financial incentive to provide low-quality care for minimum effort and minimum cost.

Prospective reimbursement can take two forms. With *global budgeting* the size of the budget paid to the hospital is set prospectively across the whole range of treatments provided. It is unrelated to the actual costs incurred and to workload. This provides a financial incentive to constrain total expenditure $(= W \times AC)$. Global budgeting gives overall expenditure control to the third-party payer, but because the way in which the global budget is distributed throughout the hospital is not specified, the allocation of the global budget within the hospital may not be efficient. The size of the global budget might be set historically with an additional adjustment made each year to account for inflation and changes in case-mix, or it might be set according to a resource allocation formula based on the size of the need-weighted population served by the provider. In the latter case, the incentives of the global budget will depend on the precise components of the formula.

With prospectively set cost per case, the amount paid per case $S \times I$ is determined before treatment is provided. By setting the costs per case prospectively, reimbursement is divorced from the costs incurred (AC) or the services provided per case (S), which generates incentives for cost containment. Total reimbursement can still be increased by increasing workload. So, unlike global budgeting, this method does not provide overall expenditure control to the third-party payer.

An example of prospectively set costs per case is the diagnostic-related groups (DRG) pricing scheme introduced into the Medicare system in the USA in 1984, and subsequently used in a number of other countries (see Boxes 6.5 and 6.6). Under this scheme, DRG payments are based on average costs per case in each diagnostic group derived from a sample of hospitals. Total reimbursement achieved by a hospital is given by $R = W \times DRG$, where DRG is the DRG-based prospective payment.

BOX 6.5   Fee-for-service versus prospective costs per case in European and Central Asian Countries

During the 1990s and early 2000s, many European and Central Asian countries moved away from funding hospitals using global budgets. Instead, they paid hospitals using either fee-for-service (FFS) or prospective costs per case using Diagnosis Related Groups (DRGs) or similar mechanisms. Moreno-Serra and Wagstaff (2010) used data from 1990–2004 for 28 countries to look at the impact that this had on hospital performance, including admissions, length of stay, numbers of beds, bed occupancy, cost per admission and quality. They also looked at the impact on total spending and mortality amenable to medical care.

They hypothesised that DRGs would increase admissions more than FFS, since FFS hospitals can earn more from existing patients than DRG hospitals by conducting more tests on them. It was also expected that DRG hospitals' average length of stay and cost of admissions would fall, as hospitals can keep cost savings that they make. Total health expenditure was expected to increase under both FFS and DRGs. The impact of the changes on mortality, quality of care or total hospital costs was uncertain.

They used regression analysis to look at the impact of changes in the payment methods upon hospital performance, expenditure and mortality. The underlying economic model was defined as Yit = f(Xit, FFSit, DRGit) for country i at period t, where Yit was either hospital performance, expenditure or mortality, Xit were independent variables that influence these outcomes and FFSit and DRGit were indicators for FFS and DRG. They specified an error term that included country- and time-specific effects and used a difference-in-difference regression model that looked at the impact of how the variables changed over time. They tested the robustness of their results by checking for reverse causality – that a country might change its payment system in response to poor hospital performance.

They found that total hospital spending increased under both FFS and DRGs but it was unclear if this was due to an increase in costs per admission or in administration costs. The impact upon hospital performance differed between payment methods: FFS increased admissions and DRGs had no effect; FFS had no effect on average length of stay but DRGs decreased it. DRGs appeared to have a beneficial effect on mortality amenable to medical care.

BOX 6.6   Healthcare Resource Groups (HRGs) in the NHS

Healthcare Resource Groups (HRGs) have been developed in the UK as a standardised way of classifying health care activities. They consist of defined categories of clinically similar treatments that consume roughly equal amounts of health care resources. They are very similar to DRGs in concept, structure and methods of development, but their top-level classification is based on clinical specialties, very broadly defined, rather than disease categories. These are called 'Chapters' and, for health care activities that can be classified, the HRG4 classification introduced in 2007 defines 20 of them. HRG4 defines more than 1 400 groups.

HRGs are used for three main purposes in the NHS. They have been used as the basis of Reference Costs since 2007, and for both Payment by Results and Programme Budgets since 2009. Reference Costs, which have been published since 1998, are an annual report of the national average unit cost of an HRG or other unit of health care activity.

Payment by results (PbR) is a prospective reimbursement system used to commission NHS-funded health care services from NHS providers. This consists of a national 'tariff' of prices for each HRG. It is based on the reference cost data, but is not simply the national average cost. PbR is the basis on which secondary care services are commissioned for patients, and it determines some of the revenues that hospitals receive from their activities. However, not all commissioning is undertaken using tariffs. The official aim of PbR is to 'provide a transparent, rules-based system for paying trusts. It will reward efficiency, support patient choice and diversity and encourage activity for sustainable waiting time reductions. Payment will be linked to activity and adjusted for casemix.'

NHS Programme Budgets (see Chapter 13) are also based on HRGs, although they have a different top-level classification, which consists of 23 healthcare programmes, based on the World Health Organisation's International Classification of Disease (ICD10).

The precise effect of this type of reimbursement will depend on the actual costs incurred by the hospital. If $DRG < AC$, hospitals will reduce AC until $DRG = AC$; hospitals have an incentive to minimise costs. If, on the other hand, $DRG > AC$, hospitals will increase costs until $DRG = AC$. They will spend more on amenities in order to improve their competitive position in the health care market, which will cause AC to rise.

Predicted effects of the DRG pricing scheme are cost shifting, patient shifting and DRG creep. Cost shifting and patient shifting are ways of circumventing the cost-minimising effects of DRG pricing by shifting patients or some of the services provided to patients out of the DRG pricing scheme and into other parts of the system not covered by DRG pricing. For example, instead of being provided on an inpatient basis, treatment might be provided on an outpatient basis where it is reimbursed retrospectively. DRG creep arises when hospitals classify cases into DRGs that carry a higher payment, indicating that they are more complicated than they really are. This might arise, for instance, when cases have multiple diagnoses.

6.5 Integration between third-party payers and health care providers

The way in which health care providers are reimbursed for the services they provide is a crucial determinant of health care costs and the quality of services provided. Retrospective reimbursement is likely to lead to an escalation in health care costs, while prospective reimbursement leads to concerns over quality and access. The problem from the point of view of the third-party payer is how best to monitor the activities of health care providers, and how to encourage them to act in a mutually beneficial way. This problem might be reduced if health care providers and third-party payers are linked in some way so that they share common goals.

There are three levels of integration between third-party payers and health care providers. In the first, the third-party payer and the health care provider are separate entities with separate aims and objectives. The goals of health care providers may not be consistent with those of insurance providers. In the second, there is selective contracting, with the third-party payer agreeing to steer people insured on their plans to selected providers and, in return, the selected providers charge lower prices to the third-party payer. Typically the third-party payer will undertake utilisation reviews to check the appropriateness of the selected providers' practices with respect to the cost and quality of care. In the third, there is vertical integration in which the insurance provider and the health care provider merge to become different parts of the same organisation. Vertical integration means that a single organisation provides health care in return for payment of an insurance premium. Because the two entities are parts of the same organisation, they have common goals with respect to the cost and quality of care. Integration between third-party payers and health care providers is a key feature of managed care.

The most straightforward type of insurance is *indemnity* insurance. This means that the insurer reimburses the patient or the health care provider for their health care expenses as these are incurred. The traditional private insurance model in the USA was that indemnity plans allowed patients to choose any provider that they wanted. This was seen as a major cause of spiralling health care costs, and other ways of arranging insurance were created to control this. Managed care organisations (MCOs) were the result. As noted, a key feature of managed care is the integration between the third-party payer and the health care provider. Typically, health care is provided by an MCO to a defined population at a fixed rate per month. The payments made by people are lower than with direct out-of-pocket payment or indemnity plans. In return for paying lower premiums, enrolees are required to receive health care from a limited number of providers with whom the MCO has negotiated lower reimbursement rates. There are three broad types of MCO, reflecting the extent of integration between third-party payers and health care providers.

6.5.1 Preferred provider organisations

In return for payment of an insurance premium, preferred provider organisations (PPOs) provide insured people with two options when they require treatment. First, they can use the PPO's preferred providers – those with which it contracts selectively in return for lower reimbursement rates. By using the preferred provider people face lower user charges, and so the reduced costs of care with the preferred provider are passed on to the insured. Secondly, people may choose to use a different provider outside the network of preferred providers but with higher user charges. Patients can choose freely which option they prefer because there is no gatekeeper to authorise the type of care selected; but there is obviously a financial incentive to use the preferred providers.

6.5.2 Health maintenance organisations

In its simplest form, the main feature of a health maintenance organisation (HMO) is that the insurance company and the health care provider vertically integrate to become different parts of the same organisation. The HMO provides health care to the insured in return for a fixed fee (insurance premium), thus combining the role of third-party payer and health care provider. Usually HMOs provide comprehensive health care but stipulate that all care is to be provided by an authorised provider integrated with the HMO in some way. HMO members are assigned a primary care physician who has a gatekeeper role and authorises any health care provided; the insured must pay an additional charge for any treatment not authorised. Box 6.7 reviews the performance of HMOs in the USA.

There are four broad types of HMO, reflecting different relationships between the third-party payer and the health care provider. In the *staff model* the HMO employs physicians directly. In the *group model* the HMO, instead of employing staff, contracts with a group practice of physicians for the provision of care. In the *network model* the HMO contracts with a network of group practices. Finally, in the case of *independent practice associations* physicians in small independent practices contract to service HMO members.

BOX 6.7 **HMO performance in the USA**

The potential advantage of HMOs over indemnity plans is that they can reduce health care costs by incentivising health care providers to charge lower prices, by encouraging patients to choose cheaper providers, and by emphasising potentially cost-saving prevention and health promotion practices. The potential disadvantages are that in seeking to reduce costs they may limit access to care and result in reduced quality.

Miller and Luft (2002) undertook a systematic review of the peer-reviewed literature from 1997 to mid-2001, to investigate various dimensions of HMO performance relative to non-HMOs in the USA. They identified 79 studies and HMO performance was judged according to whether or not the findings were favourable to HMOs relative to non-HMOs and whether or not the findings were statistically significant. The outcome measures included quality of care, access to care, patient satisfaction, prevention practices, length of hospital stay and use of expensive resources.

In general HMOs were found to be successful in reducing health care costs, evidenced by lower lengths of stay and use of expensive resources. They also tended to provide more prevention activities. In some studies HMOs resulted in lower quality and worse access, but not all, so that the overall conclusions about such effects were ambiguous. This was interpreted to mean that quality and access were not uniform and that they varied across providers, plans (HMOs and non-HMOs)+ and geographical areas. Patient satisfaction was generally lower with HMOs than with non-HMOs.

Summarising their work, Miller and Luft stated: ' . . . [I]f quality is comparable for HMO and non-HMO plans, then many HMO enrolees who have a choice among plans seem willing to accept lower satisfaction for lower out-of-pocket payments. Based on the findings from the articles reviewed here and in the past, the trade-off overall does not appear to be one of lower quality of care for lower out-of-pocket payments.'

They concluded: 'The consistently mixed quality-of-care results for HMO versus non-HMO plans over the past two decades suggests that for HMOs to meet the vision of their advocates and as a whole outperform PPO and indemnity plan quality of care, nothing less than a systematic revamping of health care information systems, incentives, and clinical processes may be required. It remains to be seen whether such a revamping will occur.'

6.5.3 Point-of-service plans

Point-of-service (POS) plans are a mixture of PPOs and HMOs. As with PPOs, in return for payment of an insurance premium patients have two options when they require treatment: use the preferred provider network with lower user charges; or use non-networked providers on less favourable terms. Unlike PPOs, however, POS plans employ primary care physician gatekeepers who authorise any health care provided by the preferred provider network. In this way, POS plans are like HMOs.

6.6 Health care financing systems

Different countries have adopted very different health care financing systems. In fact, it is arguable that the arrangements for financing of health care are more variable between different countries than the financing of any other good or service. In this section we return to the three main options for health care financing identified at the beginning of this chapter: private health insurance, social health insurance and taxation. For each system we summarise their main features and outline the mechanisms that have been developed to correct for some of the market failures. More details can be found in texts such as Mossialos *et al.* (2002).

Private health insurance has all the main features of the basic insurance model developed in the first part of this chapter. People enter into contracts with insurance providers voluntarily, and pay premiums out of their own pocket or are paid by their employers as part of their salary package or both. Private health insurance is usually supplied by profit-making companies, though it can also be offered by public bodies or by not-for-profit organisations. The size of the insurance premium is usually based on the risk status of the insured person. Patients may be required to pay user charges, in the form of co-payments or deductibles, to cover all or part of the costs of their health care. Private health insurance can be substitutive, when it provides the only form of insurance cover for someone; complementary, when it provides cover for health care that is excluded or not fully covered by the compulsory insurance system; or supplementary, when its role is to increase subscriber choice of provider and improve access. Private health insurance can be provided via indemnity plans or MCOs.

Social insurance is based on the notion of 'solidarity', whereby workers, employers and government each contribute to the financing of health care by paying into a social insurance fund. Payments by employees can be fixed, or related to the size of their income, but are not related to individual risk. The government might set the size of the contribution, or it might be set by an association of funds or by individual funds. There may be upper and lower income thresholds above and below which contributions are not levied. Many countries finance their social insurance funds by means of a hypothecated pay-roll tax, each provider paying an amount related to the number of people they employ. The funds are usually independent of direct government control. Membership may be assigned according to occupation or region of residence, or people may be free to choose a fund. Children are covered through their parents' funds, and husbands and wives who do not work are covered by their spouses' funds. Contributions can be made into social health insurance funds for retired and unemployed people either by the state, or via pension funds and unemployment funds.

Taxation-based systems usually cover the whole population. Finance for health care is mainly taken from taxes, which are collected by the government at the local, regional or national levels. They can be general (tax revenues are pooled together and allocated according to budgetary decisions made by the government) or hypothecated (earmarked specifically to pay for health care); direct (levied on people or providers) or indirect (determined by the amount of consumption); compulsory or non-compulsory; and based or not based on ability to pay. This means that a person's payments for health care are not related to their risks.

Table 6.1 summarises the key features of each system and the mechanisms available in each system for dealing with health insurance market failures. The mechanisms adopted to deal with moral hazard are similar in all systems, whilst the mechanisms adopted to deal with adverse selection and incomplete coverage are very different. Compulsory insurance is used by social insurance and taxation to combat adverse selection and incomplete coverage. Private insurance relies instead on experience rating to address adverse selection and a mix of retrospective reimbursement and selective contracting and vertical integration to deal with incomplete coverage.

TABLE 6.1 Key features of insurance-based health care financing systems

	Private health insurance	Social health insurance	Taxation
Key features	1. Insurance is voluntary 2. Premiums are paid by the insured, their employer or both 3. Premiums are based on individual risk status 4. Insurance providers may be profit maximisers or have goals other than profit maximisation 5. Insurance provision may be via indemnity plans or MCOs	1. Insurance is compulsory for all or part of the population 2. Premiums are usually paid in the form of a hypothecated payroll tax 3. Payments are related to ability to pay, usually as a proportion of income; they are not related to individual risk 4. Payments are made into a social insurance fund	1. Insurance is compulsory for the whole population. 2. Premiums are paid in the form of tax payments made to the government 3. Payments are related to ability to pay; they are not related to individual risk 4. Taxes can be: direct or indirect; general or hypothecated; set locally, regionally or nationally
Countries with predominantly this system type	USA	France, Germany, Luxembourg, the Netherlands	Denmark, Finland, Ireland, Italy, Norway, Portugal, Spain, Sweden, UK
Dealing with adverse selection	Experience rating	Compulsory insurance	Compulsory insurance
Dealing with moral hazard	1. Co-insurance 2. Deductibles 3. No-claims bonuses 4. Retrospective reimbursement 5. Selective contracting and vertical integration between third-party payers and health care providers	1. Co-insurance 2. Deductibles 3. Retrospective reimbursement 4. Selective contracting and vertical integration between third-party payers and health care providers	1. Co-insurance 2. Deductibles 3. Retrospective reimbursement 4. Selective contracting and vertical integration between third-party payers and health care providers

Dealing with non-price competition	1. Co-insurance 2. Deductibles 3. No-claims bonuses 4. Retrospective reimbursement 5. Selective contracting and vertical integration between third-party payers and health care providers	1. Co-insurance 2. Deductibles 3. Retrospective reimbursement 4. Selective contracting and vertical integration between third-party payers and health care providers	1. Co-insurance 2. Deductibles 3. Retrospective reimbursement 4. Selective contracting and vertical integration between third-party payers and health care providers
Dealing with incomplete coverage	1. Retrospective reimbursement 2. Selective contracting and vertical integration between third-party payers and health care providers	Compulsory insurance in which payments are related to ability to pay	Compulsory insurance in which payments are related to ability to pay

Most health care systems are a mix of the types discussed above, and so cross-country comparisons are unlikely to be able to isolate the success or failure of a particular system of financing. The World Health Organisation (WHO) monitors the performance of different health care systems and aims to make comparisons. Such comparisons are inhibited by comparability of data sources and objective measures of success. Box 6.8 reports on an analysis of the WHO data that compares the performance of OECD and non-OECD countries. This is essentially a technical assessment of health care systems' performance. A different approach is to ask what the public think about them. Box 6.9 discusses a survey that has been carried out using that approach. Taken at face value, the findings suggest that the type of health care financing system has little bearing on overall satisfaction, though it does influence the causes of dissatisfaction.

BOX 6.8   **The performance of health care systems: comparing OECD and non-OECD countries**

In 2000, the World Health Organisation (WHO) developed an international 'league table' of health system performance. They measured how well each country performed on improving health, variations in health amongst the population, responsiveness to patients and financing. The impact on health was measured using Disability Adjusted Life Years (DALYs), which are described in Chapter 11. A composite of DALYs and the distribution of health was created, using weights from a survey of WHO staff and people who completed a questionnaire on the WHO website. The WHO rankings have been criticised for many reasons, including their focus on current outcomes rather than improvements over time.

Hollingsworth and Wildman (2003) used the WHO data to compare the performance of the health systems of 140 countries in 1993–1997. They adopted a health production approach, as described in Chapter 2, to assess the efficiency of countries in producing Disability Adjusted Life Expectancy (DALE) over time. The underlying economic model was defined as $Yit = f(Xit, Vit)$ for country i at period t, where Yit is health measured by DALE, Xit are independent variables, included health expenditure and schooling, and Vit is the degree of inefficiency. A Farrell measure of efficiency (see Chapter 3) was used, which takes values between 0 and 1, where 1 means maximum efficiency. This was estimated using Data Envelopment Analysis and Stochastic Frontier Analysis.

The authors observed that there are systematic differences between the health systems of OECD and non-OECD countries, reflected in very different levels of efficiency. The overall average was 0.815, but for OECD countries it was 0.919 and for non-OECD countries it was 0.784, although they reported some specification problems with their analyses of OECD country data which might lead to some inaccuracy. They also found that non-OECD countries were improving their efficiency more quickly. Non-OECD countries experienced an average 4% increase in efficiency over the time period compared to an average increase of 2% in OECD countries.

BOX 6.9   **The performance of health care systems: The public's view**

Most health care systems are financed from a variety of sources, including taxation, social health insurance, private health insurance and out-of-pocket payments. The top panel in Table 6.2 shows the sources of health expenditure in five countries: Australia, Canada, New Zealand, UK and USA. Each has a mix of public and private funding sources. The first four are predominantly tax-based, with a high proportion of public expenditure and a low proportion of social security expenditure, which includes social health insurance. The USA is financed mainly from private sources, such as out-of-pocket expenditure and private health insurance plans.

Because most countries rely on a mix of revenue sources, it is difficult to evaluate a country's health care system performance based simply on the sort of health care financing system that it has. Bearing this in mind, Blendon *et al.* (2003) interviewed by telephone 750–844 'sicker adults' in each country during March–May 2002. Their views were elicited on a variety of issues relating to their satisfaction with the health system in their country and the major problems associated with it.

A large minority of respondents in every country had negative views about their health care system. The proportion saying that they were 'not very' or 'not at all' satisfied ranged from 31% in the UK to 48% in New Zealand. The proportion reporting that they were 'very satisfied' was smaller than 25% in every country.

When respondents were asked to list the two biggest problems facing their health care system there were marked differences between countries. Unsurprisingly for a predominantly private health insurance system, the high cost of health care and inadequate coverage of services were major concerns in the USA. These were far less important in the other countries. Instead, inadequate government funding was identified as a problem, which is also unsurprising in predominantly publicly funded systems. Consistent with these findings, when asked what was the single most important thing the government could do to improve care, respondents in all countries except the USA said increased public spending on health care. In the USA, the government policy endorsed most frequently was to improve coverage of services or people.

Clearly, there were differences in responses related to the way in which each health care system is financed, but the authors concluded: 'Interestingly, despite clear structural differences among the systems, findings in all five countries reveal consistent dissatisfaction among surveyed populations with general health system quality.'

| TABLE 6.2 | Health system financing and public satisfaction | | | | |

	Australia	Canada	New Zealand	UK	USA
National Health Accounts					
Total expenditure on health as % GDP	9.5	9.6	8.5	7.7	14.6
GDP per person in international dollars	28 277	30 429	21 943	27 959	36 056
Public expenditure on health as % total expenditure on health	67.9	69.9	77.9	83.4	44.9
Private expenditure on health as % total expenditure on health	32.1	30.1	22.1	16.6	55.1
Social security expenditure on health as % public expenditure on health	0	2.1	0	0	30.8
Out-of-pocket expenditure on health as% private expenditure on health	61.4	50.3	72.6	55.9	25.4
Prepaid plans as % private expenditure on health	22.7	42.1	25.9	18.6	65.7
Satisfaction with health system (%)					
Very satisfied	15	21	14	25	18
Fairly satisfied	48	41	36	41	36
Not very satisfied	21	23	32	21	25
Not at all satisfied	14	13	16	10	19

Sources: National Health Accounts: WHO (2006). Satisfaction with health system: Blendon *et al.* (2003).

Summary

1. At the individual level, ill health is usually unpredictable. This means that the demand for many types of health care is uncertain and that consumers typically operate under conditions of uncertainty. Health care expenditures may be 'catastrophic' if they require individuals to spend a significant proportion of their income on health care as a result of unforeseen or unexpected illness.
2. Problems arising from the existence of uncertainty may be addressed by health insurance which is a contract between an insurance provider and an individual who considers

themself to be at risk of ill health. When an individual buys health insurance they enter into an agreement with the insurer to pay an agreed price, called an insurance premium, in exchange for a payout to be made to the insured should they become ill.

3. Individuals choose to buy health insurance because they are risk averse. This means that they will refuse a fair gamble (a gamble which, on average, will make exactly zero profit). The amount of money an individual is prepared to pay for insurance is equal to the fair premium, which is their expected loss if uninsured, plus a risk premium which reflects their degree of risk aversion.

4. Insurance companies are able to supply health insurance because they can pool risks across a large number of insured individuals. The total premium charged by insurance providers is equal to the fair premium plus a loading factor, which covers the insurance provider's administration costs and the profit it needs to earn for each insured individual to remain in the market.

5. Adverse selection is a source of insurance market failure and arises because of the asymmetry of information between individuals who wish to buy insurance and the insurance provider. Because of this asymmetry the insurance provider may set a community rate for insurance which will be more attractive to high-risk individuals. This will mean that people with low risks will choose not to buy insurance, and premiums can spiral until the insurance market collapses. Adverse selection may be addressed by experience rating and compulsory insurance.

6. Moral hazard is a problem of excess use of health care. It arises when it is possible to alter the probability of illness or the size of the payout required by the insurance provider. Moral hazard may be reduced by co-insurance, deductibles and no-claims bonuses.

7. Non-price competition arises when health care providers compete for patients not on the basis of price but on other factors such as comfort, available facilities and the quality of food. This will cause health care costs to rise.

8. Incomplete health insurance coverage is likely to be a problem for low-income groups and for high-risk groups even if health insurance is charged at the fair premium rate.

9. The method of reimbursement relates to the way in which health care providers are paid for the services they provide. Reimbursement may be retrospective or prospective. Retrospective reimbursement gives weak incentives for cost containment. Prospective reimbursement can take two forms: global budgeting and prospectively set costs per case.

10. There are three levels of integration between third-party payers and health care providers: they can be separate entities; there can be selective contracting; or there can be vertical integration.

11. Managed care organisations have arisen predominantly in the private health insurance sector in the US health care system as a means of controlling spiralling health care costs. A key feature of managed care is the integration between the third-party payer and the health care provider. There are three broad types of managed care organisation: preferred provider organisations; health maintenance organisations; and point of service plans.

12. With private health insurance people enter into contracts with insurance providers voluntarily, and pay premiums out of their own pocket or are paid by their employers as part of their salary package or both. Private health insurance is usually supplied by

profit-making companies, though it can also be offered by public bodies or by not-for-profit organisations.

13. In the case of social insurance workers, employers and government each contribute to the financing of health care by paying into a social insurance fund. Payments by employees can be fixed, or related to the size of their income, but are not related to individual risk. The government might set the size of the contribution, or it might be set by an association of insurance funds or by individual funds.

14. Taxation-based systems usually cover the whole population. Finance for health care is mainly taken from taxes, which are collected by the government at the local, regional or national levels. They can be general (tax revenues are pooled together and allocated according to budgetary decisions made by the government) or hypothecated (earmarked specifically to pay for health care); direct (levied on people or providers) or indirect (determined by the amount of consumption); compulsory or non-compulsory; and based or not based on ability to pay.

CHAPTER 7

Equity in health care

7.1 Introduction

The way in which health care systems are organised and funded is, as we have shown in Chapters 5 and 6, important for efficiency. It also has important implications for the way that health care is distributed among people. The aim of this chapter is to consider equity – that is, fairness – in relation to the distribution of health care and the financing of health care.

Equity is an important policy objective in almost every health care system (Box 7.1 illustrates its importance to the NHS in the UK). However, what is actually meant by equity might well differ between countries. The precise meaning and importance of equity at the health system level will depend upon factors such as cultural beliefs and attitudes.

While there is no uniquely correct way of defining equity, it is informative nonetheless to consider it in a systematic way. A useful distinction, which will be made frequently throughout this chapter, is between horizontal and vertical equity. Horizontal equity refers to the equal treatment of equals, for example, the extent to which those who are equal with respect to needs for health care have equal access to health care. Vertical equity refers to the unequal treatment of unequals, for example, the extent to which those who are unequal with respect to income differ with respect to how much they have to contribute towards the costs of health care. We will also develop a taxonomy of other equity concepts, and we will describe how equity might be measured, with respect to both finance and distribution.

As noted in Chapter 1, the analysis of equity has both positive and normative aspects. Positive analysis is commonly undertaken to describe or measure the distribution of health and of health care use, and of the way in which payments for health care are shared between different people in society. We will show in this chapter how economists undertake analyses of this kind. As we shall also see, economists usually analyse equity with respect to some measure of equality, such as whether people with the same ability to pay for health care make equal payments, or whether people with equal needs for health care have equal utilisation.

BOX 7.1   The equity foundations of the UK NHS

In discussing the establishment of the NHS, Whitehead (1994) argued that its introduction in 1948 grew out of a realisation by the government that the pre-NHS system was 'inequitable, inefficient, and near to financial collapse'. In the 1930s, only 43% of the population were covered by the national insurance scheme, mainly men in manual and low-paid occupations, and covered only for GP services. Around 21 million people were not covered by any health insurance, and faced potentially catastrophic expenditure should they become ill. Additionally, there was an uneven distribution of services, with deprived areas in particular being poorly served in terms of the quantity and quality of available health services. According to Whitehead:

> Against this background a wide consensus formed in the 1940s about the need to build a more equitable service and what the principles and values of such a service should be. The concept of equity in the NHS articulated by Aneurin Bevan, the minister of health responsible for introducing the NHS, was multifaceted, incorporating the following principles:
>
> **A service for everyone:** Everyone was to be included in the scheme as of right, without having to undergo a means test or any other test of eligibility.
>
> **Sharing financial costs and free at the point of use:** In the words of Bevan: 'It has been the firm conclusion of all parties that money ought not to be permitted to stand in the way of obtaining an efficient health service.' The method of funding chosen, through general taxation, was linked to the ability to pay.
>
> **Comprehensive in range:** There was a clear commitment to extend coverage – to preventive, treatment, and rehabilitation services, covering mental as well as physical health, chronic as well as acute care.
>
> **Geographical equality:** With the intention of creating 'a national service, responsive to local needs', came a commitment to improve the geographical spread of services.
>
> **The same high standard of care for everyone:** The Royal Commission [Merrison, 1979] emphasised that this principle must be based on levelling up, not levelling down: 'The aim must be to raise standards in areas where there are deficiencies but not at the expense of places where services are already good.'
>
> **Selection on the basis of need for health care, not financial position in situations of scarcity:** People had the right to expect that no one would be able to gain access to a service ahead of others, by money or social influence.
>
> **The encouragement of a non-exploitative ethos:** To be achieved by maintaining high ethical standards and by minimising incentives for making profits from patients.
>
> (Whitehead, 1994)

Clearly, equity considerations played a key role in the establishment of the NHS and equity continues to be an important objective for the NHS today.

Normative analyses are needed to make judgements about which equalities define equity, and which inequalities define inequity. For example, are inequalities in payments for health care, or in health care use or in health, across income groups, inequitable?

We begin by looking at equity in the finance of health care; whether or not the way in which health care is paid for is fair. For example, do certain people in society, such as those who are poor, pay more for health care than they ought to? In the second part of the chapter we focus on distribution, which considers various equity principles and how they affect the distribution of health and health care. For example, do some people receive more health care than they ought to?

7.2 Equity in the finance of health care

The literature on equity in the finance of health care has focused largely on the extent to which health care is financed according to ability to pay, and in particular on whether people with different levels of income make appropriately different payments, which is a vertical equity concern. Much less attention has been paid to horizontal equity, which considers the extent to which people with the same income make the same payments.

7.2.1 Vertical equity

The extent to which payments for health care vary by income can be measured by the progressivity of the health care financing system. The principle of progressivity in this context can be seen with reference to the hypothetical example in Table 7.1. Column 1 shows income deciles in a hypothetical population. The first decile shows the income and amount spent financing health care for the poorest 10% of the population. The second income decile shows the amounts for the second poorest 10% of the population, and so on. Column 2 shows the mean annual income across everyone in each income decile. This shows that the poorest 10% of people earn a mean annual income of £2 000, while the richest 10% earn a mean annual income of £100 000. Columns 3 to 5 show three hypothetical scenarios examining the amount of money that people in each decile spend on health care, with the proportion of their income that this represents in parentheses.

In a *progressive* financing system, the proportion of income that is used to pay for health care rises as income rises. This is shown in column 3. In a *regressive* financing system (column 4), the proportion of income that is used to pay for health care falls as income rises. In a *proportional* financing system the proportion of income paid does not vary with the level of income (column 5). Note that it is the *proportion* of income that is spent on health care that is relevant for determining the progressivity of the health care financing system, not the actual amount of income that is spent. Column 4, for example, demonstrates a regressive system even though rich people spend more money on health care than poor people. Economics can

| TABLE 7.1 | Amount and proportion of income spent on health care, by income decile | | |

| Income decile | Mean annual income (£) | Annual amount spent paying for health care (%) | | |
		Progressive	Regressive	Proportional
1	2 000	160 (8)	340 (17)	240 (12)
2	5 000	450 (9)	800 (16)	600 (12)
3	9 000	900 (10)	1 350 (15)	1 080 (12)
4	14 000	1 540 (11)	1 960 (14)	1 680 (12)
5	20 000	2 400 (12)	2 600 (13)	2 400 (12)
6	27 000	3 510 (13)	3 240 (12)	3 240 (12)
7	35 000	4 900 (14)	3 850 (11)	4 200 (12)
8	45 000	6 750 (15)	4 500 (10)	5 400 (12)
9	65 000	10 400 (16)	5 850 (9)	7 800 (12)
10	100 000	17 000 (17)	8 000 (8)	12 000 (12)

describe a system in terms of vertical equity, but statements about the fairness of these types of financing system rely on value judgements about fairness.

7.2.2 Kakwani's progressivity index

One way in which the progressivity of health care financing can be measured is Kakwani's progressivity index (Kakwani, 1977). This measures the extent to which health care finance departs from proportionality. The basic ideas can be illustrated with reference to Figure 7.1, which shows concentration curves for income and for payments for health care.

The curve CC_{YY} is the prepayment income concentration curve, which is sometimes referred to as the *Lorenz curve* for income. It plots the cumulative proportion of the population, ranked according to income (Y), against the cumulative proportion of income (Y). The shape of CC_{YY} measures the degree of inequality in the distribution of income. If income were equally distributed throughout the population – if everyone earned the same income – then CC_{YY} would coincide with the 45° line, which delineates equality. By definition of the x-axis,

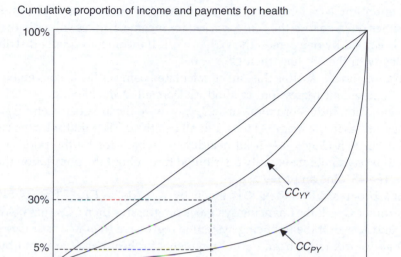

Cumulative proportion of income and payments for health

Figure 7.1 Concentration curves for income and for payments on health care

CC_{YY} must lie on or below the 45° line. The further the curve is below the line of equality the more concentrated the distribution of income is among the rich. In Figure 7.1, CC_{YY} indicates that the poorest 50% of the population earn 30% of total income.

CC_{PY} is the payment concentration curve. This plots the cumulative proportion of the population ranked according to prepayment income (Y), against the cumulative proportion of health care payments (P). The shape of CC_{PY} measures inequality in the distribution of payments for health care. If payments were equally distributed throughout the population then CC_{PY} would coincide with the 45° line. If health care payments were concentrated among the rich (poor), then CC_{PY} would lie below (above) the line of equality. The further the curve is below (above) the line of equality the more concentrated health care payments are among the rich (poor). In Figure 7.1, the CC_{PY} curve indicates that the poorest 50% of the population contribute 5% of the total payments for health care.

If payments as a proportion of income are constant across the income distribution, so that the source of health care finance is proportional, then CC_{YY} and CC_{PY} coincide. If payments as a proportion of income rise with income – that is, payments are progressive – CC_{PY} lies below CC_{YY}. If payments as a proportion of income fall with income, if they are regressive, CC_{PY} lies above CC_{YY}. As shown in Figure 7.1, CC_{PY} lies below CC_{YY}, which indicates that the financing system is progressive: the poorest 50% of the population earn 30% of income but contribute only 5% of payments for health care. Therefore, the richest 50% of the population earn 70% of total income and contribute 95% of all payments for health care. Payments for health care must therefore account for a larger proportion of income of the richest 50% of the population than they do of the poorest 50% and the health care financing system is progressive.

The concentration *index* for income, CI_{YY}, is twice the area between CC_{YY} and the 45° line. CI_{YY} is sometimes referred to as the *Gini coefficient* for income. It takes values in the range 0 to 1. If all income is earned by one person then $CI_{YY} = +1$. If income is equally distributed so that CC_{YY} coincides with the 45° line, then $CI_{YY} = 0$.

Concentration indices such as this can be calculated using either a 'convenient covariance' formula or a 'convenient regression' method (O'Donnell *et al.*, 2008).

The concentration index for payments, CI_{PY}, is twice the area between CC_{PY} and the 45° line. CI_{PY} takes values in the range -1 to $+1$. If all health care is paid for by the richest person in the population then $CI_{PY} = +1$. If all health care is paid for by the poorest person then $CI_{PY} = -1$, and if payments are equally distributed throughout the population then CC_{PY} will coincide with the 45° line and $CI_{PY} = 0$.

Kakwani's progressivity index K is given by $K = CI_{PY} - CI_{YY}$. This is twice the area between CC_{YY} and CC_{PY}. If the financing system is progressive then CC_{PY} lies below CC_{YY}, and $CI_{PY} > CI_{YY}$, and $K > 0$. If the financing system is regressive then $K < 0$. If it is proportional then $K = 0$. Values of K range from -2 (all payments for health care are paid by the poorest person, and all income is earned by a single person) to $+1$ (all payments for health care are paid by the richest person, and income is equally distributed).

The overall index for a financing system consisting of more than one source of finance is the weighted average of the indices for the individual sources, where the weights are the proportions of each source of total health expenditure. This means that the progressivity of the health care financing system depends on the proportion of total health expenditure raised from each source of finance and the progressivity of each source. Another feature of K is that it is possible for a source of finance to be progressive (or regressive) at one income level but then regressive (or progressive) at another income level. The implication is that CC_{YY} and CC_{PY} will cross. Calculating K as the difference between CI_{PY} and CI_{YY} implies that the effects at different income levels will offset one another.

Box 7.2 discusses the progressivity of health care finance measured in a number of countries and compares this to the mix of health care financing methods in those countries.

BOX 7.2   Progressivity of health care finance

Wagstaff *et al.* (1999) investigated the progressivity of health care finance in 13 countries. Data on prepayment income, direct out-of-pocket payments on health care and payments for private health insurance were collected primarily from household surveys in each country. Data on social health insurance payments and tax-based payments were either obtained from the same surveys or computed using data on the incidence of social health insurance payments and direct and indirect taxes from tax files combined with the household survey data on income.

Progressivity indices for total payments for health care in 12 of the countries, combining tax-based payments, social health insurance payments, private health insurance and direct out-of-pocket payments are shown below.

Country	K
Switzerland	−0.1402
US	−0.1303
Netherlands	−0.0703
Germany	−0.0452
Portugal	−0.0445
Sweden	−0.0158
Denmark	−0.0047
Spain	0.0004
France	0.0012
Finland	0.0181
Italy	0.0413
UK	0.0518

Source: Wagstaff *et al.* (1999).

The authors compared these results with details on the mix of health care financing methods in the 12 countries. They found that in those countries whose health care system is financed predominantly via social health insurance (France, Germany and the Netherlands) health care finance is either proportional (K is close to zero) or regressive. In countries with a predominantly tax-based system (Denmark, Finland, Spain, Sweden and the UK) the health care financing system is either proportional or progressive. The main exception is Portugal, where total payments are regressive due to a large proportion of direct out-of-pocket payments. In Switzerland and the USA, where there is a greater reliance on private health insurance, the financing system overall is highly regressive. In Italy, where the health care system is financed by an equal mix of taxation and social health insurance, total payments are progressive.

7.2.3 Horizontal equity

Horizontal equity in health care financing is defined by comparing what people could pay for health care with what they actually pay. There is horizontal inequity if people with the same ability to pay for health care, for example the same income, pay different amounts for it.

The reasons for horizontal inequity depend on the type of health care financing system. In a tax-based system horizontal inequity will arise with direct taxation if local taxes vary across regions. It arises with indirect taxation if people in the same income group consume different amounts of taxable goods. With social health insurance there is horizontal inequity if households with similar incomes are members of different social health insurance schemes with different payment schedules. This might arise because they are in different occupation groups – social health insurance schemes tend to be occupation-specific. In the case of private health insurance, because it is not compulsory, people with the same income may make unequal payments if they choose to buy different levels of insurance cover. Also, people with the same income will pay different private insurance premiums if they have different risk status. With direct out-of-pocket payments, horizontal inequity can arise because of individual variation in the incidence of ill health and preferences for use of health care services across people with the same income.

Various measures of horizontal inequity in finance have been developed. One of the more commonly used was proposed by Aronson *et al.* (1994). In their approach, horizontal inequity is measured by the variation in health care payments, or in their case taxes, among groups of people or households with the same prepayment income. If there is no variation within each group, there is horizontal equity. If there is variation, there is horizontal inequity. Typically, the variation in payments for health care is measured using the concentration index for payments CC_{PY} shown in Figure 7.1 for each prepayment income group. An overall index of horizontal inequity is constructed by taking a weighted sum of these concentration indices across all the groups.

Little empirical work has been undertaken to investigate horizontal inequity in health care finance using measures such as these. This is because they are cumbersome to compute, requiring many concentration indices for payments, one for each income group (Wagstaff and van Doorslaer, 1997). In one of the few studies to attempt an analysis of horizontal inequity in health care finance, van Doorslaer *et al.* (1999) analyse health care financing mixes in 12 OECD countries and decompose overall inequality in health care payments into a vertical inequity component, a horizontal inequity component and a re-ranking component, which accounts for the extent to which a financing system causes people to move up or down the income distribution. The findings show that vertical inequity is much more important in explaining inequality in health care payments than horizontal inequity and re-ranking, but that their relative importance varies by the type of finance. For example, tax-based payments and social health insurance payments tend to have less horizontal inequity than private health insurance payments and direct out-of-pocket payments.

7.3 Equity in distribution

In addition to equity in finance, there usually exists within most health care systems a concern that health care is distributed in an equitable way. In this section we consider this in more detail. The first question we ask is what is the 'distribuendum' – that is, the thing that we want to distribute fairly? Three plausible candidates are health care, health and utility.

7.3.1 Equity in the distribution of health care, of health or of utility?

Health economists are interested in the health care sector of the economy, for example, in the optimal way of organising health care systems and of producing specific health care goods and services. This interest in health care leads understandably to a view that it is equity in the distribution of *health care* that should be the focus of equity in distribution.

However, and in keeping with Grossman's (1972) model, health care services are demanded largely because of their effect on *health*. This explains why, for instance, health economists are interested not just in the supply of health care discussed in Chapter 4, but also in its impact on the health of patients (see Chapter 11, which looks specifically at measuring and valuing health care output). This suggests that it is health – not health care – that should be the focus of equity in distribution. Proponents of this view include Williams and Cookson (2000), who argue that equity in health is a more fundamental objective than equity in health care, and that focusing on health care ignores all other possible ways for improving health.

Pursuing the line of reasoning that health care is a means to an end and not an end in itself, it is the case that many health care services have as their output things other than improvements in health. For example, a health education programme that increases awareness of the symptoms of meningitis aims, among other things, to provide information to reassure people about their health, though it may not influence their health directly; *in vitro* fertilisation enables infertile couples to have the opportunity to experience parenthood; tattoo removal provides the opportunity to avoid social stigmatism, Viagra^{TM} provides the opportunity to enjoy increased sexual pleasure, and dental veneers provide the opportunity to improve one's appearance. In these cases, the goal is to improve utility rather than to improve health. If we take the view that the appropriate distribuendum is determined by the goal of health care, then equity in distribution might plausibly be couched in terms of utility.

Whether the focus should be on health or utility depends on whether we believe that resource allocation should depend only on the utility obtained by people – a stance known as welfarism – or whether it should also depend on factors other than utility, such as health, which is associated with extra-welfarism. In Chapter 8 we compare and contrast welfarism and extra-welfarism in more detail.

7.3.2 Some concepts of equity

Having discussed what it is that we want to distribute fairly, another relevant question is what is the appropriate concept of equity to use in order to achieve this? As we mentioned at the start of the chapter, there are many concepts of equity that could be pursued; these are limited only by our capacity to think about the different ways in which resources could be allocated. It is unsurprising therefore that so many concepts of equity are discussed in the literature. In this section we will focus on the concepts that are commonly mooted by health economists. These are utilitarianism, equal health, equal expenditure, equal access, equal use, maximin and the fair innings.

It is worth bearing in mind that some of these may constrain the distribuendum. For example, Williams and Cookson (2000), who advocate equity in the distribution of health, show that 'the principle of equal access to health care places ethical constraints on the health possibility set: it rules out all attainable health outcomes that require unequal access to health care'. An example in the case of physiotherapy services is that equity in the distribution of health might be achieved only by limiting access to those with the most severe musculoskeletal problems, which is at odds with the principle of equal access.

Utilitarianism is the view that the most desirable states of the world are those that maximise society's welfare. With strict utilitarianism, society's welfare is the equal-weighted sum of the utilities of every member of society. Weighted utilitarianism allows differential weights to be applied to the utilities of different people or groups of people. Utilitarianism has a long history in philosophy dating back to Jeremy Bentham and John Stuart Mill in the eighteenth and nineteenth centuries. The principle is consistent with our discussion of demand in Chapter 2, where we assumed, at least at the outset, that the consumers of a good are utility maximisers. Restated, a policy of strict utilitarianism would aim to distribute health care in such a manner that the greatest good was achieved for the greatest number of people. One implication is that it might increase inequality, which is at variance with many other equity concepts that aim for equality in some dimension.

For example, suppose a policy maker has the option of introducing a public health campaign that would increase physical activity levels in the general population. Research suggests that the campaign would reduce slightly the prevalence of obesity and hence provide a small positive effect on health for a large proportion of the population. To fund the programme, the policy maker would have to stop funding an expensive ultra-orphan drug that treats paroxysmal nocturnal haemoglobinuria (PNH), which is a potentially life-threatening condition that affects around one or two people per million each year. After applying a principle of strict utilitarianism, the policy maker chooses to fund the public education campaign – the sum of the small improvements in health over a large number of people is greater than the sum of the substantial loss of health experienced by the small number with PNH. While society's welfare has increased, there is an increase in inequality because the health of the majority improves at the expense of those with PNH. Thus, while strict utilitarianism treats everybody equally in terms of how they contribute to social welfare, it may exacerbate inequality in outcomes. These inequalities may be vitiated by placing more weight on certain people in society, for example those with PNH. In this case the policy maker may be less likely to choose the public health campaign and there is less inequality. A more formal description of utilitarianism, in which we construct social welfare functions (SWFs) for both strict and weighted utilitarianism, is provided in Chapter 9.

The concept of *equal health*, where health is measured for example in terms of quality-adjusted life years (see Chapters 10 and 11) or some other measure of mortality and morbidity, is closely related to the principle of *reducing inequalities* in health, and might be applied within age and sex groups. One feature of this concept is that achieving equal health may involve imposing restrictions on how people live their lives. For instance, smoking cigarettes is unlikely to be consistent with equal health. Another feature is that the influence of health care on health is limited. Other factors such as diet, lifestyle, education, economic activity and housing are equally or perhaps more important determinants of health. Hence, it becomes difficult to answer the question of how best to allocate scarce health care resources to achieve equal health, which is often the concern of health economists.

In the case of *equal expenditure* each person receives the same share of health care spending. As it stands this ignores the distribution of need across society (see Chapter 1 for a more detailed discussion of how economists define this) but it could be amended to equal expenditure for equal need. This is similar to *equal use* for equal need because it ignores preferences for health and for health care and, in the case of risky health care programmes, it ignores attitudes to risk. To illustrate, suppose two people have the same need for a crown to be fitted on one of their teeth. One person dislikes going to the dentist but the other does not. With equal use for equal need the aim would be for both of them to visit the dentist and get a crown fitted. An alternative is to focus on *equal access* for equal need, in which people with equal needs have the same *opportunity* to access health care. With this concept, people in equal need may legitimately have unequal use owing to different preferences or attitudes to risk; the person who does not like going to the dentist might legitimately not do so.

Equal access for equal need is frequently cited as an appropriate equity principle (see for example Mooney, 1983, and Mooney *et al.*, 1991), though it is difficult to formulate a usable definition of equal access. One option is that the two people needing crowns described above have equal access if the costs incurred by them in receiving treatment are valued equally – that is, if they face the same access costs. These costs include travel costs and time costs as well as monetary costs arising directly for health care. These will depend on geographical factors (travel distances, travel times, availability of transport), waiting times for treatment, and information known by patients. Equal access should also account for differences in income or some other measure of ability to pay, since this is also a determinant of access (Olson and Rodgers, 1991). Note that this means that access is both a supply-side and a demand-side phenomenon. The consequence is that while one person might legitimately visit the dentist and the other might not, with the principle of equal access it would be unacceptable if it were for reasons other than preferences or risk aversion – for example, if one person was better informed than another about dental services on offer, was more proficient at accessing dental care, or incurred lower costs. Because access is difficult to measure, most empirical studies tend to focus on equal use for equal need (see Section 7.3.3).

The concept of *maximin* was introduced in the context of game theory in Chapter 4. Simply put, the maximin principle is that when making choices, the preferred option is the one whose worst outcome is least bad. This idea was developed into a concept of equity based on distributive justice by Rawls (1971). He identified equitable behaviour as that which would be chosen by people if they were placed under a 'veil of ignorance'. Under this veil, every person is ignorant of the position they will have in society. They will not know, for instance, whether they will be rich or poor, or healthy or unhealthy. Rawls argued that, placed in this situation, people would adopt a maximin principle: a risk-minimising strategy that maximises the position of the least well off. This principle is also sometimes referred to as the *difference principle*. Applied simply to health care, it would mean that health care is distributed to maximise the health of the most ill people in society. The Rawlsian social welfare function is discussed in more detail in Chapter 9. An opposing view to that of Rawls was put forward by Nozick (1974), who argued that any distribution of goods and services such as health care is acceptable as long as it comes about in a free exchange between consenting adults and is made from a 'just' starting position. With this *libertarian* view the distribution is acceptable even if large inequalities emerge from the process. This is in direct contrast to Rawls' *egalitarian* view that inequalities in distribution must benefit the least well off.

The final concept we consider is the *fair innings* approach, introduced by Harris (1985) and advocated more recently by Williams (1997). This is based on the idea that everyone is entitled to some common quantity of lifetime health measured, for example, in terms of quality-adjusted life years. Anyone failing to achieve this has been 'cheated', while anyone getting more than this is 'living on borrowed time' (Williams, 1997). To operationalise the principle, Williams proposes that health care services for people facing less than a fair innings should be valued more highly than for people expecting a fair innings or more. He demonstrates how weights might be computed for different population groups to accomplish this. Williams shows that the fair innings principle is particularly relevant to the issue of differential treatment of the young and the old, though it also applies to other population groups, distinguished for example by socioeconomic status. He concludes: 'The analysis suggests that this notion of intergenerational equity requires greater discrimination against the elderly than would be dictated simply by efficiency objectives' (Williams, 1997).

7.3.3 Measuring equity in distribution

While there are many theoretical concepts of equity in distribution, the measurement of equity requires an empirically testable definition. To this end the literature on equity measurement focuses mainly on two concepts. The first is horizontal inequity, and in particular whether people with the same need for health care have the same use of health care services. As we shall see, far less attention has been paid to vertical equity, which in this context is usually interpreted to mean whether people with different levels of ill health have appropriately different levels of use. The second concept that is often the focus of empirical analysis is equal health, and in particular, the extent to which inequalities in health vary systematically with socioeconomic status.

In order to investigate horizontal and vertical equity in health care use, positive analysis is required to identify the factors that determine the use of health care services. Normative analysis is then required to distinguish which of these factors *ought* to affect use and which ones ought not to. Factors which ought to affect use are referred to as *need variables* and those which ought not to are *non-need variables*. Using this distinction it is possible to generate more practical definitions of horizontal and vertical inequity and relate them to inequality. There is inequality when people have different levels of health care use. There is horizontal inequity when use is affected by non-need variables. This means that people with the same need consume different amounts of care. There is vertical equity when people with different needs consume appropriately different amounts of health care.

7.3.4 Horizontal inequity

Most empirical studies of factors affecting the use of health services find that it is determined by morbidity, age, gender, income and other measures of socioeconomic status, ethnicity and supply. They typically use regression analysis to measure the impact of these factors on use, and examine the effect of each factor after controlling for the other factors. Making normative judgements about whether these factors are need or non-need variables allows us to test for, to identify, horizontal inequity. Most studies tend to classify socioeconomic status and ethnicity as non-need variables.

In the case of income, if we believe that use ought not to vary by income and it does, this indicates horizontal inequity with respect to income. If, after controlling for differences in need, income is positively correlated with use – that is, the rich have more use than the poor – there is pro-rich horizontal inequity. Conversely, if the poor have greater use there is pro-poor horizontal inequity. Analogous arguments apply for other measures of socioeconomic status, for example education, economic activity and social class.

With ethnicity, suppose we make a simple distinction between white and non-white ethnic groups. If whites have more use than non-whites after controlling for need then there is pro-white horizontal inequity. Conversely, if non-whites have more use than whites there is pro-non-white horizontal inequity. This ignores cultural differences in attitudes to use. Some evidence on this is provided in Box 7.3, which examines evidence of inequity in the use of health care by income and ethnic groups in the NHS in England.

BOX 7.3   Inequity and inequality in the use of health care in England

Morris *et al.* (2005) undertook a regression-based analysis of the determinants of health care use in England. The analysis was based on data from three years (1998–2000) of the Health Survey for England, which contained comprehensive individual level data on the determinants of four types of NHS use: GP consultations; outpatient visits; day case treatment; and inpatient stays. Factors affecting use were morbidity, age, gender, income, education, economic activity, social class, ethnicity and supply. The authors found that morbidity, measured using a number of measures including self-assessed general health, limiting long-standing illness, and types of illness, had the expected positive effects on all forms of use.

The estimated effects of income and ethnicity on selected measures of use were:

	GP visits	Outpatient visits	Inpatient stays
Income	ns	+ve	ns
Ethnic group			
Black Caribbean	ns	ns	ns
Black African	ns	ns	ns
Black Other	ns	ns	ns
Indian	+ve	ns	ns
Pakistani	ns	−ve	ns
Bangladeshi	ns	−ve	ns
Chinese	ns	−ve	−ve
Other	ns	−ve	ns

ns = not significantly different from 0.
Source: Morris *et al.* (2005).

Controlling for morbidity and the other factors, income has a positive effect on outpatient visits, that is, the rich were more likely to have an outpatient visit than the poor. But it does not have a significant effect on GP consultations or on inpatient stays. Relative to the white ethnic group, those in the Indian group are more likely to visit a GP. Those in the Pakistani, Bangladeshi, Chinese and Other groups were less likely to have an outpatient visit than whites, and those in the Chinese group were less likely to have an inpatient stay.

Overall, the analysis provides evidence of inequality in the use of health care services with respect to income and ethnicity. In particular, some non-white groups have lower than expected use of certain types of hospital services. The interpretation is complicated by potentially unobserved cultural differences, which may affect the use of health services. The authors argued that these factors might be expected to have a smaller impact on hospital services than GP visits because doctors exert more influence over hospital utilisation than over GP utilisation. If so, there is evidence of pro-white horizontal inequity in the case of hospital services.

We have focused so far on how to identify horizontal inequity. The *extent* of horizontal inequity can be quantified using concentration indices for actual and for needed health care. The basic ideas are illustrated using Figure 7.2.

The curve CC_{MY} is the health care concentration curve. This plots the cumulative proportion of the population, ranked according to income (Y), against the cumulative proportion of health or medical care (M) received. The shape of CC_{MY} measures the degree of inequality in the distribution of health care across income groups. If everyone received the same health care then CC_{MY} would coincide with the 45° line. If health care is concentrated among the rich (poor),

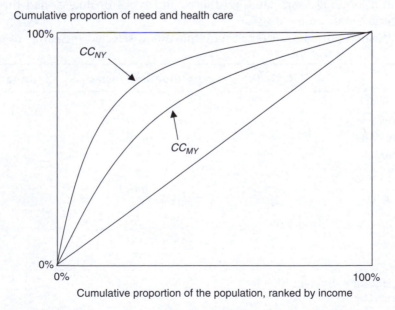

Figure 7.2 Concentration curves for need and for health care

then CC_{MY} would lie below (above) the line of equality. The further the curve is below (above) the line of equality the more concentrated health care is among the rich (poor). The concentration index for health care, CI_{MY}, is twice the size of the area between CC_{MY} and the 45° line. CI_{MY} takes values in the range -1 to $+1$. If all health care was received by the richest person in the population, then $CI_{MY} = +1$. If all health care was received by the poorest person then $CI_{MY} = -1$. If health care was equally distributed throughout the population then $CI_{MY} = 0$.

CC_{MY} and CI_{MY} provide evidence on income-related *inequality* in health care use but say very little about income-related *inequity* because they do not account for differences in needs for health care, which may vary by income. If poorer people consumed more health care this is evidence of inequality in health care use but it may not be inequitable if the poor may have greater needs.

Wagstaff and van Doorslaer (2000a) proposed measuring horizontal inequity in health care use (*HI*) as the difference between the extent of inequality in actual use (CI_{MY}) and inequality in use if everyone with the same needs was treated equally (CI_{NY}). Hence, $HI = CI_{MY} - CI_{NY}$.

CI_{NY} is based on predicted values of health care use, usually obtained using regression analysis. These values are calculated as the expected amount of health care a person would receive if they were on average treated as others with the same need characteristics. This is related to the concentration curve CC_{NY} in Figure 7.2, which plots the cumulative proportion of the population ranked according to income against the cumulative proportion of predicted health care use when everyone with the same needs receives the same treatment. It is defined analogously to the health care concentration curve, and may lie on, above or below the 45° line. CC_{NY} is sometimes referred to as the need-expected or need-predicted concentration curve and CI_{NY} the need-expected or need-predicted concentration index.

HI is twice the area between CC_{MY} and CC_{NY}. If there is pro-poor horizontal inequity then CC_{MY} lies above CC_{NY}, and $CI_{MY} < CI_{NY}$, and $HI < 0$. If there is pro-rich horizontal inequity then $CI_{MY} > CI_{NY}$ and $HI > 0$. If there is horizontal equity then $HI = 0$. Because CI_{MY} and CI_{NY} are related, values of *HI* range from -1 to $+1$. The curves in Figure 7.2 show pro-rich horizontal inequity.

HI measures horizontal inequity 'on balance' (Wagstaff and Van Doorslaer, 2000b) in the sense that if for some types of need there is pro-rich horizontal inequity but for others there is pro-poor horizontal inequity then CC_{MY} and CC_{NY} cross. The two effects will offset one another in the index.

Box 7.4 discusses the construction of *HI* indices in more detail and presents results for 12 European countries.

| BOX 7.4 | **Horizontal inequity in health care use in Europe** |

In horizontal inequity studies health care needs are often controlled for using indirect standardisation. This involves a regression model using individual level data:

$$M_i = \alpha + \sum_{j=1}^{J} \beta_j N_{ij} + \sum_{k=1}^{K} \delta_k Z_{ik} + \varepsilon_i$$

where i indexes individuals, N is a set of J needs indicators, Z is a set of K non-needs indicators, α, β, and δ are coefficients to be estimated and ε is an error term. Testing for the statistical significance of the non-need variables tests for horizontal inequity. There is horizontal inequity if $\delta \neq 0$ (see Box 7.3). Indirect standardising for health care needs gives the need-expected or need-predicted level of utilisation:

$$\hat{M}_i = \hat{\alpha} + \sum_{j=1}^{J} \hat{\beta}_j N_{ij} + \sum_{k=1}^{K} \hat{\delta}_k \overline{Z}_{ik}$$

$\hat{M}$ is the expected amount of health care a person would receive if they were treated in the same way as others with the same need characteristics, on average. The effect of the non-need variables is neutralized by setting them equal to a constant, usually the mean $\overline{Z}$. The concentration curve based on $\hat{M}$ is the need-expected or need-predicted concentration curve CC_{NY} in Figure 7.2, and the related concentration index CI_{NY} is used to calculate HI.

The regression model can also be used to decompose inequality in health care use. Wagstaff *et al.* (2003) proposed the following decomposition:

$$CI_{MY} = \sum_{j=1}^{J} \left(\frac{\hat{\beta}_j \overline{N}_j}{\overline{M}} \right) CI_{N_j Y} + \sum_{k=1}^{K} \left(\frac{\hat{\delta}_k \overline{Z}_k}{\overline{M}} \right) CI_{Z_k Y} + \frac{GC_\varepsilon}{\overline{M}}$$

where the bars represent mean values of M, N and Z, CI_{NY} and CI_{ZY} are concentration indices for N and Z, respectively, defined analogously to CI_{MY}, and $GC_\varepsilon / \overline{M}$ is the generalized concentration index for the error term. CI_{MY} can therefore be decomposed into two components, one deterministic, shown by the first two terms on the right hand side of the decomposition equation, equal to the weighted sum of income-related inequality in the need and non-need variables with the weights given by the elasticity of health care use with respect to each of these variables, and the other random. When the regression model is linear, HI can also be calculated as CI_{MY} minus the contribution of the needs variables in the decomposition equation.

More sophisticated methods have been devised to account for measures of health care use that require non-linear regression models and for different ranges of values for the health care use variable. Studies have combined data on the probability of visits and the number of visits, estimated inequity using panel data, and calculated standard errors around concentration indices and their decompositions.

Van Doorslaer *et al.* (2004) investigated horizontal inequity in GP and specialist visits in 12 European countries using individual level survey data from the *European Community Household Panel*. The results are summarized in the table, capturing both the probability of each type of visit, and the number of visits. The results are evidence of pro-*poor* horizontal inequity with respect to GP visits, but pro-*rich* horizontal inequity with respect to specialist visits.

Country	GP visits		Specialist visits	
	CI_{MY}	HI	CI_{MY}	HI
Austria	−0.0499*	0.0146	0.0345	0.0740*
Belgium	−0.1145*	−0.0508*	−0.0269	0.0255
Denmark	−0.0831*	−0.0008	0.0223	0.0844*
Germany	−0.0636*	−0.0268*	0.0158	0.0517*
Greece	−0.1258*	−0.0308*	−0.0418*	0.0492*
Ireland	−0.1323*	−0.0696*	0.0770*	0.1388*
Italy	−0.0649*	−0.0349*	0.0179	0.0537*
Luxembourg	−0.0918*	−0.0406*	−0.0704*	−0.0282
Netherlands	−0.0535*	−0.0113	−0.0178	0.0413*
Portugal	−0.0692*	0.0051	0.0971*	0.1604*
Spain	−0.0906*	−0.0492*	0.0267	0.0714*
UK	−0.1006*	−0.0240*	−0.0234	0.0524*

* P-value <0.05
Source: van Doorslaer et al. (2004)

The authors found that for GP visits the most important variables contributing to the pro-poor distribution were education, retirement and non-participation in the labour force. In the case of specialist visits income was the most important determinant.

7.3.5 Vertical equity

Vertical equity considers the extent to which people with different needs for health care have appropriately different levels of use. Testing for vertical inequity requires strong judgements about the way health care use ought to vary across people with different levels of need. This implies normative statements about the relative merits of the effect of health care on people with different levels of need, and positive statements about the effects of this. As a consequence, most empirical studies of equity in the distribution of health care have tended to focus on horizontal inequity using the methods outlined in the previous section.

As noted by Abasolo et al. (2001), a necessary but not sufficient test for vertical equity is whether higher levels of need – usually represented by more severe morbidity – are associated with higher levels of use. For this test, information on appropriate use at different morbidity levels is not required; all that is needed is that those with greater morbidity receive more health care. Further decisions about vertical inequity are not possible without information or normative judgements concerning the appropriate level of use at different levels of need.

While measuring vertical inequity in the distribution of health care is difficult for this reason, focusing solely on horizontal inequity ignores the possibility that different amounts of health care received by people with different needs is inappropriate, which is what vertical inequity considers. As van Doorslaer *et al.* (2000) put it, this assumes that 'on average the system gets it right'. This is particularly problematic when examining horizontal inequity between regions or time periods, as Sutton (2002) notes: '[i]n international comparisons the vertical equity assumption becomes "on average the system gets it right, possibly in different ways". In time series comparisons this means "on average, the system gets it right each year, possibly in different ways".'

In one of the few studies to test for and measure vertical inequity, Sutton (2002) analysed the relationship between health status and use of GP services at different levels of health status among health survey respondents in Scotland. He found a generally negative correlation: those with higher health status had lower use, but the relationship was unexpectedly positive at low levels of health status. Taking the normative view that the appropriate negative linear relationship between health status and health care use at the higher levels of health status should apply across the whole range of health status, this provided a method of testing for vertical inequity and measuring its extent. He measured socioeconomic-related vertical inequity, the results indicating pro-rich vertical inequity. More specifically, the 'divergence between the current allocation of health care and the target allocation of health care therefore falls disproportionately on the poor, although the estimate of vertical inequity is not significant' (Sutton, 2002). Sutton concludes: 'The results of this study are consistent with the widespread concern that the high primary care needs of some people are "squeezed" by the less important demands of others' (Sutton, 2002).

7.3.6 Inequalities in health

As discussed in Section 7.3.1, it has been argued that concerns about the distribution of health care arise from more deep-seated concerns about the distribution of health. Therefore, in a discussion about measuring equity in distribution it is useful to examine the measurement of equity in the distribution of health, which focuses on health inequalities.

There is a huge literature on analysing inequalities in health, much of it emanating from the public health field. This tends to focus on testing whether ill health measured in lots of different ways varies by population groups, such as by socioeconomic status and by ethnicity. We focus here on the type of analyses that tend to be undertaken by economists. Some of the work by economists measures pure inequalities in health. This looks at inequalities in health across people irrespective of their socioeconomic status or other factors.

There is also a body of work by economists that focuses on measuring the extent of socioeconomic inequalities in health by quantifying the inequality in health between the rich and the poor. This might typically be measured using the concentration curve approach described above. A common approach is to use the ill health concentration curve (see Figure 7.3).

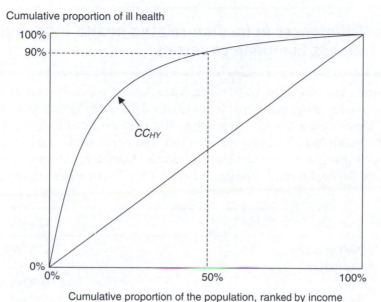

Figure 7.3 Ill health concentration curve

The *ill health* concentration curve CC_{HY} plots the cumulative proportion of the population, ranked according to income (Y), against the cumulative proportion of ill health in the population (H), measured in some way such as by the presence of disease or life expectancy. The concentration index for ill health, CI_{HY}, is twice the size of the area between CC_{HY} and the 45° line. CI_{HY} takes values in the range -1 to $+1$, depending on whether ill health is concentrated among the rich ($CI_{HY} > 0$) or among the poor ($CI_{HY} < 0$), and the degree of concentration. If everyone has the same health then CC_{HY} would coincide with the 45° line and $CI_{HY} = 0$. In Figure 7.3 the poorest 50% of the population incur 90% of ill health – there is a pro-poor distribution of ill health.

A closely related concept is the *health* concentration curve, measured analogously except that the y-axis is increasing in good health. Box 7.5 is an example of this, an analysis of income-related health inequalities across a number of European countries.

An extension to the concentration index is the *health achievement index* (Wagstaff, 2002), which is a combined measure of both the average level of health in a population as well as the extent of income-related inequality in health.

Once inequity in health care has been identified, policy makers may choose to intervene to bring about a more equitable allocation of health care services. Given the likelihood of market and government failures in health care, as discussed in Chapter 5, a more explicit method for determining what health care services should be provided may be required. In light of the discussion in this chapter, such a method would ideally allow different members of society to be weighted differently from one another in order to ensure equitable distribution (see Tsuchiya and Williams, 2001). These weights could, for example, be used in economic evaluation, as an explicit way of addressing distributional issues.

Differences in income-related health inequalities across European countries

Van Doorslaer and Koolman (2004) computed health concentration indices for 13 European countries using individual level survey data from the European Community Household Panel. A self-assessed general health question rated in five categories was converted to health 'utility' scores between zero and one, based on the Health Utilities Index Mark III using a method developed by van Doorslaer and Jones (2003).

Values of the health concentration indices for the 13 countries are reported below.

Country	CI_{HY}
Netherlands	0.0034
Germany	0.0043
Italy	0.0063
Spain	0.0066
Belgium	0.0071
Austria	0.0073
France	0.0075
Ireland	0.0077
Denmark	0.0094
Luxembourg	0.0104
Greece	0.0119
UK	0.0129
Portugal	0.0218

Source: Van Doorslaer and Koolman (2004).

In all countries CI_{HY} is positive, indicating pro-rich health inequality. Relatively high health inequality is observed in Portugal and the UK; relatively low values are observed in the Netherlands and Germany.

The authors undertook a decomposition analysis of CI_{HY} and found that income was the most important but not the only factor driving the observed health inequalities. They also found that the elasticities of the variables included in the decomposition analysis were generally more important than their unequal distribution by income in explaining differences between countries in income-related health inequality.

Summary

1. Equity is an important policy objective in almost every health care system. However, what is actually meant by equity might well differ across countries. The precise meaning and importance of it will depend on factors such as cultural beliefs and attitudes.

2. There are two main areas of health care in which issues of equity (or fairness) are likely to arise: finance and distribution.

3. A useful distinction can be made between horizontal and vertical equity. Horizontal equity refers to the equal treatment of equals. Vertical equity refers to the unequal treatment of unequals.

4. Equity in the finance of health care has focused on whether there is vertical equity in the finance of health care. This considers the extent to which people with unequal ability to pay for health care make appropriately unequal payments. This is usually measured by the extent to which the health care financing system is progressive, regressive or proportional, which refers to whether payments for health care rise or fall as a proportion of income as income rises. The progressivity of health care financing systems is usually measured using progressivity indices.

5. There usually exists within most health care systems a concern that health care is distributed in an equitable way. An important question is what is the distribuendum? That is, what is it that we want to distribute fairly? Three plausible candidates are health care, health and utility.

6. Some aims that are commonly mooted by economists to achieve equity are utilitarianism, equal health, equal expenditure, equal use, equal access, maximin and the fair innings.

7. The measurement of equity in distribution tends to focus on horizontal inequity in use, which considers the extent to which people with the same need for health care have the same use of health care services, and in measuring health inequalities.

CHAPTER 8

Health care labour markets

8.1 Labour as a factor of health care production

In Chapter 3 we examined the theory of production and noted that inputs into the production of goods and services are referred to as factors of production. These are commonly categorised into three types, labour, land or raw materials, and capital. In this chapter we look more closely at the role of labour in the production of health care.

There are many different types of health care workers. These include doctors, dentists, nurses and midwives, as well as a host of allied health professionals involved in the health care that patients receive, including pharmacists, chiropodists, radiographers, dieticians, occupational therapists, physiotherapists, paramedics, and speech, language, drama and music therapists. These workers may specialise in different therapeutic areas. For example, doctors work in such diverse specialties as anaesthesia, intensive care medicine, emergency medicine, general practice, medicine, obstetrics and gynaecology, occupational medicine, ophthalmology, paediatrics, pathology, psychiatry, public health, radiology and imaging and surgery. Health care providers also employ laboratory staff who deliver health care but who do not normally have direct contact with patients, and non-clinical staff who do not provide care but may have contact with patients although not in a clinical capacity, for example receptionists, maintenance staff, administrators, accountants, IT specialists and managers. Also, there are many workers not employed by health care providers, but who do contribute to the production of health care, including workers in the pharmaceutical and medical devices industries, as well as those providing medical supplies and capital goods.

We devote a whole chapter to this topic first because labour is very important to the health care sector. For example, salaries and wages paid to health care workers account for a substantial component of total health expenditure: the average country devotes over 40% of its government-funded health expenditure to paying its health workforce (Table 8.1), though there are regional variations. As well as being important to the health care sector, health care

TABLE 8.1	Numbers of and spending on health workers

WHO Region	Total health workforce, number, 000s	Density per 1000 population	Health service providers, number, 000s (% total)[1]	Management and support workers, 000s (% total)[2]	Percentage of government health expenditure paid to health workers[3]
Africa	1 640	2.3	1 360 (83)	280 (17)	29.5
Eastern Mediterranean	2 100	4.0	1 580 (75)	520 (25)	50.8
South East Asia	7 040	4.3	4 730 (67)	2 300 (33)	35.5
Western Pacific	10 070	5.8	7 810 (78)	2 260 (22)	45.0
Europe	16 630	18.9	11 540 (69)	5 090 (31)	42.3
Americas	21 740	24.8	12 460 (57)	9 280 (43)	49.8
World	59 220	9.3	39 470 (67)	19 750 (33)	42.2

Source: WHO (2006)

[1] Those who deliver health care, including those who do not normally have direct contact with patients (e.g., laboratory staff).
[2] Non-clinical staff who may have some contact with patients but not usually in a clinical capacity.
[3] Wages, salaries and allowances of employees as a percentage of general government health expenditure.

labour markets are also important to the economy as a whole, evidenced by their size. The WHO estimates there are around 59 million paid health workers worldwide (Table 8.1), around nine workers for every 1 000 population, with around two-thirds of the total providing health care and one third working in a non-clinical capacity.

We said previously that a market is a place where those who wish to supply goods and those who demand them are brought together in order to effect an exchange. Much of the discussion so far in the book has concerned the market for health care, which is an example of a goods market. Factor markets are those in which the factors of production are exchanged. Health care labour markets can be described and explained using similar concepts to those used to describe the market for health care. One notable difference between the two markets is that the roles of the supplier and demander are reversed. In the health care market households buy health care services either directly out of their own pocket or indirectly via a third-party payer and suppliers such as hospitals provide health care and are reimbursed for it. In health care labour markets hospitals demand labour and households supply it in return for payment in the form of salaries and wages. Generally we expect that the supply and demand curves for labour will slope the same way as for goods and services. When drawing these curves for labour, the y-axis shows the price of labour and the x-axis shows the quantity of labour. The price of labour is also referred to as the wage w and is usually measured as the annual income divided by annual hours. The quantity of labour, Q, is measured as the number of labour hours worked or the number of workers employed.

When bringing together the two sides of the health care labour market it is useful to make a similar distinction to one made in goods markets between perfect and imperfect factor markets. This provides a yardstick against which to judge the impact of imperfections in health care labour markets. These imperfections include health care workers and employers with market power, slow response of health care labour to changes in demand and supply conditions, non-maximising behaviour by health care providers and workers, and wage discrimination. We examine all of these issues in this chapter. We begin by examining the supply of and demand for health care labour.

8.2 Supply of health care labour

Supply of labour can be considered at three levels: the supply of work hours by an individual worker; the supply of workers to an individual employer; and, the total market supply of workers.

The supply curve for an individual worker depends on the relative magnitude of two effects. The substitution effect of an increase in wages is that as wages increase people tend to work more hours because time spent not working (in leisure) involves a greater sacrifice of income and consumption; hence people substitute work for leisure. The income effect is that as wages increase people feel they can afford to work less and have more leisure. It is normally assumed that the substitution effect outweighs the income effect, producing an upward sloping supply curve as shown by the curve $S_{Individual}$ in Figure 8.1(a). However the income effect might outweigh the substitution effect, especially at high wage levels. In this case the supply curve will begin to slope backwards. In Figure 8.1(a) this is shown by the backward bending supply curve S_{BB}, in which the income effect outweighs the substitution effect at wages higher than w^*.

In a perfectly competitive labour market the supply of labour to an individual employer is perfectly elastic, as shown by $S_{Employer}$ in Figure 8.1(b). The equilibrium wage w^* is determined by the intersection of the demand and supply curves across all workers and all employers in the labour market, shown in Figure 8.1(c). The employer (like each individual worker) is a wage taker (analogous to a price taker in a perfectly competitive goods market) and has no power to influence wages. Suppose a hospital wants to employ a number of temporary agency nurses and to do so goes to a nursing agency. The hospital is required to pay the hourly wage w^*; it can employ as many agency nurses as it likes at this wage, but no agency nurses will be available at a wage rate below w^* – they will all be employed elsewhere instead – and there is no incentive for the hospital to pay higher wages than w^*.

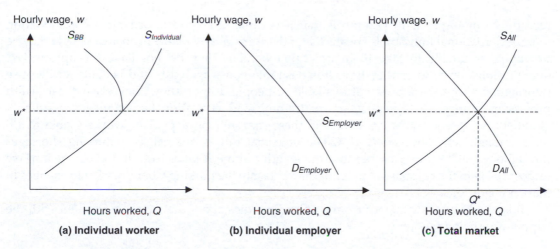

Figure 8.1 A health care labour market

Typically the total market supply curve will be upward sloping, as shown by S_{All} in Figure 8.1(c); the higher the hourly wage in a particular job the more people will want to do that job and (assuming the substitution effect is larger than the income effect) the greater the number of hours workers currently employed will work.

Total market supply depends on the hourly wage, but also on the number of people willing and able to take the job at a given wage. This will depend on the number of suitably qualified people, the non-wage costs and benefits of the job, and the wages and the non-wage costs and benefits in alternative jobs. A change in the wage rate will produce a movement along the supply curve, changes in the other aspects will shift the supply curve. As we shall see, the duration of training required to become a health professional affects the number of suitably qualified people able to enter the labour market, which can cause slow responses to changes in demand and supply conditions. Non-wage costs and benefits are important in health care because workers may choose not to leave relatively low paid jobs due to non-wage factors that affect job satisfaction.

Of particular interest to employers and wage-setting organisations is the wage elasticity of supply, defined analogously to the price elasticity of demand introduced in Chapter 2. The wage elasticity of supply measures the responsiveness of changes in supply to changes in wages. In the face of financial constraints in the health sector, if doctors' wages fall in real terms will there be a big reduction in the supply of doctors or only a small one? If nurses' wages rise in response to nursing shortages, will a lot more nursing labour become available or only a little? The degree of responsiveness depends on the mobility of health care labour – the ability and willingness of workers to move jobs. The greater the difficulties and costs of moving jobs the more immobile the labour force and the less wage elastic the labour supply.

Immobility is of two types – geographical and occupational. Workers are geographically immobile if they are unable or unwilling to move to different geographical areas to take up new jobs, maybe because of the financial costs involved or social and family ties. An example of the effect of geographical immobility is a shortage of health care workers in areas with high living costs. Finalyson *et al.* (2002) report that one reason for the difficulties in recruiting nursing staff in London is that it is difficult to find affordable accommodation there. Occupational immobility means that if there are jobs available in an area people may be unwilling or unable to take them up, either because they do not have the appropriate qualifications, or because they have less desirable non-wage costs and benefits, or because information about the jobs is not available so people do not know they exist. Most health professionals undergo several years of training and education before they are suitably qualified. So, even if jobs are available there may not be a pool of workers able to fill them immediately. Simoens *et al.* (2005) note that this is one cause of nursing shortages throughout OECD countries, because the length of time it takes to train to become a nurse imposes a lag in the response of potential entrants into the nursing labour market to changes in market conditions.

Box 8.1 discusses evidence from empirical studies about the factors associated with the supply of nursing labour.

BOX 8.1   Empirical studies of nursing labour supply

Antonazzo *et al.* (2003) reviewed 16 North American and British econometric analyses of nursing labour supply. The underlying economic model is given by $Q = f(w, V, Z, S)$, where Q is labour supply, w is wages, V is non-labour income, Z is non-wage job characteristics and S is individual worker characteristics. It is estimated empirically using regression analysis in which the dependent variable is nursing labour supply, measured in terms either of participation in the nursing labour market – a yes/no variable – or the number of hours worked or both. Models are typically run for women only and the independent variables usually include some or all of the following: own wage, husband's wage, non-labour income, age, total number of children, number of children in different age ranges, number of adults living in the household in different age groups, family attitude towards the wife working, education and area of residence. The coefficient on the own wage variable can be used to calculate the wage elasticity of supply.

Selection bias was identified as an important methodological issue. Some studies are based on working nurses. This can create selection bias, because it excludes nurses who have refused the wage offered to them and dropped out of the market. The hours of nursing work or wages for these people are not observed, but if we could they might be different to working nurses due to unobserved characteristics such as tastes for nursing work and motivation. The sample is therefore not representative of all nurses and the coefficients from a simple econometric model of hours worked may be biased and may mislead. Selection bias can be addressed using econometric techniques, probably the most widely used of which is a two-step method (Heckman, 1979). First, a regression model for the probability of working in the labour market is estimated from a sample of workers and non-workers. Non-workers might be identified as those with nursing qualifications not employed as nurses. This produces a variable measuring the propensity to work, called the inverse Mills ratio (IMR). The hours of work equation is then estimated for the sample of working nurses, incorporating the IMR.

The review's findings about the impact of wages are ambiguous. A large, positive and statistically significant association between wages and hours worked was found in five studies, a non-significant or weak association was found in four, and a significant and negative association was found in three. The more recent studies, accounting for selection bias, tended to show a non-significant relationship. Five studies analysed the correlation between wages and participation in the nursing labour market, and generally found the relationship to be non-significant.

For the other covariates, most studies found that spouse wage, household non-labour income and the presence of young children were negatively associated with nursing labour force participation and hours worked. Age and the education of the participant were generally not found to be significantly related to nursing labour supply.

8.3 Demand for health care labour

Firms employ factors of production to produce goods and services. The demand for factors of production is therefore a derived demand, for example the demand for nurses in a hospital is derived from the demand for operations at the hospital.

The demand curve for labour is typically downward sloping because the higher the wages that profit-maximising employers have to pay the lower the quantity of labour they will want to employ. This can be explained using marginal products and the law of diminishing returns, introduced in Chapter 3. The marginal product of labour MP_L is the change in output resulting from a change in the quantity of labour used, other things held constant. The marginal product of nursing labour could be measured as the increase in the number of operations a hospital can perform if the number of nurses employed were increased, holding the amount of all other inputs (for example number of doctors and health care assistants employed, number of hospital beds) constant. The law of diminishing marginal returns is that if increasing quantities of a variable factor (nurses) are applied to a given quantity of fixed factors (for example doctors, health care assistants, beds), the marginal product of the variable factor will eventually decrease. Using our example, successive increases in nursing inputs, holding other factors constant, will eventually result in smaller and smaller increases in the number of operations. Box 8.2 provides an overview of studies examining the MP_L for physicians in the USA.

Using these concepts we can derive the demand curve for health care labour. An employer will maximise its profits when the marginal cost of employing an additional unit of labour equals the marginal revenue that the worker's output earns for the firm. This is analogous to the profit maximisation level of output given by $MC = MR$ in the goods

BOX 8.2   Measuring physician productivity

Measurement of doctor productivity is useful for workforce planning, designing remuneration systems, and for workload management. Reinhardt (1972) analysed the productivity of physicians and auxiliary workers in private medical practice in the USA. The underlying economic model is $Q = f(H, X_1, X_2, \ldots, X_n)$ where Q is physician output, H is the physician labour input, and $X_1, X_2, \ldots, X_n$ are other inputs, capital inputs and other types of labour, used in the physicians' practice. This was specified so that positive rates of Q are permitted when the inputs are zero. Both increasing and decreasing marginal products (MP) over the range of inputs observed are possible. The model was estimated using regression analysis applied to cross-section data for 1965 and 1967 for self-employed physicians. Outputs were total patient visits and office visits per week and annual patient billings. Inputs were physician labour, measured as total practice hours per week, numbers of registered nurses, technicians and office aides employed in the practice, and capital equipment. Other variables likely to affect outputs were included.

There were diminishing marginal returns to factor inputs. For total patient visits, the MP of physician hours increased up to 25 hours worked per week, and declined thereafter, decreasing to zero at 110 hours per week. For patient billings these were 24 hours and 120 hours, respectively. At the sample mean of 60 hours worked per week the physician-hours elasticity of output was 0.77 for total patient visits per week, 0.67 for office visits per week and 0.52 for annual patient billings. Output increased by 5–8% for each 10% increase in physician hours, other things constant. The MP of auxiliary workers (registered nurses, technicians and office aides combined) increased up to one aide per physician then declined and fell to zero at around five. At the sample mean of two aides per physician the number-of-auxiliary-workers elasticity of output was 0.31 for total patient visits per week, 0.36 for office visits per week and 0.34 for annual patient billings.

Brown (1988) retested these results using a larger sample of USA office-based physicians from 1976, measuring output as total patient visits per week. At sample mean values of the inputs, the MP of physician hours was 2.967. The MP of hours worked by auxiliary workers ranged from 0.192 (secretarial, administrative and clerical workers) to 0.585 (registered nurses). If physicians utilise auxiliary workers efficiently, the MP per dollar spent on each input should be equal (see Chapter 3). The ratio was 0.114 for physician hours per week, and for all auxiliary workers combined it was 0.063. Only for one group of auxiliary workers – "practical nurses" – was the ratio higher (0.129). The conclusion was that practical nurses were underutilised, but that relative to physician time, all other auxiliary workers were overutilised.

Thurston and Libby (2002) estimated a more general production function, based on similar data for 1965, 1967, 1985 and 1988. They found that the MP of an additional hour of physician labour at sample mean values was 1.34 total visits per week and 0.55 office visits per week. For totals visit the MP of employing an additional auxiliary worker ranged from 6.17 (technicians/aides) to 10.75 (nurses); comparable figures for office visits were 5.95 to 7.62. In terms of capital inputs, the results suggested that it would take about $5 000 in extra spending on capital to generate one additional visit.

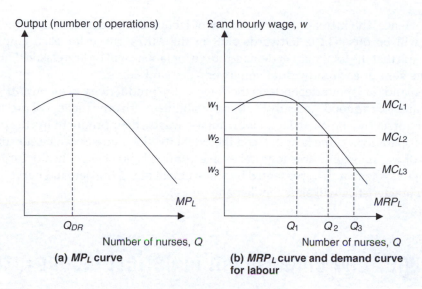

Figure 8.2 Deriving the demand curve for nursing labour

market. The marginal cost of labour MC_L is the extra cost to the employer of employing one more worker. As noted, under perfect competition the employer faces a horizontal supply curve and the additional cost of employing one more worker is the wage rate, $MC_L = w$.

The marginal revenue from employing an additional unit of labour is the marginal revenue product of labour MRP_L, which is the marginal product of labour multiplied by the marginal revenue from selling one more unit of output, $MRP_L = MP_L * MR$. If employing an extra nurse means that the hospital can provide 10 more operations per week and the hospital earns £2 000 for each operation then the extra nurse adds £20 000 to the hospital's revenue each week, which is the nurse's MRP.

An MP_L curve is shown in Figure 8.2(a). The law of diminishing marginal returns means that as more nurses are employed there will come a point when diminishing returns set in. On the figure this occurs at Q_{DR} and the MP_L curve slopes downwards beyond this point. The MRP_L curve in Figure 8.2(b) has a similar shape to the MP_L curve since it is the MP_L curve multiplied by a constant amount. Combining the marginal costs and marginal revenue of labour, the employer maximises profits when employing the number of nurses where $MC_L = w = MRP_L$.

This can be used to derive the demand curve for labour because whatever the wage the quantity of labour demanded is given by the intersection of w and MRP_L. In Figure 8.2(b) Q_1 labour is demanded at hourly wage w_1, Q_2 is demanded at w_2 and Q_3 is demanded at w_3. The MRP_L curve shows the quantity of labour employed at each wage; it is therefore the employer's demand curve for labour.

Note that the total demand curve for labour is not the sum of the demand curves for each employer. We know from Figure 8.2(b) that when wages fall an employer will employ more labour. But so will other employers in the market, and when they do this increases total output which decreases the MR from selling one more unit of output, which reduces the MRP_L for all employers. Hence, the increase in the quantity of labour demanded from a reduction in the wage rate will be offset by a leftwards shift in the MRP_L curve for each employer. The consequence is that the total market demand curve for labour will be less elastic than the curve given by the sum of each individual employer's demand curve.

The demand for labour depends on the wage w, the productivity of labour MP_L, the price of and demand for the good, and substitution possibilities with other factors of production. So, demand for nurses by a hospital depends on nurses' wages, their productivity, the price of and demand for operations at the hospital, and the extent to which nurses can be substituted with other types of worker such as less comprehensively trained and cheaper health care assistants. A change in the wage rate is represented by a movement along the demand curve, changes in the other characteristics will shift the demand curve.

8.4 Wages and employment in perfect labour markets

The assumptions of perfect labour markets are similar to those for perfect goods markets, as described in Chapter 4:

- There are many employers and workers in the labour market.
- There is freedom of entry and exit into the labour market. There are no restrictions on the occupational and geographical movement of labour – workers are free to move to other geographical areas or to other jobs with, for example, better wages or working conditions. There are no barriers to entry, for example formal registration requirements by medical and nursing professional bodies.
- Labour is homogenous – all labour of a particular type is identical, for example all doctors are equally skilled and motivated.
- There is perfect knowledge, so workers are fully aware of jobs that are available, and details of their wages and employment conditions. Similarly, employers are aware of the workforce that is available and its productivity.

The impact of the first three of these conditions is that all employers and workers are wage takers (analogous to price takers in the goods market) – neither employers nor workers can influence and so have to accept the market wage.

The resulting labour market is illustrated in Figure 8.1. Equilibrium hourly wages w^* are determined by the intersection of the total market demand and supply curves (Figure 8.1(c)). Individual employers and workers, as wage takers, have to accept these wages (Figures 8.1(a) and (b)) and demand workers who supply their time based on the market wage. If the market wage exceeds the equilibrium wage there is a surplus of workers, more people would be looking for employment than employers were willing to employ. The wage rate would fall as employers find it easy to employ workers at a lower wage. If the market wage is lower than the equilibrium wage then there would be a shortage of workers and employers would not be able to fill the vacancies they had available. The market wage would rise as employers found it necessary to increase wages to attract workers. Only at the equilibrium wage w^* are there no market forces operating to change the market wage.

8.5 Economic rent and transfer earnings

Labour earnings can be split into two elements. Transfer earnings are what workers must earn to prevent them from leaving the labour market and moving to an alternative job for example it is the minimum amount a nurse must earn to stop them from leaving the profession. Economic rent is anything earned over and above transfer earnings. For example, suppose a nurse earns £20 000 a year, could earn £18 000 if she worked in a bank, and would move into banking if her nursing salary was below £18 000. The nurse's transfer earnings are £18 000 and her economic rent is £2 000. For the nursing labour market as a whole, as shown in Figure 8.3(a), starting at point a and moving to point b, more nurses are attracted into the labour market as the hourly wage rises. As wages progressively increase new nurses enter the labour market because the wages are sufficient to persuade them to do so – these wages are entirely transfer earnings. For nurses already in the profession, with lower transfer earnings, part of the higher wages are economic rent because they are now being paid more than the minimum required to keep them in the labour market. Economic rent is the difference between the market wage and the point on the supply curve at which the worker entered the labour market. At the market wage w^* in Figure 8.3(a) the total economic rent of all nurses employed is the light shaded area above the supply curve and the dark shaded area is the sum of the transfer earnings.

The relative size of economic rent and transfer earnings depends on the wage elasticity of supply – the less elastic the supply curve the higher the ratio of economic rent to transfer

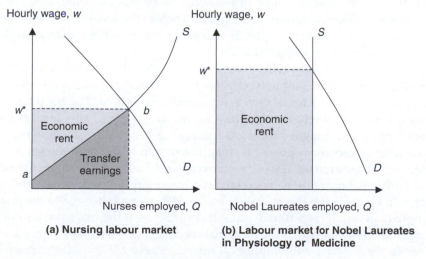

(a) Nursing labour market

(b) Labour market for Nobel Laureates in Physiology or Medicine

Figure 8.3 Economic rent and transfer earnings

earnings. In an extreme case with a totally inelastic supply curve labour supply is fixed, wages are determined entirely by demand, and all earnings are economic rent. An example is in Figure 8.3(b), which shows the labour market for Nobel Prize Winners in Physiology or Medicine of which there have been fewer than 200 since 1901.

8.6 Wage determination and employment in imperfect labour markets

In the real world the assumptions of perfect health care labour markets are unlikely to be met. Health care workers and/or employers may have market power and be able to influence wages. Training and education requirements mean that health care labour may be slow to respond to changes in demand and supply conditions causing persistent disequilibria. Employers and workers may practise non-maximising behaviour. There may be wage discrimination.

8.6.1 Employers and workers with market power

When a firm is the only employer of a certain type of labour it is a monopsony, for example in a rural area the local hospital may be the only employer of nursing labour. This position may give the hospital market power in setting wages. An oligopsony is when there are a few employers with some market power. Health care professionals may also have market power as members of trade unions or professional bodies, e.g., the British Medical Association is the professional medical association and trade union for doctors and medical students in Great Britain. When a single trade union or professional body acts on behalf of a certain type of labour it acts as a monopolist. Strong trade unions such as the BMA may also have the power to influence wages. A bilateral monopoly is said to exist when a monopsony employer faces a monopoly trade union or professional body.

First, consider a monopsony. It is a wage maker rather than a wage taker, for example a rural hospital may have sufficient market power to keep nurses' wages low because alternative employment possibilities for nurses in rural areas are limited. The hospital being a wage maker faces the market supply curve, which is upward sloping. This means that to attract more nurses it must pay a higher wage. Assuming the hospital is not able to practise wage discrimination, to attract more nurses it must not only pay the new nurses it employs the higher wage, but also the nurses already employed at the hospital. Therefore the marginal cost of hiring an additional nurse to the hospital, called the marginal factor cost MFC, exceeds the market wage. In Figure 8.4(a) this is shown by the MFC curve lying above the market supply curve. As noted, an employer will maximise its profits when the marginal cost of employing an additional unit of labour equals the marginal revenue that the worker's output earns for the firm. Therefore the hospital will employ Q_1 nurses, where $MFC = MRP_L$. From the supply curve, the wage required to employ this many nurses is w_1. If the labour market had been

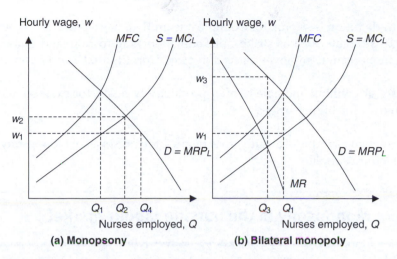

Figure 8.4 Monopsony and bilateral monopoly

perfectly competitive, the market wage and the number of nurses employed would have been set by the intersection of the demand and supply curves at w_2Q_2. The monopsony hospital has forced the wage rate to below the perfectly competitive level by restricting the number of nurses employed.

What happens when the monopsony hospital faces nurses grouped in a trade union monopoly? This is illustrated in Figure 8.4(b). The monopsony equilibrium is w_1Q_1 as before. The marginal revenue MR earned by the trade union monopolist labour supplier is derived from the MRP_L curve, which corresponds to the market demand curve under perfect competition. The profit maximising trade union will equate its marginal revenue and the marginal cost of labour supply, which is now given by the MC_L curve rather than the MFC curve. It will therefore wish Q_3 nurses to be employed, where $MR = MC_L$. The corresponding point on the demand curve gives the trade union's desired wage w_3, which is above the wage preferred by the monopsony hospital. The preferred outcomes of the monopsony hospital (w_1Q_1) and the monopoly trade union (w_3Q_3) are not mutually consistent. Therefore, there is not an equilibrium wage and level of employment in a bilateral monopoly.

Ultimately the wage rate and level of employment in a bilateral monopoly will depend on the relative bargaining power of the workers and the employers in wage negotiations. The bargaining strength of the nurses' trade union is likely to be higher in the following circumstances:

- When there is little scope for substituting other factors of production for nursing labour (e.g., health care assistants).
- When the provision of health care is unaffected by the wages paid to nurses. This might be the case if nursing labour costs are a small proportion of the total costs of providing health care so that higher wages will have little impact on the total costs of production. If nursing labour costs are a high proportion of the total costs, for example due to the size of the nursing workforce, then modest increases in wages may not be affordable.

- When the trade union is strong, for example it is unified, has significant resources, and can make effective threats such as strikes, picketing, working to rule, and non-co-operation.
- When the monopsony employer earns substantial profits that can be devoted to higher wages.
- When nurses are willing and able to offer productivity deals, for example working longer hours, in return for higher wages.

Box 8.3 gives an example of a study investigating the presence of monopsony power in the US nursing labour market.

BOX 8.3   **Monopsony in the nursing labour market**

Hirsch and Schumacher (2005) investigated monopsony in the USA nursing labour market using two approaches. The first examined the relationship between nurses' wages and employer (hospital) concentration. If markets are monopsonistic then wages are expected to decline in areas with higher hospital concentration where there are fewer employers. The second approach is based on the proportion of new nursing employees recruited from employment and from out of employment. If the proportion of new recruits from employment (from other nursing jobs) is high this suggests that nurses are mobile and monopsonistic power will be weak. If new recruits come mainly from outside employment (they were previously unemployed or from out of the labour force) this suggests there is little mobility among those in employment and employers exert monopsony power. The intuition behind this approach is that it is the ability and willingness of employees to move between employers and not market structure that affects monopsony power, and if markets are monopsonistic then wages will decline in areas where the proportion of new recruits coming from outside employment is higher.

Hirsch and Schumacher analysed data for 240 metropolitan and non-metropolitan areas in the USA from 1998–2002. They measured hospital concentration using the Herfindahl-Hirschmann Index described in Chapter 4. The second measure of monopsony, the proportion of new recruits from outside employment M, was calculated as $(u + n)/R = 1 - (e/R)$, where R is the number of newly hired nurses in each area, each of whom arrives from one of three positions, from being unemployed u, from being out of the labour force n, and from being employed as a nurse e. Relative wages were calculated for all hospital registered nurses versus the control group comprising women with an associate or baccalaureate degree employed in non-health related occupations within specified occupational groups.

They found that nurses' relative wages were not significantly related to hospital concentration, but based on longitudinal analysis they found evidence that hospital concentration reduces nurses' relative wages in the short run. They found no evidence of a significant relationship between nurses' wages and M. They concluded that in the USA there is no compelling evidence of monopsony power in nursing labour markets.

8.6.2 Labour markets slow to respond to changes in demand and supply

Market power by employers and workers is not the only cause of imperfect labour markets. Another is that health care labour may be slow to respond to changes in demand and supply conditions causing persistent disequilibria. One reason for this is that when wages are set via a process of collective bargaining, as is the case in bilateral monopoly, the wage agreement will usually last for a specific period of time, such as one year. During this period the demand and supply curves for labour may change, producing a disequilibrium that cannot be corrected until the next round of bargaining.

The length of training period to become a health professional may also make the labour market slow to respond to changes in demand and supply conditions. While health care labour markets will in principle adjust towards the market equilibrium in the long run, responses to changing market conditions are unlikely to be immediate because the training period imposes lags in the response of potential labour market entrants to changes in wages. As noted, the lags can cause cycles of shortages and surpluses of workers, and have been used to explain nursing shortages in OECD countries (Simoens *et al.* 2005).

This phenomenon has been referred to as the cobweb model because of how it appears in demand and supply diagrams – see Figure 8.5 for an example. Suppose the labour market for nurses is initially in equilibrium, shown by the intersection of the demand and supply curves D_0 and S_0 and equilibrium wage and employment $w_0 Q_0$. Demand for nursing labour increases from D_0 to D_1 because the demand for health care increases. The new market equilibrium is $w^* Q^*$. New entrants are attracted by the increase in wages following the increase in demand, but are unable to enter immediately due to the length of time it takes to train to become a nurse

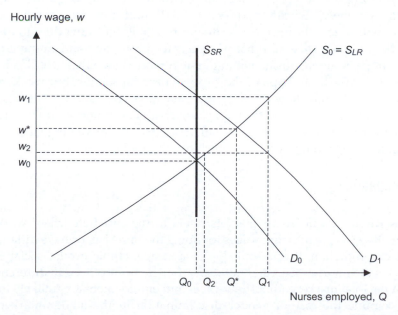

Figure 8.5 Cobweb model

(for example three years). Supply is fixed in the short-run at Q_0, the short-run supply curve is S_{SR}. For the market to clear wages increase from w_0 to w_1, given by the intersection of the demand curve and the short-run supply curve. The short-run equilibrium is w_1Q_0. Note that Q_0 is less than Q^* and this difference represents a shortage of nursing labour. On the long-run supply curve S_{LR} the employment corresponding to wage w_1 is Q_1. So when enough time has elapsed for new entrants to complete their training there will be Q_1 nurses in the labour market, which is more than Q^*, resulting in a surplus of nurses. But the quantity of nurses is now fixed at Q_1 in the short run, and for markets to clear, the wage will fall to w_2. At this wage nurses will move out of the profession, but the effect will not be immediate due to, for example, notice periods. When supply does adjust, it will adjust to Q_2, rather than Q^*. Hence, once again there will be a shortage of nurses, and the cycle will begin all over again, and will continue until the long-run equilibrium w^*Q^* is reached.

8.6.3 Non-maximising behaviour

Another source of imperfect health care labour markets is that neither employers nor workers are rational economic maximisers. Employers may not be profit maximisers. As we have seen in Chapter 4 there are alternatives to profit maximisation in health care. In these cases, the demand for labour will not be at the profit-maximising level defined above, and the perfectly competitive equilibrium will not be achieved.

Not all workers will be rational economic maximisers either. Rational workers will not necessarily aim to maximise their wages. They will work in jobs that maximise their utility, which is a function of wages and also non-wage costs and benefits. For example, job satisfaction is an important factor explaining retention in the nursing profession (see Yildiz *et al.* 2009 for a review). Shields and Ward (2001) find that nurses who report overall dissatisfaction with their jobs have a 65% higher probability of intending to quit than those reporting to be satisfied. They find that prospects for promotion and training opportunities have a strong impact on job satisfaction in nursing, more than either workload or wages. As noted such factors affect the shape of the supply curve for labour. But workers may not be rational, and give little thought to the wage and non-wage costs and benefits of different jobs. They may stay in their current job through sheer apathy and inertia. In this case the supply curve for labour may simply not be a good analytical tool for modelling labour supply and a perfectly competitive labour market equilibrium will not be achieved.

8.6.4 Discrimination

Economic discrimination in labour markets refers to the situation where workers who are equally productive receive different wages for doing the same job, or have different chances of employment or promotion. It can occur by gender, age, ethnic group, social class or other factors. It affects the hourly wages and numbers of workers employed in different groups, and means that in the total market equilibrium wages and employment are unlikely to be achieved.

Let us examine the case of gender discrimination in the labour market for doctors. Assume that male and female doctors are equally productive, shown by the curves MRP_F and

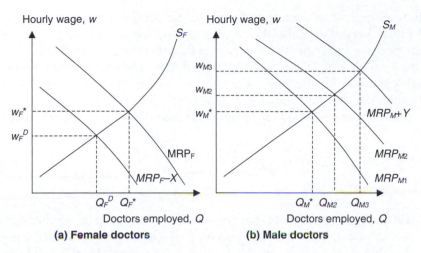

Figure 8.6 Labour market discrimination

MRP_{M1} in Figure 8.6. If there is no discrimination female doctors would be paid wages $w_F^* w_F^*$ and Q_F^* would be employed. For male doctors the equilibrium is $w_M^* Q_M^*$. Suppose now that employers discriminate against female doctors. This shows as hospitals employing female doctors using a lower MRP curve $MRP_F - X$, where X represents the extent of discrimination. Employment of female doctors will therefore be at the lower level Q_F^D and wages will be lower at w_F^D. Negative discrimination against female doctors also affects male doctors. Because fewer female doctors are being employed there will be fewer doctors employed in total and therefore the MRP of male doctors will increase. In Figure 8.6(b) the productivity of male doctors shifts to MRP_{M2}, increasing the employment and wages of male doctors to $w_{M2} Q_{M2}$.

In addition to there being negative discrimination against female doctors employers may discriminate positively in favour of male doctors. The hospital will employ male doctors along a higher MRP curve $MRP_M + Y$, where Y represents the extent of discrimination. This will increase the wage and employment of male doctors further to w_{M3} and Q_{M3}.

Box 8.4 describes an empirical approach to measuring wage discrimination and an application to data for general practitioners in England.

BOX 8.4   Gender discrimination in doctors' wages

A common method used to investigate wage discrimination is to decompose mean wage differentials between groups into differences in their characteristics and in the returns to the characteristics, using a method proposed by Blinder (1973) and Oaxaca (1973). This involves estimating separate wage equations for male and female doctors:

$$\log y_i^j = \alpha^j + x_i^j \beta^j + \varepsilon_i^j, \quad j = 1, 2$$

where i indexes individual doctors and j indexes gender ($j = 1$ for male doctors, $j = 2$ for female doctors). $\log y$ is the natural logarithm of wages, α is a constant term, x is a set of individual, practice and patient characteristics that affect wages, β is a set of coefficients relating the x variables to wages and ε is an error term. The equation is estimated using individual level data for doctors using least squares regression, so the estimated fit passes through the sample mean, $\overline{\log y}_{ij} = \hat{\alpha}^j + \overline{x}_i^j \hat{\beta}_i^j$.

The difference in wages, D, is decomposed into the following components:

$$D = \overline{\log y}^1 - \overline{\log y}^2 = (\hat{\alpha}^1 - \hat{\alpha}^2) + \underbrace{(\overline{x}^1 - \overline{x}^2)\beta^*}_{E} + \underbrace{\left[\overline{x}^1\left(\hat{\beta}^1 - \beta^*\right) + \overline{x}^2\left(\beta^* - \hat{\beta}^2\right)\right]}_{U}$$

where β^* is the set of coefficients that would be obtained if male and female doctors were treated identically. The second term on the right hand side of this equation E is the part of D due to differences in characteristics (the x variables), it is the explained part of the observed differential. E provides information about the differences between the characteristics of male and female doctors that affect wages, for example if male doctors have more years of experience or see more patients. The third term is the unexplained component U based on the returns to the characteristics. It has two elements. The first measures the extent to which the coefficients for male doctors are greater than those of the appropriate comparator group, and the second measures differences in coefficients between the comparator group and female doctors. U provides information about differences in the impact of these characteristics on wages, e.g., if the returns to years of experience or list size differ for male and female doctors. The first term $(\hat{\alpha}^1 - \hat{\alpha}^2)$ is the part of D arising from differences in the constant terms. This is presented separately from the other components of the decomposition because it includes both differences in unobserved characteristics and in the effect of these on wages. Assuming that the x variables fully explain doctors' productivity, U/D or $((\hat{\alpha}^1 - \hat{\alpha}^2) + U)/D$ can be interpreted as measures of discrimination.

Oaxaca (1973) suggests that β^* could be either $\hat{\beta}^1$ or $\hat{\beta}^2$. Other specifications have also been proposed. If $\beta^* = \hat{\beta}^1$ then male doctors are assumed to be not discriminated against, their returns to characteristics are appropriate. The same applies for females if $\beta^* = \hat{\beta}^2$.

Gravelle et al. (2011) used this approach to analyse gender discrimination in general practitioners' pay in England in 2008. The annual income of female GPs was 70% of those of male GPs and hourly wages were 89%. Using a model of income controlling for hours they found that about two-thirds of the difference in mean incomes between male and female GPs was unexplained. They used other tests for discrimination by comparing male and female incomes in single- and mixed-gender practices, based on the proportion of male and female GPs in each practice and the senior GP's gender. The senior GP's gender had no effect on the incomes of male or female GPs. GPs had smaller incomes where the proportion of female GPs was higher but there were no significant differences in the effect on male and female GPs. The authors concluded that there is weak support for the existence of GP gender discrimination.

8.7 Health care labour market shortages

A number of definitions of labour shortages exist. One is a needs-based shortage, based on a value judgement about how much health care people should receive and a calculation of how many workers are needed to provide that care. For example, the WHO (2006) estimated a critical worldwide shortage of 2.4 million doctors, nurses and midwives and 4.3 million health workers in total using this approach. The figures were calculated based on the population density of health workers required to ensure 80% of births in every country are attended by appropriately skilled health workers. Needs-based measures such as this are unrelated to the operation of the labour market and whether or not it is working efficiently.

An economic shortage exists when the quantity of labour demanded by employers exceeds the supply of it at the existing market price. There are two types of economic shortage (see Yett, 1970, for a discussion). The first is an equilibrium shortage, which arises with monopsony or oligopsony. This is shown in Figure 8.4(a) in the labour market for nurses. According to the monopsony equilibrium, the preferred wage and employment of the monopsony employer are w_1 and Q_1 both of which are lower than the perfectly competitive equilibrium. At the monopsony equilibrium wage the hospital would like to employ Q_4 nurses but it is only able to recruit Q_1. There is a shortage of workers. This is an equilibrium shortage in the sense that there are no market forces causing wages to rise. The shortage does not represent an excess demand and will not exert an upward pressure on wages.

A dynamic shortage exists when demand for workers increases over time, and employers try to employ additional workers at the market wage but there are no workers available. The reason for this type of shortage is that market responses to changes in demand are not immediate because of the length of training period to become a health professional. This was discussed previously and explained using the cobweb model.

The demand for health care workers is expected to increase in future due to rising incomes, continual technological change and ageing populations. There are concerns that the health care labour force will not expand to match the increase in demand – e.g., due to the demographics of the labour market many health professionals will reach retirement age and fewer young people will enter the workforce (Simoens *et al.*, 2005). A recent report published by the OECD suggested four main options to close the gap between the demand for and supply of health workers over the next two decades (OECD, 2008). The first option was to train more health care workers within each country, the second to improve the retention and delay the retirement of existing health workers, the third to raise productivity of existing health workers and the fourth to recruit health workers internationally from other countries.

Summary

1. Salaries and wages paid to health care workers account for a substantial component of total health expenditure: the average country devotes over 40% of its government-funded

health expenditure to paying its health workforce. There are around 59 million paid health workers worldwide.

2. Supply of labour can be considered at three levels: the supply of work hours by an individual worker; the supply of workers to an individual employer; and the total market supply of workers. Typically the total market supply curve will be upward sloping. Total market supply depends on the hourly wage, but also on the number of people willing and able to take the job at a given wage. This will depend on the number of suitably qualified people, the non-wage costs and benefits of the job, and the wages and the non-wage costs and benefits in alternative jobs.

3. The wage elasticity of supply measures the responsiveness of changes in supply to changes in wages. The degree of responsiveness depends on the mobility of health care labour – the ability and willingness of workers to move jobs. Immobility is of two types, geographical and occupational.

4. The demand for factors of production is a derived demand. The demand curve for labour is typically downward sloping because the higher the wages that profit-maximising employers have to pay the lower the quantity of labour they will want to employ. The marginal revenue product of labour curve shows the quantity of labour employed at each wage; it is therefore the employer's demand curve for labour. The demand for labour depends on the hourly wage, the productivity of labour, the price of and demand for the good, and substitution possibilities with other factors of production.

5. In perfectly competitive labour markets all employers and workers are wage takers – neither employers nor workers can influence and so have to accept the market wage. Equilibrium hourly wages are determined by the intersection of the total market demand and supply curves.

6. Transfer earnings are what workers must earn to prevent them from leaving the labour market and moving to an alternative job. Economic rent is anything earned over and above transfer earnings.

7. In the real world the assumptions of perfect health care labour markets are unlikely to be met. Health care workers and employers may have market power and be able to influence wages. Training and education requirements mean that health care labour may be slow to respond to changes in demand and supply conditions causing persistent disequilibria. Employers and workers may practise non-maximising behaviour. There may be wage discrimination.

8. When a firm is the only employer of a certain type of labour it is a monopsony. This may give the employer market power in setting wages. Health care professionals may also have market power as members of trade unions or professional bodies. A bilateral monopoly is said to exist when a monopsony employer faces a monopoly trade union or professional body.

9. Imperfect labour markets exist because health care labour may be slow to respond to changes in demand and supply conditions causing persistent disequilibria. One reason for this is the length of training period to become a health professional.

10. Another source of imperfect health care labour markets is if employers and/or workers are not rational economic maximisers.

11. Economic discrimination in labour markets refers to the situation where workers who are equally productive receive different wages for doing the same job, or have different chances of employment or promotion. It can occur by gender, age, ethnic group, social class or other factors.

12. Needs-based shortages of health care labour are based on value judgements about how much health care people should receive and a calculation of how many workers are needed to provide that care. Economic shortages exist when the quantity of labour demanded by employers exceeds the supply of it at the existing market price. There are two types of economic shortage. An equilibrium shortage arises with monopsony. A dynamic shortage exists when demand for workers increases over time, and employers try to employ additional workers at the market wage but there are no workers available.

CHAPTER 9

Welfarist and non-welfarist foundations of economic evaluation

9.1 The normative economics foundations of economic evaluation

In Chapter 1, we drew a distinction between positive and normative economics. The former is descriptive or predictive in nature. Economic analysis describes trends in economic variables, generates testable hypotheses about the relationships between them and is then able to explain and predict future trends. However, many of the questions that health economics seeks to address are also concerned with making judgements about the relative desirability of alternative ways of delivering health care. Chapters 9–13 of this book are concerned with how economics is used to evaluate the benefits and costs of alternative uses of resources in the health care sector.

Economic evaluation describes a broad set of analytical approaches used to describe and compare the benefits and costs of competing uses of resources. It is normative in two respects. Most obviously, to conclude that one treatment option is better value for money than another, having weighed up both the benefits and costs, is either explicitly or implicitly prescriptive. Although economists can occasionally be seen actively to promote or oppose a particular option, most emphasise that their role is to provide evidence to inform decisions, rather than to make them. Restricting the role of the economist to describing the benefits and costs of alternatives does not, however, avoid value judgements. Although the methods of economic evaluation we describe in Chapters 10–13 are highly technical, involving sophisticated modelling and statistical procedures, underlying this quantitative toolkit are views on what constitutes a cost, what is a benefit and how these things are to be valued.

The theory and practice of economic evaluation is therefore inescapably normative in nature. Economic evaluation is crucially concerned with how benefits are to be measured and valued – and the economist's notion of cost is the value of other opportunities forgone. Further, given that increasing the benefits enjoyed by one person or persons involves sacrificing benefits to other persons, conclusions about the desirability of any given option invokes value judgements about the extent to which such trade-offs are acceptable and desirable.

The aim of this chapter is to explain the value judgements that underpin the principles and practice of economic evaluation, to show the role that these play in providing the theoretical foundations of economic evaluation methods, and to assess critically their defensibility as a basis for social choices.

Normative economics is often, in the mainstream economics literature, taken as synonymous with welfare economics (for example, Boadway and Bruce, 1984; Johansson, 1991). Here we distinguish between two normative economics approaches – welfarism and non-welfarism – which are evident in the practice of economic evaluation of health care. The term 'welfarist' was first used by Sen (1977) as a means of distinguishing the traditional normative economics approach to social choices from contemporary critical non-welfarist positions on it (see Section 9.9). We conclude the chapter by considering whether or not these normative positions can be reconciled, and by re-iterating the implications of the analyst's normative position for the science of economic evaluation.

9.2 Welfare economics

Welfare economics, or welfarism, is generally defined as the systematic analysis of the social desirability of any set of arrangements, for example a state of the world or allocation of resources, solely in terms of the utility obtained by individual people.

Welfare economics is the principal normative tradition in economics. Its aim is to devise a set of rules – essentially, value judgements – that can be used to achieve a logical and consistent ranking of all alternative social states, for example how scarce health care resources are allocated, between which we might choose. Of course, there are many ways in which this might be achieved: we could delegate decision making to politicians, and rely upon their judgements about what is best for society, or an autocrat could make these choices on society's behalf. The distinctive approach taken by welfare economics in assessing the relative desirability of states is traditionally characterised by the following three arguments.

First, welfare economics is based on individualism. The only relevant information in making social choices is the views of the individual people affected by those choices. Each person is deemed to be the best judge of their own welfare, and to behave in a manner that is utility maximising. The effects of social choices are therefore considered to be most appropriately measured by considering the impact on individual people as they see it themselves. This impact is captured by changes in their utility, any given state of the world being considered is assessed in terms of their own evaluation of whether it makes them better, worse or equally well off as in other states of the world. In welfare economics, social welfare – a measure of the well-being of society as a whole – is therefore exclusively a product of the utilities of individual members of society. Judgements by others, for example experts such as health care professionals, and paternalistic views of what is good for people are deemed irrelevant.

Secondly, given its basis in consumer choice theory, welfare economics is consequentialist. It traditionally only takes into account the outcomes for people, in terms of their consumption of specific types and quantities of goods and services and the consequent utility obtained. The utility associated with the consumption of goods and services is considered neutral to the process, be it a market, political or other process, of choosing or receiving those goods. Utility is generated only from consumption – our own consumption and, where there are caring externalities, the consumption of others whom we care about.

Thirdly, an objective of welfare economics is to devise a decision rule that allows us completely and consistently to rank all states of the world, and to base this ranking strictly on the consequences, in utility terms, for each person. Given this, the principal challenge in welfare economics is to propose a defensible basis for aggregating peoples' preferences. Inevitably, we confront situations where the relative desirability of states depends upon what sort of trade-offs between peoples' utilities we deem acceptable. There is no objective way of dealing with such trade-offs. The basic judgement used in welfare economics, and its defining feature as a normative framework for social choice, is the Pareto principle.

9.3 The Pareto principle

Since a value judgement is necessary, it seems reasonable to suggest that the best value judgement to use is that which would command widest support – that is, one with which most of us would agree. A value judgement with this characteristic is described as weak because the view that it represents is relatively uncontentious. The value judgement that lies at the heart of welfare economics was proposed by Pareto in 1906 (Busino, 1987).

Paretian concepts are especially important to economic evaluation and resource allocation decisions. They provide a basis for judging a given state of affairs to be optimal or not, and for ranking states relative to each other, by reference to the utility obtained by each person in each state. The theoretical basis of Paretian analysis is consumer choice theory (see Chapter 2). This requires that each person can consider a set of states of the world – effectively, bundles of goods – and consistently rank them, meaning that they have stable and transitive preferences. A goal of Paretian analysis, and indeed of welfare economics generally, is to aggregate these preferences to produce a social welfare ordering (SWO). This is a complete and consistent ranking of all possible states in terms of their social desirability.

As well as defining optimality, Paretian analysis provides a set of related concepts that are important in judgements about social welfare, such as the notion of Pareto improvements. For example, a change in the state of the world that increases the utility of all affected people is a weak Pareto improvement. A change in the state of the world that increases the utility of at least one person, and does not decrease the utility of anyone else is a strong Pareto improvement. Paretian concepts play a crucial role in economics – for example, they provide a means of judging efficiency in production (as we saw in Chapter 3) and provide the basis

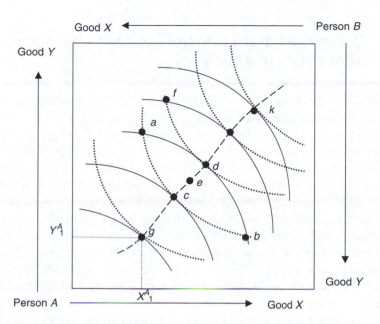

Figure 9.1 The Pareto principle demonstrated using an Edgeworth box

for the conclusion that competitive markets generate socially optimal outcomes (as we saw in Chapter 5).

Figure 9.1 illustrates the Pareto principle, using a geometric representation of the possibilities for allocating a fixed total quantity of two goods, X and Y, between two people, A and B. This is known as an Edgeworth box (or sometimes as an Edgeworth–Bowley box). It is constructed from the indifference curve maps of two people, as introduced in Chapter 2, where the walls of the box are the axes for person A and person B, respectively. Both people are shown simultaneously, by rotating the indifference map of person B 180° onto that of person A. The length of the X-axis shows us the total quantity of good X available; the length of the Y-axis shows us the total quantity of good Y available. Each and every point within the box is a feasible allocation of these quantities of the two goods between the two people. Choose any point within this box: it represents a unique allocation of quantities of goods X and Y between person A and person B. For example, at point g, person A receives X^A_1 units of good X and Y^A_1 units of good Y. The quantity of X received by person B at point g is whatever is left over, that is the difference between the total quantity of good X available and that consumed by person A (X^A_1); the same is true for good Y. Associated with every point within the space defined by the walls of the Edgeworth box is an indifference curve for both person A and person B. This shows us the utility they each experience from consuming the exact bundle of goods X and Y represented by that point. Points lying to the north-east in this box will be preferred, that is ranked more highly, by person A than points lying in the south-west, as they are associated with higher utility; the opposite applies to person B.

The Pareto principle offers a means of identifying which of these points can be considered socially better than another, by reference to the utility of each person. Examples of each of the following Paretian concepts are provided in Box 9.1.

BOX 9.1   Using the Pareto principle to rank alternative allocations of goods

---

Figure 9.1 shows a fixed quantity of two goods X and Y to be allocated between two people. For simplicity, imagine that this is a pure exchange economy – for example a room containing two people, and a given number of units of good X and good Y. Starting from any allocation of these goods between them, such as that shown by point a, the persons can change what goods they have by choosing to exchange the goods with the other person. What can we say about the overall social welfare arising from the alternative allocations of goods that might arise in this situation? One might have an ethical view on this: egalitarians, for example, might argue that the only correct allocation is that each person gets exactly half each of the quantities of X and Y. The welfare economics approach to judging social welfare, by contrast, focuses on the utility each person enjoys from the consumption of these two goods. If, for example, one of these people happened to have very strong preferences for good X and the other for good Y, then an equal allocation of the goods is clearly not going to maximise either their individual or joint welfare.

If we start at point a, it is possible for voluntary exchange to take place between the two people such that we shift to point b. Both person A and person B are on the same indifference curve at a as at b – that is, both A and B experience exactly the same level of utility at a as they do at b. Because each of them would be just as well off after as before this reallocation, points a and b are *Pareto indifferent*. In terms of overall social welfare, the two points are identical and would be ranked equally.

Starting again from point a, reallocating goods between A and B such that we shift to point e would enable *both* people to shift onto an indifference curve farther from their origin – that is, both of them experience higher utility as a result of this new allocation of goods. This is a *weak Pareto improvement*. In terms of social welfare, e is therefore Pareto superior to point a.

Starting again from point a, reallocating goods between person A and person B such that we shift to point c is a *strong Pareto improvement*: person A is on the same indifference curve at c as at a, but person B has shifted to a higher level of utility. One person is better off and the other is no worse off. In terms of overall social welfare, c is also Pareto superior to a.

Regardless of what the starting point is, Pareto improvements will always be possible, so long as there is a different marginal rate of substitution of X for Y ($MRS_{X,Y}$) for different people. Points where the slopes of each person's indifference curves are equal, that is, where $MRS_{X,Y} = MRS_{X,Y}$, are *Pareto efficient* or *Pareto optimal*. In Figure 9.1, there are multiple Pareto optimal allocations – these have been connected with a broken line, known as a *contract curve*. Once one has arrived at a Pareto optimal allocation of goods, further exchanges of goods can only improve one person's utility by *reducing* the utility of the other. Such changes are *Pareto non-comparable*. It is not possible, using the Pareto principle, to rank states of the world in which one person is made better off and the other made worse off. To do this requires us to invoke a stronger value judgement.

If, by shifting from one point to another, the utility of both people is increased, this is a weak Pareto improvement. We would say such a change is a good thing using the Paretian value judgement, and the latter point is therefore Pareto superior to the former. The 'weak' refers to the unobjectionable value judgement invoked in deciding that the new resource allocation is better than the initial one. Who would disagree, given that both people are better off?

If, by shifting from one point to another, one person is made better off, and the other person is no worse off, that is they remain on the same level of utility, this is a strong Pareto improvement. We would conclude that this change is also a good thing, and that the latter point is Pareto superior to the former. The word 'strong' alerts us to the somewhat stronger value judgement involved.

Once all such improvements have been exhausted, we have reached an allocation of goods which is Pareto efficient or Pareto optimal. However, this is not a unique point; there are many possible Pareto optimal allocations. It is easy to spot Pareto optimal allocations in an Edgeworth box. In Figure 9.1, these are the points at which the two peoples' indifference curves are tangent to each other. At such points, the $MRS_{X,Y}$ – the slope of the indifference curve – is identical for both people. Recall from Chapter 2 that the $MRS_{X,Y}$ might also be thought of in terms of the ratio of MU_X/MU_Y. Thus, wherever this ratio is different between people, the addition to satisfaction that is derived from the consumption of X relative to Y is different between each person. The implication is that, wherever this ratio is different between people, there will be scope to improve the utility of at least one person, without reducing that of another, simply by reallocating the endowments of goods X and Y between them.

Hence, an allocation of goods is Pareto optimal if an increase in one person's utility can only be achieved by reducing the utility of at least one other person.

While a weak value judgement, the Paretian approach to social ranking of states is nevertheless a judgement – it cannot be disproved, but we might disapprove of it. For example, what if the richest person in society were able to increase their utility, while the poor continued to have the same level of utility as before: is this change a good thing? Although a Pareto improvement, this would conflict with both egalitarian and Rawlsian perspectives on equity (see Chapter 7). Similarly, a government policy that reduces poverty may be highly desirable, but if it involves a sacrifice by the rich, no matter how small, it will not be a Pareto improvement (Hammond, 1996).

Further, some Pareto optimal points represent wildly uneven allocations of goods between the two people and, more importantly from the welfarist perspective, very different levels of utility. Pareto optimal points close to A's origin (for example, point g in Figure 9.1) indicate low levels of utility for A, and high levels of utility for person B; Pareto optimal points close to B's origin (for example, point k) indicate low utility for B and high utility for A. The Pareto principle itself offers us no means of comparing these allocations with each other.

An important limitation of the Pareto principle is, therefore, that it does not provide any means of ranking Pareto optimal states, and that it is neutral to the kinds of distributional concerns that we discussed in Chapter 7. As Tsuchiya and Williams (2001) note, 'A "Pareto improvement" is not concerned with who is better off, or about the relative size of people's gains, but only that there are no losers.'

Box 9.1 demonstrates that what constitutes a Pareto improvement depends on what the starting point – the current state of the world – is. Given a point such as a, we can identify a set of points, lying along and within the lens-shaped space defined by the indifference curves for person A and B passing through a, that would yield either strong or weak Pareto improvements, including the points lying along the line between d and c, which are Pareto optimal. But we cannot compare a point such as a with a point such as g, even though g is Pareto optimal and a is not. Thus, the Pareto principle does not allow us to compare any pair of states of the world that involve trade-offs between people's well-being.

This is obviously a rather fundamental problem. The advantage of the Paretian approach is that the value judgement it embodies is relatively weak; and that it involves minimal informational requirements, requiring only that people can rank the options – bundles of commodities – presented to them. But these advantages come at the expense of its being 'useless as a criterion for social choices in many, if not all, real-world situations' (Johansson, 1991). This point is illustrated nicely by a series of columns in the *Journal of Economic Perspectives* in the late 1980s which considered the question 'Are There Pareto Improvements?'. Some contributors concluded there are no examples of Pareto improvements in real life, although one economist, Barry Nalebuff, claimed to have found one: allowing a left-hand turn at a red traffic light! (Although even that could be disputed.) Clearly, if welfare economics is to provide a practical guide to resource allocation in health care, where most decisions are not of the free-left-hand-turn variety, it needs to go beyond the Pareto principle.

9.4 Potential Pareto improvements

We have pointed out that, as well as being neutral to distributional equity, an important limitation of the Pareto principle is that it can produce only a partial ranking of social states. The Pareto criterion cannot cope with mixed outcomes, where one person's utility is increased but another's decreased. Consequently, with reference to the points in Figure 9.1:

- it cannot rank all non-optimal points against each other, for example points a and f;
- it does not allow us to rank all Pareto non-optimal points against all Pareto optimal points, for example points f and c; and,
- it cannot rank Pareto optimal points against each other, for example points d and c.

The second of these problems can be addressed if we allow the possibility of compensatory monetary transfers between those who gain and those who lose. Compensation tests were independently proposed by Kaldor (1939) and Hicks (1939); although frequently conflated, they comprise slightly different means of judging the social desirability of two states.

Imagine that we are contemplating a policy that involves one health authority being allocated an additional £3 million by the government, and another losing £2 million. What can welfare economics tell us about the relative desirability of the state of the world brought about by this policy, compared with the *status quo*? Hicks suggests assessing the desirability of the reallocation by the government by examining the extent to which those who lose would be prepared to bribe those who gain not to make the change. If the policy were implemented, the losing health authority would be £2 million worse off, so they will be prepared to spend up to that amount to avoid the policy. In this instance, the gaining health authority will not be prepared to accept the bribe, as it is less than the gain that they stand to make (£3 million): they would be worse off accepting the bribe (£2 million − £3 million = −£1 million). On the basis of these gains and losses, as assessed by each person themselves, the policy is judged socially desirable and should go ahead. In Kaldor's version of the compensation test, if those who gain can potentially fully compensate those who lose (£2 million), such that the losers are no worse off (−£2 million + £2 million = £0) and the gainers can still be better off (by £3 million − £2 million = £1 million) than before the policy then, again, the policy is judged to be desirable.

The monetary assessments of benefit and loss referred to in this example are not based on accounting procedures or some objective assessment of benefit and loss. Rather, they are defined in a very specific way that enables us to link utility, which is an intangible concept that is difficult directly to measure, and money, which is easy to measure. Following Hicks (1939), benefit (loss) may be defined as the maximum (minimum) amount of money that must be taken away from (given to) a person such that they are as well off after the change as before it. We return to these concepts in Section 9.5, and give a more formal exposition of them. For those who lose, this represents the monetary compensation they must receive, were the policy to proceed, such that they return to the same level of utility they had *before* the policy. For those who gain, this represents the amount of money that must be taken away from them, were the policy to proceed, such that their utility returns to its pre-policy level.

In essence, the compensation tests simply involve adding up the monetary losses and gains assessed in this manner; if their sum is positive the policy is recommended for implementation, and if negative it is rejected. The compensation tests preserve the spirit of the Pareto principle. If those who gain do so to such an extent that they could hypothetically fully compensate those who lose and still be better off themselves, this is a strong potential Pareto improvement. If those who gain do so to such an extent that they could hypothetically make a payment to the losers which is greater than the amount the losers require as full compensation, and still be better off themselves, then both could be made better off, which is a weak potential Pareto improvement.

Figure 9.2 illustrates the compensation tests using a utility possibilities frontier (UPF). A UPF plots the pairs of individual utility levels associated with any allocation of goods within the Edgeworth box. The labelled points in Figure 9.2 correspond to those in the Edgeworth box of Figure 9.1. Any point off the contract curve in Figure 9.1, such as point *a*, is a non-optimal allocation of goods and will lie inside the frontier in Figure 9.2. Thus, from point *a*, a shift to either *c* or *d* will be a strong Pareto improvement, and a shift to *e* a weak Pareto improvement. Pareto optimal points – those lying along the contract curve in Figure 9.1 – create the frontier. The UPF has a negative slope: from any Pareto optimal allocation of goods, an increase in one person's utility cannot be achieved without making the other person worse off. Given that this analysis does not require a cardinal measure of utility, we cannot impose any requirement for this function to be strictly convex or concave; thus it is shown here as a non-monotonic, but decreasing, function. The compensation tests enable any point *within* the UPF, for example

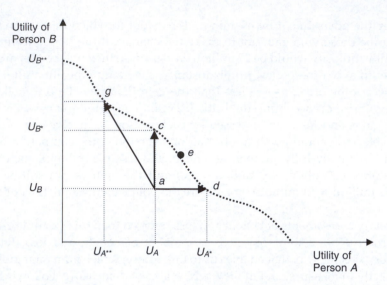

Figure 9.2 Potential Pareto improvements demonstrated using a utility possibilities frontier

point *a*, to be ranked against any point *on* the UPF, for example point *g*, that is they address the second type of non-comparability noted earlier. A shift from *a* to *g* does not *in itself* improve social welfare, but the improvement in overall efficiency associated with that change would enable transfers to take place between *A* and *B* such that a movement to a point such as *c* is possible.

There are a number of problems with compensation tests. First, while the compensation tests allow the identification of potential Pareto improvements, the compensation remains potential rather than being realised. The tests require only that compensation be hypothetically possible, but actual money transfers are not required to take place. This is important, because a shift from point *a* to point *g*, which would be deemed socially desirable using the compensation tests, may not in practice be accompanied by compensation for *A*. Implementing this policy without compensation involves a redistribution of wealth or well-being in favour of *B*, at *A*'s expense. The rationale for this, as explained by Boadway and Bruce (1984) is that:

> The purpose of considering hypothetical redistribution is to try and separate the *efficiency* and *equity* aspects of the policy change under consideration. It is argued that whether or not the redistribution is actually carried out is an important but *separate* decision.

Some economists have pointed out that to distinguish between efficiency and equity in this way is somewhat disingenuous, given the expressly normative purpose of welfare economics (for example Little, 1957).

Secondly, compensation may be possible, but may be costly to negotiate and organise. If redistribution is costly, then the identification of potential Pareto improvements that can be achieved by cost-free lump-sum transfers is, arguably, not very helpful in a practical decision-making context.

Thirdly, the use of money as a metric with which to represent the corresponding changes in utility for gainers and losers depends on each unit of this metric (£1) corresponding to equal increments of total utility for each person involved. Imagine a situation where there are identical gains and losses in utility terms, but where those who lose have low incomes and those who gain have high incomes. If we believe that income, like goods, is subject to diminishing marginal utility, the addition to utility obtained from each additional £1 of income is likely to be higher for a low-income person than for a high-income person. The consequence is that the amount of money required fully to compensate the loser for their utility loss from this change will be lower than the amount of money required to compensate the gainer for forgoing the change. Although in terms of utility the gains and losses are identical, the compensation test would deem this policy to be desirable.

Fourthly, there is a theoretical possibility that a change in the state of the world and a reversal of that change might both appear to be socially desirable using the compensation tests. Scitovsky (1941) therefore suggested a qualification, whereby a change in the state of the world is desirable if and only if it is associated with a potential Pareto improvement, and a return to the original state of the world is not.

Finally, while compensation tests allow any non-optimal states to be ranked vis-à-vis any optimal state, they do *not* allow Pareto optimal states to be ranked against each other or for non-optimal states to be ranked against each other. The identification of Pareto improvements and potential Pareto improvements is not sufficient to obtain a complete and consistent ranking of all states of the world; that is, to obtain an SWO.

9.5 Social welfare functions

The welfare economics approach to social choices might be thought of as a hierarchy of value judgements. Starting with the weakest value judgement, the Pareto criterion can rank many states of the world, but there remain many that cannot be ranked. Further rankings can be obtained using compensation tests, but not for Pareto optimal states. Ranking of alternative Pareto optimal allocations requires us to invoke still stronger value judgements than those represented by the compensation tests.

So far, we have considered the SWO only in ordinal terms, that is, as a social ranking of states of the world. Moreover, it is based upon information on the manner in which individual members of society rank those states. If, however, we had some means of measuring each person's utility, social welfare could also be measured by aggregating these individual utilities in some way. This would allow us to represent the SWO as a social welfare function (SWF), where society's welfare is measured in real numbers as a function of its members' individual utilities. Early economists concerned with these issues, such as Jeremy Bentham and John Stuart Mill, tended to think about utility in very concrete terms that were potentially measurable. Bentham, for example, refers to hypothetical units of measurement called 'hedons', denoting pleasure and deriving from the word 'hedonist'; others have described utility in notional units of 'utils'.

The most general formulation of this is known as the Bergson or Bergson–Samuelson SWF. The level of social welfare (W) associated with any given state of the world (x) is a function of the utility obtained by each iperson $U_A, \ldots, U_n$ in that state:

$$W(x) = f(U_{A(x)}, U_{B(x)}, U_{C(x)}, \ldots, U_{n(x)}) \qquad (9.1)$$

This is not constrained to have a particular functional form – that is, the mathematical relationships between the variables are left unspecified. Therefore, this SWF does not specify exactly the nature of the trade-offs we are prepared to accept between, for example, U_A and U_B, but it does have some useful properties. First, the only determinants of W are the utilities of individual people – thus, it is a welfarist approach. Secondly, other things being equal, W is increasing in each person's utility, so it is consistent with the Pareto criterion. For example, in Figure 9.3, as the utility of person B increases from U_B to $U_{B'}$ to $U_{B''}$, and the utility of A remains unchanged at U_A, social welfare increases from W_1 to W_2 to W_3. Any curve, such as W_1, shows the various combinations of U_B and U_A that yield identical levels of social welfare and between which society will therefore be indifferent. We would generally expect this curve to have a negative slope: if we increase U_A, U_B must be reduced for society overall to remain just as well off as before. Thus, the SWF can be thought of as society's indifference curve, explicitly showing the manner in which the utility of society's members are aggregated to determine the well-being of society as a whole. Social welfare curves farther from the origin represent higher levels of social welfare.

The Bergson SWF is often drawn, as in Figure 9.3, as convex. This is not a requirement of the Bergson SWF; instead it reflects a particular view about the way that people's utilities are aggregated. Implicitly, inequality in the utility levels obtained by people is regarded as being socially undesirable to some extent, but not completely abhorrent. A convex SWF implies that

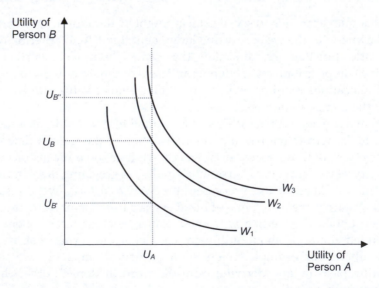

Figure 9.3 The social welfare function

successive increases in the utility of one person, holding that of others constant, confer diminishing marginal increases in society's welfare. Another way to express this is that the slope of the social welfare function, $-\Delta U_B/\Delta U_A$, which is the amount by which person B's utility must decrease given an increase in person A's utility for social welfare to remain constant, is decreasing.

Assuming that this semi-egalitarian ethic is a reasonable representation of society's preferences over the utilities of its members, the SWO, which is the ultimate goal of welfare economics, can be re-cast as a simple optimisation problem. This is solved by selecting from the UPF the pair of utilities that maximises society's welfare.

This can be seen in Figure 9.4, which combines the UPF introduced in Figure 9.2 with society's preferences over people's utilities, shown by the SWF in Figure 9.3. Points within the UPF, such as a, are not efficient: Pareto improvements are possible by movements to d, c or e. Points such as x are more desirable than any of points a–g, but are not feasible to achieve, given the underlying endowments of resources and existing technology. Points g, c, e and d all lie along the UPF: they are all Pareto optimal and neither the Pareto principle nor compensation tests can rank them. However, given the stronger value judgement captured by the SWF, clearly point c is the best distribution of utility between A and B, as it generates the highest possible level of social welfare (W_3). All of points g, c, e and d are optimal in the Pareto sense, but, according to the SWF, c is the *optimum optimorum* – the best of the best. At this point, the utilities of person A and person B are U_{A^*} and U_{B^*} respectively. This is also referred to as the 'bliss point' or, in Pareto's own language, as the point of 'maximum ophelimity'.

Given that the SWF encapsulates society's view about the trade-offs between people's utility that are acceptable, exactly what shape it is depends entirely on our views on equity and distributive justice. Utilitarians, as we saw in Chapter 7, advocate an ethical position whereby states of the world deemed most desirable are those which generate 'the greatest good for the

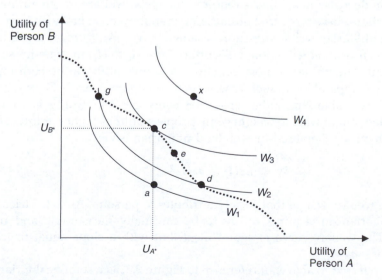

Figure 9.4 Maximising social welfare

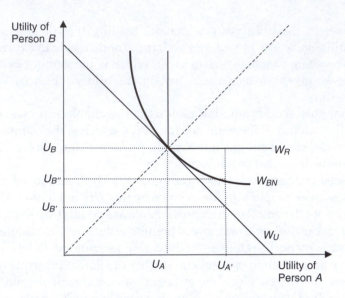

Figure 9.5 Utilitarian, Bernoulli-Nash and Rawlsian social welfare functions

greatest number', that is they maximise the sum of the utilities of members of society. This yields an SWF given by

$$W = (U_A + U_B + \ldots + U_n) \tag{9.2}$$

Given that the utilitarian's measure of the social welfare in any given state is simply the sum of individual utilities, this implies a 1:1 relationship between an increase in utility of one person and the decrease in another's required for social welfare to remain unchanged. The slope of the welfare curve for a strict utilitarian is therefore constant and always equal to –1. In Figure 9.5, the utilitarian welfare function is shown by W_U. An increase in A's utility from U_A to $U_{A'}$ requires an *identical* reduction in B's utility from U_B to $U_{B'}$ in order for social welfare to remain constant. The utilitarian position clearly requires utility to be both measurable and interpersonally comparable for such assessments to be possible.

This SWF is egalitarian in the sense that every person's utility is weighted equally. However, society might want to weight some people's utilities higher or lower than others. In this case, we have a generalised or weighted utilitarian SWF:

$$W = (a_A U_A + a_B U_B + \ldots + a_n U_n) \tag{9.3}$$

where a_i is the welfare weight that society attributes to person i. As with strict utilitarianism, weighted utilitarianism requires utility to be cardinally measurable and interpersonally comparable. The welfare curve is again linear, but with a slope equal to the ratio of the weights, that is $-a_A/a_B$.

What we referred to above, in reference to Figure 9.3, as a semi-egalitarian ethic implies that an increase in A's utility from U_A to $U_{A'}$ requires a smaller reduction in B's utility, in comparison with the utilitarian SWF, from U_B to $U_{B'}$, in order for social welfare to remain constant. This concave social welfare function, the properties of which we have already described, is sometimes referred to as the Bernoulli-Nash SWF. It represents social welfare as the product of individual people's utility functions:

$$W = ((U_A)(U_B) \ldots (U_n)) \tag{9.4}$$

This function, shown in Figure 9.5 as W_{BN}, in effect places a lower weight on the utility of those with high levels of utility. The state of the world selected by maximising it is also known as a Nash solution, because it can be derived from the bargaining theory of John Nash. It reflects what may be viewed as a fair rule by players in a bargaining game (see Section 4.3.6). It is the only rule that satisfies all of these four axioms: no interpersonal utility comparisons; independence of irrelevant alternatives; symmetrical treatment of all players; and the strong Pareto criterion.

An alternative to these SWFs is the maximin SWF, where society's welfare is measured by the minimum utility level, that is, the level obtained by its worst-off member:

$$W = \min(U_A, U_B, \ldots U_n) \tag{9.5}$$

Often referred to as the Rawlsian SWF, following Rawls' (1971) *Theory of Justice*, the implied welfare curves are shown by W_R in Figure 9.5. Given any initial unequal distribution of utility in favour of one person, an increase in the utility of that person will increase society's welfare up to the point where utilities are strictly equal. Beyond that point, further increases in that person's utility will not increase social welfare – only equal increases in utility for both people will do so. For example, an increase in A's utility from U_A to $U_{A'}$ leaves W unchanged – because $U_A = U_B$, the increase in A's utility confers no improvement in social welfare, so no reduction in B's utility is required for social welfare to remain constant. The Rawlsian SWF in Figure 9.5 thus treats the utility of person A and person B as perfect complements in the SWF. It is also called the Maximin SWF, because the social choices suggested by such a SWF would involve maximising the position of the worst-off person.

Each of these SWFs rests upon strong value judgements. In essence, an SWF is an explicit statement of ethical beliefs about what is socially good and optimal.

While these are the specific functional forms commonly found in the literature, there clearly exists a wide range of other, distinctive ethical positions and divergent views on what constitutes social equity. Many of these – for example Nozick's (1974) *Theory of Entitlement*, in the libertarian tradition, and Roemer's (1998) writing on *Equality of Opportunity* – cannot be captured as SWFs because the views they present pertain to the fairness of the *process* by which various distributions of goods or utility arise. Welfarism restricts its consideration to the *consequences* in terms of individual peoples' utility, and is neutral to the process by which those are achieved. Thus, although the particular shape and functional form of the SWF must reflect a particular ethical stance, not every ethical stance is capable of being rendered as an SWF. Furthermore, which SWFs are candidates for making social choices is, in practice, constrained by the extent to which we can measure and compare individual people's utility.

9.6 Measurability and comparability of utility

Imagine that we had at our disposal a dependable measuring rod for utility that gave us valid measures of change in any one person's utility and that each number on that measuring rod represented the same level of utility across all people. Further imagine that we could agree on our ethical position as a society, so we can construct an SWF to aggregate those utilities. Also imagine that we all agreed that welfarism is the right way to make social choices: for any given decision all we are concerned with is the effect of the quantities of goods and services consumed and their consequences for individual utilities. In these circumstances, every social decision could be made by feeding the corresponding utilities into the SWF. The SWO is complete and consistent, and the decisions that maximise welfare would be readily obtained.

The real world is, of course, rather different. In practice, attempts to construct SWFs are constrained by our ability to measure utility. In the absence of a cardinal measure of utility, it might only be possible to measure peoples' preferences on an ordinal scale. Such assessments of utility may not be comparable between different people.

For cases where information on preferences is restricted to their ranking of states, Arrow (1951) reported an extraordinary finding. A complete and consistent SWO can only be achieved if we allow one arbitrarily chosen person's preferences to dominate every choice – this person is sometimes called a dictator, though this is not meant in the pejorative real-world sense. If we rule out the dictatorship option on the grounds that it is an undesirable way to make social choices, then Arrow's result is that it is impossible to produce a complete and consistent SWO. Arrow called this a 'possibility theorem', but it is usually referred to as Arrow's impossibility theorem, because that is a more useful description. Of course, in the unlikely case where all members of a society had exactly the same preferences, a social ranking would simply be the ranking common to all of them – in accordance with the weak Pareto criterion. However, in any situation where people's preferences conflict, so that they have different rankings of states, these cannot be reconciled to produce a consistent social ranking. The simplest illustration of the problem, which was used by Arrow in his 1972 Nobel Prize acceptance speech, is provided by a majority voting system.

Imagine that there are three states of the world: x, y and z, which voters are asked to rank. One-third of the voters (group 1) rank these states x, y, z: that is, x is their first, most preferred choice, followed by y, and z is their least preferred option. One-third of the voters (group 2) have the ranking y, z, x; and one-third (group 3) have the ranking z, x, y.

Now consider the ranking of the states generated by a majority vote. Two-thirds of the voters (group 1 and group 3) prefer x to y, outweighing group 2's preferences. And the majority of the voters (group 1 and group 2) prefer y to z, outweighing group 3's preferences. Given that the majority prefers x to y, and the majority also prefers y to z, one might therefore logically expect that the majority prefers x to z. Instead, and paradoxically, the majority (group 2 and group 3) prefers z to x. The social ordering of these states generated by the majority vote is intransitive, that is to say logically inconsistent. While this majority vote example provides something of the flavour of the theorem, it is not a proof of it.

Arrow (1972) concludes: 'The philosophical and distributive implications of the paradox of social choice are still not clear. Certainly, there is no simple way out.'

How might we get around Arrow's finding? One way would be to improve the information available for making social choices – effectively, to develop the cardinal measures of utility that Bentham and Mill once imagined possible. Sen (1970) demonstrated that even if cardinal measures were invented that were meaningful representations of any one given person's utility, unless these are interpersonally comparable, the dictatorship result persists. Boadway and Bruce (1984) outline the range of welfare functions that are possible under different assumptions about the degree of measurement and inter personal comparability. Interestingly, health economics is unique among economics subdisciplines in that it has devoted considerable efforts to the development and use of measures of health-related utility that are both cardinal and interpersonally comparable. This research poses considerable challenges; we discuss the theory and methods in detail in Chapter 12. Another option is to relax the requirements of welfarism – for example, to allow arguments other than individual utility to influence social decision making. We turn to these non-welfarist and extra-welfarist approaches in Section 9.8.

9.7 The application of welfare economics

The welfare economics theory we have described so far provides the principal theoretical foundations for economic evaluation. In this section we show how this theory translates into the practice of cost–benefit analysis, which is defined formally in the next chapter. In addition, we outline how the theory has been developed to measure changes in welfare that arise when the equilibrium quantity of good is not Pareto optimal. In a practical exercise, decision makers cannot directly observe or compare the individual utilities that are central to the welfare economics approach. Thus, the application of welfare economics relies on the use of money as a proxy for utility.

We introduced the notion of compensating payments in Section 9.4 in relation to Hicks' compensation tests; here we provide a more formal exposition, drawing on Johansson (1995). The basic framework for welfare economics, as we have emphasised, is consumer choice theory: each person is assumed to maximise their utility. They have a limited after-tax income, y, that they wish to spend on n different goods, the consumed quantities of which are denoted by $x = (x_1, x_2, \ldots, x_n)$. Each of these n goods has an associated price denoted by $p = (p_1, p_2, \ldots, p_n)$. The objective is to maximise their utility, subject to their income. Their utility (U) is a function both of the goods they consume (x) and their health status, denoted by z, which we assume can be measured as a single number on a 0–1 scale. Formally, the utility function is given by $U = U(x, z)$ and the maximisation problem is to maximise $U = U(x, z)$ subject to $px \leq y$.

Using this framework we can construct measures of welfare change using money as the metric for comparison. Note that by including health status z in the utility function we can quantify welfare changes arising from a change in health status, which in turn might arise

TABLE 9.1	Compensating and equivalent variations for gains and losses

	For a gain arising from a change in the state of the world:	For a loss arising from a change in the state of the world:
CV	The amount of income that would have to be *taken away* from someone *following* this change, in order that they return to their *original* level of utility.	The amount of money that must be *given* to someone *following* this change, in order that they return to their *original* level of utility.
EV	The amount of income that would have to be given to someone *before* this change, that would increase their utility to the *new* (higher) levels they would obtain were the policy to proceed.	The amount of money that would have to be taken away from someone *before* this change that would give a reduction in their utility to the *new* (lower) level they would experience if the policy were to proceed.

from health care. Hicks (1939) proposed two distinct means of using money to measure changes in utility: the compensating variation (*CV*) and the equivalent variation (*EV*). Each can be applied to the assessment of either gains or losses, as summarised in Table 9.1.

In essence, the *CV* approach seeks monetary amounts that represent the impact on a person of any given change considered *ex post*, relative to their *initial* levels of utility. The *EV* approach seeks monetary amounts that represent the impact on a person of any given change considered *ex ante*, relative to the *new* levels of utility that the change is anticipated to bring. Chapter 11 will explain the practical methods and research instruments used by economists to elicit measures of *CV* and *EV*; here we focus on their theoretical rationale and derivation.

To estimate these two money measures of a change in health we need to construct the *indirect utility function*. We know from the above maximisation problem that x is constrained by the person's income and prices, that is, $x = x(p, y)$. Substituting this into the utility function gives the following expression for the indirect utility function V:

$$V = U[x(p, y), z] = V(p, y, z) \tag{9.6}$$

This states that indirect utility is a function of prices (p), post-tax income (y) and health status (z).

A change in health status, such as might result from receiving health care, will change the person's utility. The change in utility (ΔV) following a change in health status is given by

$$\Delta V = V(p, y, z_1) - V(p, y, z_0) \tag{9.7}$$

where subscript 0 denotes the person's initial level of health (state 0) and subscript 1 denotes the person's final level of health (state 1). Prices and income are assumed to remain constant. ΔV is positive if $z_1 > z_0$, that is, if health status is improved. We want to value in monetary terms the change in utility (ΔV) arising from a change in health.

If health improves, the CV is the maximum amount of money that can be taken from the person after that improvement, leaving them just as well off as they were before the improvement:

$$V(p, y - CV, z_1) = V(p, y, z_0) = U_0 \qquad (9.8)$$

This is called the *willingness to pay* for an improvement in health. U_0 is the person's level of utility before the improvement in health (in state 0). If health deteriorates, CV is the minimum amount of money that must be given to the person to compensate for their loss in health.

With a potential improvement in health, the EV is the minimum amount of money that must be given to a person to make them as well off as they would have been after the improvement in health:

$$V(p, y + EV, z_0) = V(p, y, z_1) = U_1 \qquad (9.9)$$

This is called the *willingness to accept* for not receiving an improvement in health. U_1 is the person level of utility after the health improvement (in state 1). If health deteriorates, EV is the maximum amount of money the person is willing to pay to prevent the deterioration.

Note that the CV for a given *improvement* in health is equal to the EV associated with the exactly opposite *deterioration* in health provided that there are no income effects.

These measures of CV and EV provide us with an observable measure of the value of changes in health status reflecting corresponding changes in a person's utility. However, the use of these measures in social decision making requires a means of aggregating them to construct a measure of social welfare (W). A generalised utilitarian social welfare function would be one where social welfare in state i (W_i) is given by

$$W_i = \sum_{j=1}^{N} a_j V_{ij}(p, y, z) \qquad (9.10)$$

where a_j is the constant welfare weight that society attributes to person j, V is the level of utility experienced by person j in state i, which is a function of p, y and z, and there are N people in society.

Imagine that there is a health care programme that increases the health status (z) of people who receive it but also decreases the health status of other people who do not receive it, because it reduces the quantity of other types of health care programmes available to them. We want to offer a recommendation about whether this programme should be introduced. In a welfarist framework this involves determining whether or not social welfare increases with a move from state 0 to state 1, that is, whether or not ΔW, the change in social welfare, is positive or negative. ΔW is given by

$$\Delta W = W_1 - W_0 = \sum_{j=1}^{N} a_j V_{1j}(p, y, z_1) - \sum_{j=1}^{N} a_j V_{0j}(p, y, z_0) \qquad (9.11)$$

If it is positive, the recommendation is to proceed with this programme; if it is negative, the recommendation is not to proceed.

Unfortunately, the change in social welfare is unobservable. There is no way of directly observing the sign and magnitude of ΔW. However, we can attempt indirectly to capture the nature of the social welfare change by using the measures of CV and/or EV described above. By modifying slightly equations (9.8) and (9.9), we obtain the following:

$$CV : V_{1j}(p, y - CV, z_1) = V_{0j}(p, y, z_0) \qquad (9.12)$$

$$EV : V_{0j}(p, y + EV, z_0) = V_{1j}(p, y, z_1) \qquad (9.13)$$

We concentrate on CV here, but the following applies equally to EV. Substituting equation (9.12) into equation (9.11) yields

$$\Delta W = \sum_{j=1}^{N} a_j V_{1j}(p, y, z_1) - \sum_{j=1}^{N} a_j V_{1j}(p, y - CV, z_1) = \sum_{j=1}^{N} a_j v_j CV_j \qquad (9.14)$$

where v_j is the marginal utility of income of person j given by

$$v_j = \frac{\partial V_j(p, y, z)}{\partial y_j} \qquad (9.15)$$

We can see that CV and EV provide us with part of the information necessary to determine whether or not a project that improves people's health will lead to an improvement in social welfare. However, it is also clear, for example from equation (9.14), that knowing the CV and EV alone is not all that is required to make an assessment. What we also require is information on a_j, the welfare weight that society places on each person and v_j, the marginal utility of income of person j. Multiplying a_j, by v_j gives us the *marginal social utility of income* for each person.

We require information on a_j, because, as we have already discussed, we cannot achieve an SWO without the decision maker, for example the government, making value judgements about the way in which trade-offs between people are to be handled. The welfare weights are value judgements – essentially, statements of ethics – that are used to describe the relative importance the decision maker puts on welfare changes obtained by different people in the move from state 0 to state 1 and which are to be included in the aggregation process.

The marginal utility of income, shown in equation (9.15), tells us the rate at which a change in income (y) for each person is translated into a change in their utility (V). This explains how money measures of the change in health (CV or EV) convert into a change in utility. Unfortunately, this is unlikely to be constant across people. As we have already noted, it is generally argued that there is a diminishing marginal utility of income: as people become richer, successive increases in income yield smaller additions to total utility.

To understand the importance of these concepts, consider the following example. Imagine a society with two people, David and Nick. A health care programme is introduced which benefits David, because he receives it and it increases his health status. However, it is detrimental to Nick, because introducing it means that other health care programmes from which Nick obtained some benefits have been curtailed. We elicit from David and Nick their *CV* for the new health care programme and we have also somehow obtained estimates of *a* and *v*:

	David	Nick
CV	+10	−5
a	1	2
v	1	1.5

The sum of these *CV*s $(10 + -5 = 5)$ is positive so, using a simple compensation test criterion, the new health care programme should be implemented. However, the values for *a* tell us that society places a greater weight on Nick's welfare. Additionally Nick's marginal utility of income is greater than David's. Under these assumptions, the change in welfare from the health care programme is actually negative $(\Delta W = (1 \times 1 \times 10) + (2 \times 1.5 \times -5) = -5)$, and therefore the programme should not be implemented. The health care programme, because of its detrimental effect on Nick, actually reduces social welfare. This example highlights the perils of inferring conclusions about the desirability of a project from simply summing up money measures of changes in utility.

The problem is that the marginal social utility of income is generally unobservable. Therefore, the problem remains that it is difficult to assess the desirability of a change in social states whereby some people are made better off and others are made worse off. Unless one is prepared to adopt some rough and approximate approach it is not possible accurately to aggregate welfare changes across people from money measures of changes in health. For convenience, it is commonly assumed in cost–benefit analyses of health care programmes that equal weight should be given to welfare changes for people and that the marginal utility of income across people is constant. That such strong assumptions are used in the application of welfare economics underlines the importance of caution both in the interpretation of results and in making recommendations.

9.8 Non-welfarism

We have so far in this chapter given an overview of the welfare economics foundations of economic evaluation. It is evident that there remain unresolved difficulties in the ability of welfare economics to provide a comprehensive guide to decision making and, in particular, to address the issue that lies at the heart of social choices: the means by which conflicts in preferences and trade-offs between people are to be managed. In this section we expand on the limitations and critiques of welfarism that relate specifically to decisions regarding health care, and discuss the attempts to develop alternative non-welfarist normative frameworks to guide economic evaluation.

Non-welfarism is any normative framework for social decision making that rejects welfarism. There is no single theoretical non-welfarist paradigm; non-welfarism is consistent with a diverse set of theoretical perspectives and propositions.

Welfare economics is often asserted to be the theoretically correct approach to social choices and decision making. Its alleged superiority arises from its basis in the axioms of microeconomic theory, in particular consumer choice theory, and because its central tenets are systematically described and its conclusions derived formally. By contrast, non-welfa-rist approaches are sometimes dismissed as comprising a 'practical, but not very well formulated collection of rules of thumb' (see Tsuchiya and Williams, 2001). The arguments against using welfare economics as a basis for economic evaluation of health care are as follows.

The underlying paradigm of rational choice and utility maximising behaviour is irrelevant to health and health care behaviours

Welfare economics is viewed by some as 'less relevant to the particular context and back-ground of health care resource allocation, where the objectives of the players do not entirely agree with those upheld by standard theory' (Tsuchiya and Williams, 2001).

Thus, one of welfare economics' main strengths – its basis in microeconomic theory – is disputed in the health sector. The assumptions and models that are used to represent consumer behaviour might be argued to be less relevant to, or at least to provide poor predictions of, individual behaviour with respect to health and health care. These concerns are captured nicely by Culyer (1989), who argued that the implications of welfare economics for policy decisions 'hinge on judgements about the empirical significance of consumer rationality, the "purity" of the agency relationship, the nature of any externalities, the extent of adverse selection, moral hazard, supplier-induced demand, unnecessary premium loading under insurance, and the empirical validity of the neoclassical behavioural model that, in its normative version, is welfarism's centrepiece'. Given that market failures in health care are such that most health care systems reject the use of markets as the sole means of funding health care (see Chapter 5), is it appropriate to rely on market theories of consumer behaviour and value to provide the basis for allocating resources in non-market settings?

Welfarism assumes social welfare is determined only by utility from commodities

Critics, for example Mooney and Russell (2003), assert that welfare economics is too restrictive in its approach to social choices because its assessment is based traditionally only on individual people's utility from consumption. It seems reasonable to suggest that things other than individual utility from consumption might matter in social decision making – and that therefore welfare economics is simply too limited in scope to deal with factors we know to be important.

However, although much of welfare economics does indeed model social choices in this manner, this may be for expositional simplicity or parsimony in modelling rather than from necessity; welfarism is capable of accommodating any source of individual utility. Indeed it is possible to point to contributions to the welfare economics literature that depart from the simple focus on a person's utility from their consumption. For example, Culyer (1976) uses a welfare economics framework to analyse the effects of 'caring externalities', where utility is a function both of one's own consumption *and* the consumption of others one cares about; see Chapter 5 for a more detailed exposition. Further, Culyer (1989) points to a long tradition of attempts to incorporate non-individualistic approaches into the standard welfare economics framework. This dates back to Bergson's original paper (from 1938) on the SWF, which included unspecified terms in the social welfare function that could be used to represent things other than individual utility that might matter in social choices. It also includes Culyer's own work, which attempted to incorporate Musgrave's notion of merit goods into an orthodox welfare economics framework (Culyer, 1971).

Similarly if, as suggested in Chapter 2, the demand for health care is a derived demand, that is the increase in utility arises from the improvement in health rather than the consumption of health care per se, its benefits are nevertheless able to be represented by effects on utility (Birch and Donaldson, 2003). All the derived demand relationship implies is that it is health, rather than health *care*, which is the source of utility; that utility is therefore a function both of the consumption of goods and services *and* health; and that, as demonstrated by Johansson (1995) and described in Section 9.7, this should be reflected in the SWF. Allowing health to determine utility is entirely possible within a welfare economics framework.

Welfare economics' basis in individualism excludes community values

Regardless of whether utility is permitted to arise only from commodities, or from other sources, the underlying framework of welfare economics is nevertheless firmly rooted in the notion that people are utility maximisers. This precludes the idea that people might voluntarily be interested in contributing to some common good, which lowers their own utility. Sen (1977) describes this type of behaviour as 'counterpreferential' – for example our obligations and commitments to others. Thus the utilitarian ethic of welfare economics cannot cope with things such as a commitment to community values and community well-being (Mooney and Russell, 2003).

Utility is fundamentally flawed as a measure of individual well-being

Perhaps the strongest challenge to welfare economics arises from questions about the ability of its basic building-block, utility, to capture well-being meaningfully. The most compelling and well-known arguments on these issues are made by Sen (1985). His basic assertion is that people differ with respect to their ability to convert commodities into well-being. Sen argued that utility has two main problems: physical condition neglect and valuation neglect. A person who suffers from physical condition neglect 'can still be high up in the scale of happiness and desire fulfilment if he or she has learned to have "realistic" desires and to take pleasure in small mercies'. Valuation neglect arises because 'valuing is not the same thing as desiring and the strength of desire is influenced by considerations of realism in one's circumstances'. Measuring social welfare with respect to individual utilities will therefore be misleading, because a person's assessment of their well-being and utility is affected by their characteristics as people.

Sen described two aspects to these characteristics: *functionings* (what a person manages to be) and *capabilities* (the freedoms that a person has to make choices). Because these characteristics are potentially important influences on a person's assessment of well-being, information on them should be admitted into the process of comparing social states. This is known as *extra-welfarism* – terms extra to utility are included in the SWF. It does not exclude individual utilities from judgements about social welfare, as in non-welfarism. Instead it supplements these with additional information about each state, for example preferences regarding the process by which goods are chosen or consumed, or characteristics of each person.

Sen's extra-welfarist approach to social choices has received particular attention in relation to choices in the health sector and has, arguably, been developed more in relation to health care decisions than in any other realm of social decision making. Drawing on the arguments of Sen, Culyer (1989) advocated a general notion of 'characteristics of people' as pertinent to decisions about health care. The characteristics argued to be potentially relevant to social choices include a broad set of factors: a person's 'genetic endowment of health, their relative deprivation independently of the absolute consumption of commodities or the characteristics of commodities; their moral "worth" and "deservingness"; whether or not they are in pain, or stigmatised by society'. Other characteristics could include the nature of relationships between people; for example 'the quality of friendships; community support for someone when in need; social isolation; or changes in them, such as becoming (as distinct from being) a cripple' (Culyer, 1989).

Significantly, only some of these characteristics of people will be 'deemed relevant' (Culyer, 1989); the selection of relevant characteristics, from the menu above, is asserted to be 'related to the concept of need'. Given that the health characteristics are relevant because they are a way of describing deprivation, health care commodities are needed because they can help relieve that deprivation. In other words, health care is a means to an end. Essentially, Culyer extended Sen's very broad notion of particular characteristics to even more general notions of characteristics, but then narrowed the focus to one particular characteristic pertinent to decision making in health care: *health* (Culyer, 1989). So, the extra-welfarist position that has emerged is that health is included in the SWF. Brouwer et al. (2008) compared and contrasted the main differences between welfarism and extra-welfarism, summarised in Table 9.2.

Extra-welfarism does not necessarily imply that utility is cast aside – both sets of information can inform social choices. This suggests the following SWF:

$$W = f(U_A, H_A, U_B, H_B, \ldots, U_n, H_n) \tag{9.16}$$

TABLE 9.2	**Main differences between welfarism and extra-welfarism**	
	Welfarism	Extra-welfarism
Relevant outcome	Only individual utility	May include individual utility as well as extra measures and indicators of well-being, such as health or health gain, distribution of health of health gain, patient satisfaction or caregiver burden
Source of valuation of relevant outcomes	The affected person	May be the affected person, but could also be an expert, representative sample of general public or decision maker
Weighting of relevant outcomes	Sometimes weighted according to the distribution of individual utilities	Allowed and often considered important as a means of incorporating equity considerations. Weights may be based on a variety of considerations, such as wealth or need
Intertemporal comparability of relevant outcomes	Some comparisons are theoretically possible through the social welfare function	Explicit comparisons made though not normally in terms of utility, but in terms of characteristics such as health

Source: Brouwer *et al.* (2008)

The difference between this and the SWFs described in equations (9.1) to (9.5) is that health may be included, alongside other commodities, as an argument in a person's utility function, but social welfare is determined strictly from utilities. In equation (9.16), health enters the social welfare function *directly*, as an additional argument. Health is included not because it is a source of utility, but because it describes a characteristic of people argued to be of importance to decisions about how to allocate health care resources.

McGuire (2001) speculated that, given an SWF such as this, it might be possible to impose Pareto optimality as a normative goal on the goods sector and a competing maximand on the health sector – most obviously, the maximisation of health. There are two complications to this approach. First, utility levels and health levels are unlikely to be independent. Secondly, resources used in the health sector will be drawn from the goods sector. Given these interdependencies between health and utility, identification of an overall optimal resource allocation will be theoretically challenging – and remains to be addressed.

As we have described it, the term extra-welfarism makes sense – it implies there is something extra being taken into account alongside utility. However, in practice extra-welfarism has come to be associated with a very specific interpretation of the broad possibilities inherent in Sen's position. The set of techniques of economic evaluation which constitute *applied* extra-welfarism use health not to *supplement* utility but to *substitute* for it. That is, these economic evaluation approaches focus entirely on the maximisation of health – and this has been to the exclusion of non-health-related utility, such as that derived from the process of care rather than its outcome. The benefits of health care programmes are measured and valued as changes in *health*. Thus both welfarism and extra-welfarism have been subject to the criticism that they ignore preferences over processes that are valued in themselves rather than being instrumental to some outcome, either improved utility in welfare economics or improved health in extra-welfarism (Mooney and Russell, 2003).

Given that, in practice, extra-welfarism has come to be synonymous with the maximisation of health, it is interesting to consider how this position arose. Where did health as a maximand come from? The relevant passages from Culyer's influential (1989) paper set out the rationale in terms of need, as described above. But Culyer did not see health as completely ousting welfare; one possibility is that the focus on health emerged as a pragmatic response to methodological challenges in evaluation, as the theory of extra-welfarism itself does not justify it. Further, a problem with Culyer's rationale for selecting health as the only relevant characteristic of people is that it relies upon some external judgement about what is deemed relevant – and the sources of these external judgements, and on what authority they are based, are unclear.

It is important to note that what has become the orthodox approach to economic evaluation under extra-welfarism has emerged through practice rather than being *required* by it as a normative framework. This includes not just the focus on health, but also the rejection of individualism: the values attached to health are those of the community, not of the individual recipients of treatment.

It is tempting, given that the normative framework for extra-welfarism in health care was first set out in Culyer's writings in the late 1980s, to view extra welfarism as an *ex post* rationalisation for practical techniques of economic evaluation that had been applied since the late 1960s and were incompatible with traditional welfarist approaches.

The distinction between non-welfarism and extra-welfarism is rather tenuous and possibly overdrawn. For example, Tsuchiya and Williams (2001) reject the term extra-welfarism and categorise all competing normative approaches as being essentially non-welfarist. And while non-welfarism might be interpreted as an approach whereby information on utilities is rejected in favour of something else – health – it then seems odd that many non-welfarists strongly advocate the use of utility-based measures, such as standard gamble (see Chapter 11), as the means by which health is measured and valued (Parkin and Devlin, 2006). Finally, it is interesting to note that, given that these extra-welfarist or non-welfarist approaches arise from Sen's critique of social choices based on *utility*, Sen has also argued that making social choices about health care by relying on measures of self-reported *health* might be extremely misleading for similar reasons (Sen, 2002). We return to issues of measuring and valuing the outcomes from health care in Chapter 11.

9.9 Is there a link between welfarism and non-welfarism?

Given that economic evaluation in health care has come to be dominated by applications of extra-welfarism, there is a growing body of research investigating the extent to which such evaluations, based on the maximisation of health approach, will be equivalent to or consistent with economic evaluations following the welfarist tradition (Johannesson, 1995; Birch and Donaldson, 2003; Dolan and Edlin, 2002).

There are two crucial issues. The first is the extent to which the measures of health that are used – which we describe in detail in Chapter 11 – might be considered in themselves to constitute measures of utility. The second is whether or not the allocation of resources achieved using the principle of maximising health is compatible with a Pareto optimal allocation of resources in the economy more generally. The consensus is that very restrictive conditions need to be met if this equivalence is to be established. How one interprets this depends very much on whether one views the issue from a welfarist or a non-welfarist perspective. For example, Tsuchiya and Williams (2001) comment that 'if the objective is to work within a welfarist framework, then this is bad news ... however, for non-welfarists, whose objective is not to reproduce the results of standard welfarist full-scale cost benefit analysis, this demonstration of non-equivalence is a great relief!'.

We return to these issues in Chapter 13 after establishing the concepts and methods of economic evaluation in detail in Chapters 10–12.

Economic evaluation cannot be undertaken in a value-free manner. The appropriate value judgements to use for this purpose are a matter of some contention, with equally strong advocates for both welfarist and non-welfarist positions and no assurance that they are consistent or can be reconciled. These are non-trivial issues, with important implications for the way in which we approach the allocation of scarce resources in health care. There remains no consensus on the basic questions: What are we trying to maximise? How do we weigh up one person's loss with another's gain?

How, then, is economic evaluation to proceed? One solution is to take a pragmatic approach. Rather than searching for an elusive one-size-fits-all theoretical gold standard, Tsuchiya and Williams (2001) argue that the purpose of economic evaluation is to help people make specific decisions, and that therefore the policy context should determine the approach to be used in evaluation. However, this conclusion is itself a reflection of the authors' own extra-welfarist position.

Given the lack of consensus, economists have a duty to be explicit about the value judgements they adopt in their analysis, and to communicate clearly to decision makers the

effect of value judgements on both the results from economic analysis and the recommendations either stated or implied in them. As Fuchs (1998) states:

> Economics is 'the science of means, not of ends' . . . [I]t can tell us the consequences of
> various alternatives, but it cannot make those choices for us. These limitations will be
> with us always, for economics can never replace morals or ethics.

Summary

1. Economic evaluation describes a broad set of analytical approaches used to describe and
   compare the benefits and costs of competing uses of resources.
2. Welfare economics (or welfarism) is the systematic analysis of the social desirability of any
   set of arrangements (for example, a state of the world, or resource allocation) solely in
   terms of the utility obtained by people. Welfarism is based on individualism and
   consequentialism.
3. A basic value judgement used in welfare economics is the Pareto principle. A change in the
   state of the world that increases the utility of all affected people is a weak Pareto
   improvement. A change in the state of the world that increases the utility of at least
   one person, and does not decrease the utility of anyone else is a strong Pareto improvement. A state of the world in which no feasible Pareto improvement is possible is Pareto
   efficient or Pareto optimal. A state is Pareto optimal if an increase in one person's utility
   can only be achieved by reducing the utility of at least one other person.
4. It is not possible, using the Pareto principle, to rank states of the world where one person is
   made better off and the other made worse off. To do so requires us to invoke a stronger
   value judgement. This problem is called Pareto non-comparability.
5. One consequence of Pareto non-comparability is that the Pareto principle is unable to rank
   all Pareto non-optimal points against all Pareto optimal points. Compensation tests, such
   as those derived by Kaldor and by Hicks, can be used in these cases.
6. A complete social welfare ordering might be obtained using social welfare functions
   (SWFs), which provide a direct way of aggregating individual utilities to obtain a value for
   social welfare. Common SWFs are the Bergson (or Bergson–Samuelson) SWF, the utilitarian and generalised utilitarian SWFs, the Rawls (or maximin) SWF and the Nash SWF.
7. SWFs can be combined with utility possibility frontiers (UPFs) to identify the combination
   of individual utilities that will maximise social welfare (the bliss point).
8. Different SWFs rely on different assumptions concerning the measurability and comparability of individual utility. If utility is only measurable on an ordinal scale and if it is non-
   comparable, then the Arrow possibility theorem states that a complete and consistent
   social welfare ordering may only be obtained with a dictatorship. If we rule dictatorship as
   being an undesirable way to make social choices, then Arrow's result is that any attempt to
   produce a complete and consistent SWO is impossible.

9. Decision makers cannot directly observe or compare the individual utilities that are central to welfare economics. Thus, the application of welfare economics relies on the use of money as a proxy for utility. Two money measures of changes in utility are the compensating variation (*CV*) and the equivalent variation (*EV*).

10. The *CV* and *EV* can be aggregated to determine whether a policy has a positive or negative effect on social welfare. This requires additional information on the form of the SWF, the welfare weight that society places on each person and the marginal utility of income.

11. Criticisms of welfarism in health care are that the underlying paradigm of rational choice and utility-maximising behaviour is irrelevant to health and health care behaviours; that welfarism assumes that social welfare is determined only by utility from commodities; that welfare economics' basis in individualism excludes community values; and that utility is fundamentally flawed as a measure of individual well-being.

12. Non-welfarism is any normative framework for social decision making that rejects welfarism. There is no single theoretical non-welfarist paradigm; non-welfarism is consistent with a diverse set of theoretical perspectives and propositions.

13. Extra-welfarism can be defined as any approach to social choice that admits arguments other than individual utilities into the social welfare function. It does not necessarily exclude individual utilities from judgements about social welfare, as in non-welfarism, but supplements these with additional information about each state, for example preferences regarding the process by which goods are chosen or consumed or characteristics of each person. In health care an obvious supplement is health.

CHAPTER 10

Principles of economic evaluation in health care

10.1 What is economic evaluation?

Economic analysis helps us to understand the world by describing and explaining economic behaviour. One of the main reasons why this is valuable is that it provides information that will be of help to people in making decisions about the allocation of scarce resources. Economic evaluation (or economic appraisal) is specifically about the provision of such information. It seeks to create, in the context of non-market provision of goods and services, information to inform choices; information that in other areas of the economy would be generated by the interplay of market forces. It is a structured approach to help decision makers choose between alternative ways of using resources.

Chapter 9 introduced economic evaluation using a highly theoretical approach, to emphasise that it has a strong intellectual basis. However, economic evaluation is quintessentially an applied technique, arguably the main practical contribution that economics makes to decision making in health services; the remaining chapters deal with how it is carried out in practice. This chapter forms a bridge between the two, by setting out the principles derived from the theory that guide the practice.

The general term used for this sort of analysis in economics is *cost–benefit analysis* (CBA), and this term remains the most accurate and useful way of describing it. Its basis is the common-sense notion that a decision about whether or not to do something should depend on a weighing up of its advantages and disadvantages – comparing its benefits with its costs. From an economics perspective, this means comparing like with like, because benefits and costs are closely related concepts. Costs measure the value of scarce resources used in terms of opportunity costs, which are the benefits that could otherwise be obtained with those resources. Cost–benefit analysis is therefore simply a comparison of the benefits of one use of scarce resources with those from another. This approach and the systematic way of thinking that it promotes are at least as important as the techniques of economic evaluation.

The original purpose of cost–benefit analysis, which remains the focus of its application in most non-market areas of the economy, is *investment appraisal*. This specifically aims to mimic the investment decisions that would be taken if a large-scale capital project were undertaken in a private market, except that the context is public rather than private. It has therefore been used for many years to appraise such public sector projects as dams, bridges, reservoirs, motorways and airports. It is a straightforward extension to apply the same techniques to hospitals and other health facilities, and to large-scale capital investments such as diagnostic imaging and information technology systems.

However, the predominant use of economic evaluation in health care is not for such large-scale capital projects and indeed its most widespread use is not for investment at all. Rather, it is used to provide information on which products – health care interventions – should be provided by health services for consumption by patients. This has led to the development of a distinctive set of techniques, which have been strongly influenced by the existence of established non-economics techniques used in the evaluation of health care interventions. From the economics point of view, health care is just a special case; but from the medical point of view, economics is just an additional evaluative technique.

Simply providing information on costs and benefits is in itself not evaluative. Rather, in economic evaluation this information is structured in such a way as to enable alternative uses of resources to be judged. There are many criteria that might be used for such judgements. Many of these are important, but are not especially economics based – for example, whether or not the use of resources is ethical and respects human dignity. The criteria that are the focus of economic analysis are efficiency and equity; economic evaluation in health care should in theory regard these as equally important, but in practice efficiency is dealt with far more often and with greater attention to precise numerical estimates.

In private health care markets, efficiency is largely left to market forces, with the assumption that, in a competitive market, profit-making health care organisations have incentives to minimise costs and provide the services that their patients desire. In publicly provided health programmes, market forces might be weak or there might be none at all. Economic evaluation is largely concerned with measuring efficiency in areas where there is public involvement and there are no markets to generate the kind of information – for example, prices and profits – that enable us to judge this. However, it is also likely that public services have different goals from private services. For example, public health organisations might wish to maximise health rather than profits and might also wish to take into account equity as well as efficiency. Economic evaluation – which is concerned with the public context – must therefore take such wider goals into account.

10.2 The economics foundations of economic evaluation

10.2.1 Cost–benefit analysis

At its simplest, cost–benefit analysis (CBA) is simply an inventory of all costs and benefits, whatever they are and whoever incurs them; this forms a balance sheet in which they are weighed up against each other. This is only possible if all costs and benefits are measured in the same unit; the obvious one is money as the measure of value most used in modern economies. Monetary costs are viewed as a measure of the value of the resources used in an activity; and monetary benefits are viewed as a measure of the value that is placed upon the output of that activity.

It has been recognised that some types of costs and benefits can be measured, but not in terms of money – these are traditionally known as incommensurable items. For example, in evaluating a hospital service, we may have measures of patients' satisfaction with their care in terms of the percentages who are satisfied or not with aspects of it such as standards of cleanliness, but we do not have any measures of the monetary value of changes in satisfaction. Yet other types of costs and benefits may be known or suspected to exist but cannot be quantified at all – traditionally these are known as intangibles. For example, dealing with mental illness in the community rather than in institutions may promote a sense of independence among patients, which is clearly a benefit but is hard to quantify.

The identification of incommensurable and intangible items is context specific and refers to problems of measurement, not to the item itself. Measurement techniques improve. It is increasingly possible to place plausible money values on items once regarded as incommensurable, and many items once regarded as intangible – such as pain and suffering – can now be quantified. For example, subjective feelings such as happiness used to be regarded as entirely intangible, but there is now a large research effort in this area which has quantified this concept (Layard, 2005). For example, Oswald and Powdthavee (2007) used the General Health Questionnaire (GHQ-12) developed by Goldberg *et al.* (1997) as a measure of happiness to demonstrate the negative effects of obesity. Box 10.1 describes a cost–benefit analysis comparing two types of endoscopy for people with suspected airways cancer, which highlights some of the challenges involved in measuring costs and benefits.

BOX 10.1   A cost–benefit analysis of tele-endoscopy clinics for people with suspected airways cancer in Scotland

Van der Pol and McKenzie (2010) undertook a cost–benefit analysis of tele-endoscopy clinics in a remote location in Scotland. The patients were adults with symptoms suggesting the presence of cancer of the airways. The evaluation compared tele-endoscopy conducted at a remote clinic in the Shetland Islands with conventional endoscopy conducted at hospital on the mainland in Aberdeen. Patients at the remote clinic had their endoscopy performed by an anaesthetist or surgeon, and videoconferencing was used to send images to and communicate with a consultant in Aberdeen.

The authors collected data on the preferences of patients for the two options using a discrete choice experiment (DCE; see Chapter 11). The outcomes of interest were those attributes of the clinics that were considered to be important by the patients. These were the type of service (face-to-face or telemedicine), one-way drive time (30 minutes or less, 30 to 60 minutes, 60 to 90 minutes or two to four hours), the waiting time (4, 7, 13 or 18 weeks), and the costs (zero, £90, £180 or £300). The benefits of the tele-endoscopy and mainland clinics were valued in monetary terms, using willingness-to-pay values calculated from the DCE. The cost data were collected for both options in terms of staff, capital and disposable equipment, and travel costs, which were met by the health service.

The mean cost per patient was lower for the tele-endoscopy clinic (£353) than for the mainland clinic (£381) due to the lower travel cost. The Willingness To Pay (WTP) values for the two types of clinics are summarised in the table. These ranged from £125 to £403 depending on the type of clinic and the waiting time. With equal waiting times, the WTP values were higher for the tele-endoscopy clinic than for the mainland clinic.

	Waiting time (weeks)				
	1	4	7	13	18
WTP					
Tele-endoscopy clinic	£403	£359	£316	£228	£156
Mainland clinic	£372	£329	£285	£198	£125
Net benefit (WTP – cost)					
Tele-endoscopy clinic	£49	£6	−£38	−£125	−£198
Mainland clinic	−£6	−£50	-£94	−£181	−£254

Assuming equal waiting times, the net benefit (WTP minus cost) of the tele-endoscopy clinic was larger than that of the mainland clinic, suggesting that the tele-endoscopy clinic was the preferred option. However, if the waiting time for the mainland clinic was 1 week and for the tele-endoscopy clinic 7 weeks, the net benefit for the mainland clinic would be higher. The authors calculate that tele-endoscopy is preferred as long as the additional waiting time for tele-endoscopy clinics compared to the mainland clinic was no more than 3.8 weeks.

The question of how costs and benefits are to be measured and weighed against each other is obviously a fundamental issue, and indeed forms the main body of work on the topic. The answers to this question are often pragmatic, but they also have very strong guides from theory. However, there are two slightly different intellectual bases for cost–benefit analysis. The first arises from the origins of cost–benefit analysis as a tool used in planning and management of public services. Historically, it was one the key contributions of economics to a multidisciplinary movement (Lyden and Miller, 1972) that also produced Programme Budgeting, which is described in Chapter 13. This tradition, called by Sugden and Williams (1978) the *decision-making approach*, recognises the legitimacy of decision makers appointed by society as the source of many decisions about how costs and benefits are to be measured and weighed. The aim of CBA is to help to maximise the achievement of the decision maker's goals – which is similar to the very general definition of efficiency given in Chapter 1.

The second intellectual basis, which appeared around the same time as the public sector planning movement (Mishan, 1971), regards CBA as applied welfare economics and therefore attempts to operationalise the welfarist analysis discussed in Chapter 9. This provides a very strong guide to issues of measurement and weighing up of different costs and benefits, such as the necessity to, for example, identify all costs as social marginal costs and to employ a social welfare function to aggregate benefits. This tradition, called by Sugden and Williams (1978) the *Paretian approach*, regards economic analysis as providing an independent point of view on public sector decisions, taking the perspective of society as a whole and restricting its interest to efficiency issues. The aim of CBA is to identify Pareto improvements or potential Pareto improvements – which is consistent with the more technical economics definitions of efficiency discussed in Chapters 5 and 9.

What of the non-welfarist approach? It is clearly not entirely consistent with the Paretian approach, since it involves a different notion of what constitutes a benefit. However, non-welfarists regard the definition of what constitutes a benefit as being socially determined, rather than determined by decision makers. It is therefore consistent with the view embodied in the Paretian approach that economic analysis should provide an independent view, based on socially determined objectives, rather than simply serving decision makers who can impose their own objectives. But it could equally be regarded as consistent with a decision-making approach in which the decision maker is an idealised entity who takes a societal perspective, rather than a real one who might in practice have a more restricted view.

The identification of potential Pareto improvements is of course not a simple matter, and in practice neither is the identification of all costs and benefits relevant to any sort of decision maker, real or societal. For that reason, many support economic evaluation as a useful technique even where it falls short of being a full cost–benefit analysis, as it provides at least some useful information. A *partial cost–benefit analysis* usually means that some aspects of cost or benefit have been identified but not valued, and the usefulness of the information depends on whether we believe that if the missing elements were to be valued they would alter the balance of costs and benefits. In real economic evaluations, this is usually dealt with by *sensitivity analysis*, which will be discussed in Chapter 12.

A special case of a partial economic evaluation is where costs are valued but benefits are not. This has a justification on the grounds that it may improve some aspect of efficiency, with other aspects being left to other evaluations. For example, the aim of economic evaluation could be to improve technical efficiency or production allocative efficiency; this enables efficiency in both production and consumption to be achieved, but does not guarantee it. This justification is of course refuted by the theory of second best, described in Chapter 5, but that theory is best regarded as a warning about overconfidence in making recommendations rather than a view that inaction is best. This kind of partial efficiency is dealt with by a different type of economic evaluation known as cost-effectiveness analysis (CEA).

10.2.2 Cost-effectiveness analysis

One rationale for CEA is that whilst costs are usually measured in terms of money, it may be much more difficult to measure benefits that way. Obviously, comparison of costs and benefits that are measured in different units is not straightforward, but a theoretical basis for this can be found in the theory of production efficiency, described in Chapter 3. Recall that the isoquant identifies technically efficient points of production, measured in physical units, and a point where it is at a tangent to an isocost curve is allocatively efficient in production. Cost-effectiveness analysis tries to identify where more benefit can be produced at the same cost or a lower cost can be achieved for the same benefit. The first of these corresponds to a move to the allocatively efficient point from any other point on the same budget line, which must have lower production, and the second from any other point on the same isoquant, which must have a higher cost.

However, there are many cases where we may wish to compare alternatives in which neither benefits nor costs are held constant. In this case, a *cost-effectiveness ratio* (CER) – the cost per unit of output or effect – is calculated to compare the alternatives, with the implication that the lower the *CER* the better. However, such ratios must be used with care, as will be discussed below. Box 10.2 shows an example of a cost-effectiveness analysis of different screening strategies for chlamydia. The *CER* is expressed in terms of the cost per chlamydia infection treated.

BOX 10.2   **A cost-effectiveness analysis of different strategies for chlamydia screening and partner notification in England**

Turner *et al.* (2010) developed a model to assess the cost-effectiveness of different chlamydia screening policies in England. They compared the current screening strategy – the National Chlamydia Screening Programme (NCSP) – with increased efficacy of partner notification (from 0.4 to 0.8 partners per index case) and increased coverage of screening for men (from 8% to 24%). They calculated the direct costs of provision of each strategy and the number of infections treated. The cost per infection treated with each strategy is shown below.

Strategy	Total cost (£ million)	Cost per infection treated (£)
NCSP	46.26	506
Increased partner notification	49.57	449
Increased screening coverage for men	69.17	528

The authors concluded from this that increasing the efficacy of partner notification was cost-effective, but increasing the screening coverage for men was not. The cost per infection treated is not an incremental cost-effectiveness ratio (*ICER*) – see Section 10.5.4. Based on data reported the *ICER* for increased screening for men compared with the NCSP is an order of magnitude greater than the *ICER* for increased efficacy of partner notification compared with the NCSP, as shown below.

Strategy	Total cost (£ million)	Total numbers of infections treated
NCSP	46.26	91 438
Increased partner notification	49.57	110 306
Increased screening coverage for men	69.17	131 113

Comparison	Incremental cost	Incremental effect	ICER
Increased partner notification versus NCSP	3.31	18 868	175
Increased screening coverage for men versus NCSP	22.19	39 675	559

CBA seeks to answer whether or not a particular output is worth the cost. CEA seeks to answer the question of which among two or more alternatives provides the most output for a given cost, or the lowest cost for a given output. CBA therefore asks whether or not we should do things, while CEA asks what is the best way to do things that are worth doing. Although this sounds straightforward, the practice of economic evaluation makes it less so, particularly concerning CEA.

10.3 Economic evaluation applied to health care programmes

Many of these concepts and labels concerning efficiency and economic evaluation have become modified in their application to the economic evaluation of health care interventions. This has largely been the result of a programme of sustained research initiated by Drummond (1980), which has led to many refinements (Drummond *et al.*, 2005). This work began with the aim of classifying existing economic evaluations and continued, via improving reporting standards, to offering guidance about the conduct of evaluation using consistent methods. These modifications have been extremely useful and are largely compatible with orthodox economic theories of cost–benefit analysis, but as used in practice they have occasionally been the source of some confusion and dispute, examples of which are discussed below. As noted earlier, they have been strongly influenced by non-economic evaluation techniques and have also increasingly been influenced by concepts arising from *decision analysis* – to be discussed below – and statistical considerations.

The major preoccupation of economic evaluation in health care has been measurement of costs and benefits – what should be measured and how it should be measured – rather than the aims of the analysis. Although this focus is obviously essential in enabling applied economic analysis, it has had the unfortunate consequence that techniques such as CBA and CEA are, as we will see, defined by measurement rather than economic theory. This potentially leads to problems in interpreting and using results from such studies, since there is no guide from theory as to how we should do that.

Recall that production and cost functions, analysed in Chapter 3, relate inputs to outputs and define the efficiency aspects of the relationship. Economic evaluation essentially attempts to quantify them. If inputs and outputs are measured in 'physical' units, then we are dealing with technical efficiency. If inputs are valued and outputs remain in physical units, we have a cost function and we are dealing with production allocative efficiency, and therefore with CEA. If both inputs and outputs are valued, then we are dealing with overall allocative efficiency and therefore CBA. This measurement principle for classification of types of economic evaluation forms a valuable link between economic theory and measurement.

The literature on economic evaluation in health care does not use this measurement principle. It largely uses the term CBA to mean any comparison of costs with benefits where both are measured in money, on the pragmatic grounds that money is the only plausible measure of economic value in modern economies, rather than being defined by its aims. Similarly, CEA is used to mean any comparison of costs and benefits where benefits are measured in units other than money; it is not usually based on the theory of production and is not restricted to comparisons of alternatives that have the same cost or level of output. In fact, much of the economic evaluation literature gives the label *cost-minimisation analysis* to what was traditionally called CEA, and specifically restricts the term CEA to choices between alternatives that have similar types of effects but differing levels of effect and costs. CEA is also occasionally described as an evaluation of technical efficiency, but that is incorrect both in theory and in normal practice.

It can be difficult to specify what the appropriate measure of effect is in CEA. For example, suppose we have a comparison that involves a treatment that prevents heart disease. In one in every 20 cases of disease the person suffers a heart attack; half of those who suffer a heart attack die, which leads on average to a loss of 5 years of life. Suppose that the treatment costs £50 000 to prevent 20 cases. The *CER* could be defined as £2 500 per case prevented, £50 000 per heart attack prevented, £100 000 per death averted or £20 000 per life year saved.

In comparisons between interventions that deal with the same illness, it may not matter which of these is chosen, but care is still required to ensure that whichever measure of effect is chosen does not mislead or bias the analysis – for example, if one intervention is better at preventing non-fatal heart attacks but is worse at preventing fatal attacks, the choice of effect measure will be crucial. A more difficult issue is raised if it is recognised that the main output of health care interventions is changes in health itself, recalling that the aim of CEA is to increase output with given costs or lower costs for the same output. It follows that the measure of effect should be one which can be used for all types of illnesses and all types of health care.

The issues that arise in constructing health measures for use in economic evaluation are considered in more detail in Chapter 11. However, such indicators are usually measures of the *value* of health, although not usually expressed in money terms. As a result, a third important type of economic evaluation has arisen, called *cost–utility analysis* (CUA). This label has been given in recognition of the fact that economists often use the word utility to mean value but, as we will discuss in Chapter 11, the precise meaning of this is the subject of some dispute. In addition, the health measure usually used in CUA is gains in *quality-adjusted life years* (QALYs); this will again be discussed in detail in the next chapter, but it is essentially a composite measure of gains in life expectancy and health-related quality of life. Box 10.3 shows an example of a CUA of a cervical cancer vaccination programme.

BOX 10.3   **A cost-utility analysis of cervical cancer vaccination in preadolescent females in Canada**

Anonychuk *et al.* (2009) investigated the cost-effectiveness of vaccinating 12-year-old girls for cervical cancer. Evidence shows that some human papillomavirus (HPV) types are important causal factors for this type of cancer. The authors assess the cost-effectiveness of a vaccine for HPV 16 and HPV 18. The vaccine has also been shown to protect against other HPV types that contribute to cervical cancer and the authors investigated the impact of this cross-protection. They also estimated herd immunity effects, since by reducing the amount of HPV transmission in the population vaccination also reduces the risk of infection to non-vaccinated people.

Results were calculated for 100 000 12-year-old girls. Vaccination was calculated to prevent between 390 and 633 cases of cervical cancer, and 168 and 175 deaths, depending on whether or not herd immunity effects and cross-protection against other types of HPV were included. The costs and QALYs associated with vaccination and no vaccination are shown below.

	Non-vaccinated	Vaccinated	Difference	ICER
No herd immunity				
HPV 16/18				
Total cost (Can$)	476	739	263	
Total QALYs	30.5015	30.5098	0.0083	31 687
HPV 16/18 + cross-protection				
Total cost (Can$)	476	732	256	
Total QALYs	30.5015	30.5110	0.0095	26 947
With herd immunity				
HPV 16/18				
Total cost (Can$)	476	735	259	
Total QALYs	30.5015	30.5108	0.0093	27 849
HPV 16/18 + cross-protection				
Total cost (Can$)	476	715	239	
Total QALYs	30.5015	30.5143	0.0128	18 672

Compared with no vaccination, vaccinating 100 000 girls aged 12 years resulted in incremental costs of Can$256 to Can$263 per person and incremental QALYs gained of 0.0083 to 0.0095 per person over the lifetime of the cohort. The resulting *ICERs* – see Section 10.5.4 – for vaccination were Can$26 947 to Can$31 687 depending on whether or not cross-protection was included. The inclusion of herd immunity reduced the *ICER* by 12% to 31%. The authors concluded that the vaccine reduced cancer cases and mortality and was cost-effective.

Viewed in this way, CUA is an extended and very useful form of CEA that can be used to judge which health care interventions should be undertaken within a given health budget. However, drawing on the measurement principle discussed earlier, CUA is often regarded as a simplified form of CBA because of its valued-output basis; it requires only a money value to be placed on effects to be able to judge whether or not health interventions should be undertaken, irrespective of the budget available. This issue has led to considerable dispute about the status of CUA – is it extended CEA or restricted CBA?

Because of the particular way in which CEA has been applied in health economics, both CEA and CUA in practice usually produce estimates of the observed cost of achieving different levels of output. The difference between the two is that CEA relates to the output of particular types of health care and CUA to the output of health care as a whole, so neither is a full social CBA that takes account of the wider economy as well. However, both could be interpreted as partial CBA or form part of a full CBA. So a plausible answer is that CUA is *both* extended CEA *and* restricted CBA.

10.4 Decision rules for cost–benefit analysis

The purpose of economic evaluation is to provide information to make decisions in a structured way. An important part of that structure is to state what those decisions should be, given a particular balance of costs and benefits. These are known as *decision rules*: if we find that the costs and benefits have a particular pattern, then we should take a particular decision. Some of these rules are very simple and obvious; others are extremely complicated.

The simplest rule is the basic one for cost–benefit analysis. If the sum of the benefits of an activity is greater than the sum of its costs, then on efficiency grounds the activity should be undertaken; if costs are higher, it should not; and if they are equal it does not matter either way. Alternative ways of expressing this, which mean exactly the same thing, are that the activity should be undertaken if its *net benefit* – the difference between benefits and costs – is positive or that its *benefit/cost ratio* is greater than 1. As will be explained in Chapter 12, because costs and benefits are often incurred over time, the net benefit criterion is actually usually expressed as a *net present value*, which is the difference between all benefits and costs at all times, expressed in today's values.

This decision rule assumes that any activity that has a net benefit *can* be done. But this may not be true if only some activities can be done and there are imperfect capital markets to provide the necessary investment. For example, it may be that on cost–benefit grounds a health authority ought to build new premises for all of its general practices, new clinics for all of its community services and substantially upgrade all of its hospitals. However, it may have only limited funds available in any year to do that. As a result, it has to choose between its different investments.

If only one activity can be undertaken, then the rule is again obvious: choose the activity with the highest net benefit. Otherwise, decision making becomes far more complex. This problem is a failure of the assumption that costs fully represent opportunity costs, and account needs to be taken of the fact that the opportunity cost of each activity is that others cannot be undertaken. The aim will be to produce the greatest excess of benefits over costs from all of the projects that have the potential to produce net benefits. Unfortunately, that cannot usually be determined by a simple rule such as ranking in order of net benefit or benefit/cost ratio; but there are mathematical methods that may make it possible to find a solution that gives the optimum combination of activities.

10.5 Decision rules for cost-effectiveness and cost-utility analysis

Because CEA does not give a direct comparison between the value of effects and costs, decision rules are far more complex than for CBA and are bounded by restrictions on their applicability. The problem arises when the alternatives being appraised do not have equal costs or benefits, but instead there is a trade-off: the greater benefit that one of the alternatives has is achieved at a higher cost. The key problem is how that trade-off is to be represented, and how it can then be interpreted; essentially, encapsulating cost-effectiveness in a single index that can unambiguously be interpreted for decision-making purposes. Three approaches to this have been developed: cost-effectiveness ratios; the net benefit approach; and the probabilistic approach. A framework for investigating treatment decisions that lends itself to economic evaluation is decision analysis. This technique, which will be discussed in more detail in Chapter 12, constructs a model of decision making as a sequential process that may have several different outcomes depending on choices that are made and the results of uncertain events. What this adds to the issue of decision rules is that the values attached to costs, benefits, net benefits and *CER*s are expected values, rather than values that can be calculated with certainty. This is entirely reasonable given the uncertainty attached to medical outcomes.

10.5.1 Ratio measures

The cost-effectiveness ratio (*CER*) – the cost per unit of output or effect – is the most popular measure of an activity's cost-effectiveness, with the implication that the lower the *CER* the better. Given an activity (a health care intervention or treatment), a and its best alternative b, with costs C_a and C_b and effects E_a and E_b, respectively, the CER for activity a is

$$CER = (C_a - C_b)/(E_a - E_b) = \Delta C/\Delta E \qquad (10.1)$$

The numerator of the CER is sometimes called the incremental cost of a relative to b and the denominator is the incremental effect.

10.5.2 The cost-effectiveness plane

A useful way of showing the decision rules that apply to the CER is the *cost-effectiveness plane* (Black, 1990), shown in Figure 10.1. This diagram shows the costs and the effects of an activity compared to some alternative, with costs on the north–south axis and effects on the east–west axis. The east–west line indicates zero additional costs and the north-south line indicates zero additional effects. North of the zero additional cost line, costs are higher and to the south lower; east of the zero additional effect line, effects are higher and to the west lower. These lines divide all possible cost and effect combinations into four quadrants. To the north-west, costs are higher and effects are lower, so the activity is worse in all dimensions and is said to be *dominated* by its alternatives and should not be used on efficiency grounds. To the south-east, costs are lower and effects are greater, so the activity *dominates* its alternatives and should be used on efficiency grounds. In the other two quadrants, either greater effectiveness is gained at a higher cost, as in the north-east quadrant, or a reduction in costs is achieved at the expense of lower effects, as in the south-west quadrant. In these two quadrants, whether or not the activity should be undertaken on efficiency grounds depends on the trade-off between costs and effects.

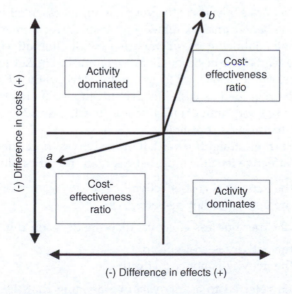

Figure 10.1 The cost-effectiveness plane

The *CER* of an activity can be represented on this diagram as the slope of a line from the origin, which represents the costs and effects of the alternative, to its cost/effect combination. Two such lines are demonstrated, one in the south-west from the origin to point *a*, and one in the north-east to point *b*. These have been depicted as rays, emphasising that all points on each line represent the same *CER*. These *CER*s are positive; those in the other two quadrants are negative.

What are the decision rules for the south-west and north-east quadrants? Without extra information on the acceptable size of the trade-off between effects and costs, we cannot say that any activities within them should be undertaken. It is tempting to conclude that if two activities have different *CER*s then the one with the lowest *CER* is more cost-effective and should be chosen. However, this is not necessarily the case. Strictly, *CER*s can be used to compare alternatives only if these can be scaled up or down to achieve the same costs or effects, without affecting the *CER*. In terms of production relationships, this requires there to be constant returns to scale and no indivisibilities.

These problems are even greater if the *CER* is based on CUA – strictly speaking, whenever the same measure of effectiveness is generic to all activities – because the scope of comparisons is then much wider. In this case, the same problems apply as with benefit/cost ratios: if it is not possible to undertake all activities, choosing them in order of *CER* from lowest to highest may not produce the combination of activities that produces the highest output from the available funds. However, as with benefit/cost ratios, it is in principle possible to determine from a complete set of cost and effect data the optimum combination of activities to maximise the improvements in health from a given health care budget or to minimise the total cost of achieving a particular level of health.

10.5.3 The cost-effectiveness threshold and acceptability

Although cost-effectiveness analysis can be very useful, its essential inability to help in the kind of choices that cost–benefit analysis allows – an absolute recommendation for a particular activity rather than one contingent on a comparison with alternatives – has proved such a strong limitation that means have been sought to overcome it. The key to this has been the *cost-effectiveness threshold* or *ceiling ratio*, which is essentially a level of the *CER* that any intervention must meet if it is to be regarded as cost-effective. It can also be interpreted as the decision maker's willingness to pay for a unit of effectiveness. In Chapter 13 we discuss approaches to identifying the cost-effectiveness threshold.

The decision rule is then straightforward. If the activity is more effective but a higher cost, then for it to be cost-effective its *CER* must be less than the threshold, R_c:

If $R_c > \Delta C/\Delta E$, the activity is cost-effective.
If $R_c < \Delta C/\Delta E$, the activity is not cost-effective.

If the activity is cheaper but less effective, then the decision rule is reversed:

If $R_c < \Delta C/\Delta E$, the activity is cost-effective.
If $R_c > \Delta C/\Delta E$, the activity is not cost-effective.

This issue is often referred to as *acceptability*, meaning that the activity is acceptable on cost-effectiveness grounds. It can be depicted using the cost-effectiveness plane, as in Figure 10.2. The four quadrants are replaced by a simple dichotomy – is the activity

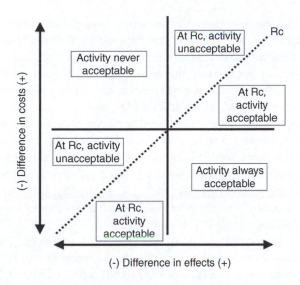

Figure 10.2 Cost-effectiveness acceptability

above the line, in which case it is not acceptable, or below the line, in which case it is? Within these halves, the only distinction, which is suppressed, is whether the activity would always be acceptable or unacceptable or its acceptability is contingent on the size of the ceiling ratio.

One of the problems with this kind of approach is that it is no longer consistent with the conventional aim of CEA. Except under special conditions, it is not consistent with output maximisation constrained by a budget. This emphasises further the issue of whether CEA and CUA are really reduced versions of CBA or are to be accepted as suitable only for a restricted range of decisions.

10.5.4 The incremental cost-effectiveness ratio

So far, we have discussed the *CER* with respect to a comparison of an activity with an alternative, without stating what that comparator is except that it should be the *best* alternative. It is useful to distinguish between a comparator that is essentially 'do nothing about the problem with which the activity deals and which incurs no costs or benefits' and one that is 'another way of doing something about that problem'. The *CER* that arises from the second of these is sometimes called an *incremental cost-effectiveness ratio* (*ICER*) and again there are arguments about the circumstances in which these two comparators should be used, assuming that they are different. However, in most cases the *ICER* is the correct measure to use.

An argument for using the *ICER* is as follows. Suppose that we have a screening programme that can be implemented using one test or two sequential tests. Because of the nature of tests, the first will pick up most of the cases of interest and the second will pick up fewer cases. In this case, the first test detects 10 cases and the second two, so the one-test screen yields 10 cases and the two-test screen yields 12 cases. The cost of each test is the same, whether it is done singly or sequentially, so carrying out two tests costs almost twice as much in total as carrying out one test, the only reduction being due to not screening those cases found in the first test. In this case, the total costs are £100 000 and £80 000, respectively, so the two-test screen costs £180 000. The *CER* for the one-test screen against 'do nothing' is £10 000 per case detected. The *CER* for the two-test screen is £15 000 per case detected. If the ceiling ratio is £35 000 per case detected, the two-test screen, although it does not have as favourable a *CER* as the one-test screen, is still at an acceptable level.

However, the proper way to view the two-test screen is that it is a one-test screen with an additional test. The extra cost of the second test converting the one-test screen to a two-test screen is £80 000 and the extra benefit is two cases; the *ICER* is therefore £40 000, which is in excess of the ceiling ratio. The two-test screen is not cost-effective. The *CER* of the two-test screen against 'do nothing' is an average of the *CER*s of the first test and the second test and is clearly misleading. Torgerson and Spencer (1995) gave more examples of potential problems of this kind that might arise if the *ICER* is not used.

Even where there is, strictly speaking, no averaging involved, the *ICER* usually gives more useful information. Suppose that we have two interventions for a particular disease: drugs and surgery. Currently, surgery is performed at a cost of £100 000 and patients live on average five years longer as a result. The *CER* is therefore £20 000 per life year gained. The drug costs £210 000 and on average patients live seven years longer. The *CER* is therefore £30 000. Comparing the two directly in an incremental analysis of drugs relative to surgery, the drug costs an additional £110 000 and gains two additional life years, giving an *ICER* of £55 000. We are using a ceiling ratio of £35 000 per life year gained. Should the drug be provided? The *ICER* gives the correct conclusion that it should not.

What if, for a different illness, there is a drug that has no alternative but has exactly the same costs and benefits as the one that the *ICER* suggested should be rejected? This second drug would be accepted, which on the face of it seems illogical. But it is simply because there is no more cost-effective way of treating patients with the second illness, while there is for the first.

A problem is that if only the *ICER* is evaluated, it must be assumed that the alternative used in the comparator is itself cost-effective; if it is not, the *ICER* may mislead. Suppose in the example above that the cost of surgery was £250 000 and the drug cost was £280 000. The *ICER* for the drug is £30 000/2, giving an acceptable £15 000. However, evaluated against no treatment, the *CER*s are £50 000 for surgery and £40 000 for the drug, neither of which is acceptable. The *ICER* and apparent cost-effectiveness of the drug is an artefact of the inefficiency of the surgical treatment currently used. The optimal solution would be to provide neither.

It is common in economic evaluations to compare more than two mutually exclusive alternatives. In this case the decision rules become even more complicated. Box 10.4 describes a study by Hallinen *et al.* (2010) which illustrates how alternative health care programmes, where each patient will receive only one of the alternative treatments, should be compared. The correct procedure is as follows:

1. Rank the options in order of increasing cost.
2. Eliminate options for which another option is cheaper and more effective, known as *simple dominance*.
3. Eliminate options where a combination of two other options is cheaper and more effective, known as *extended dominance*.

4. Calculate the incremental cost and incremental effect of each remaining option with respect to the previous option in the list.
5. Calculate *ICER*s for the remaining options.

In summary, *CER*s are valuable indicators of cost-effectiveness but they do need careful handling and are prone to misuse, particularly with an inappropriate choice of comparator. A further issue, which will be discussed in Chapter 12, is that the *CER* has many undesirable mathematical and statistical properties that add to the difficulties of using it.

BOX 10.4   **Treatment of rheumatoid arthritis in Finland**

Hallinen *et al.* (2010) investigated the cost-effectiveness of different treatment strategies for patients with rheumatoid arthritis in Finland in whom tumour necrosis factor (TNF-) inhibitors had failed. The baseline treatment was best supportive care (BSC). A number of scenarios were considered. In the first, BSC was compared against treatment with adalimumab (ADAL), abatacept (ABAT), etanercept (ETAN), infliximab (INFL) or rituximab (RTX) followed by BSC after drug treatment failure. In the second scenario, another drug treatment was added after the first when it failed followed by BSC. In the third scenario, a third drug treatment was added. All patients received methotrexate (MTX). The costs and benefits of each combination are shown below.

Scenario	Intervention	Cost (€)	Effect (QALYs)	ICER vs. intervention with lowest ICER in previous scenario*	ICER
0	*BSC*	*85 714*	*2.69*	Baseline	Baseline
1	INFL-BSC	102 558	3.15	36 121	Ext. Dom.
	RTX-BSC	*106 921*	*3.39*	*30 248*	30 248
	ADAL-BSC	111 195	3.19	50 941	Dom.
	ETAN-BSC	112 546	3.22	50 372	Dom.
	ABAT-BSC	127 580	3.31	67 003	Dom.
2	*RTX-INFL-BSC*	*120 946*	*3.77*	*37 013*	37 013
	RTX-ADAL-BSC	128 053	3.79	52 021	Ext. Dom.
	RTX-ETAN-BSC	130 258	3.83	52 698	Ext. Dom.
	RTX-ABAT-BSC	142 335	3.91	68 100	Ext. Dom.
3	RTX-INFL-ADAL-BSC	141 541	4.14	54 701	54 701
	RTX-INFL-ETAN-BSC	143 686	4.18	54 836	Ext. Dom.
	RTX-INFL-ABAT-BSC	155 493	4.26	70 616	Ext. Dom.

*Shown in bold italics
'Dom.' means that the option is eliminated by simple dominance.
'Ext. Dom.' means that the option is eliminated by extended dominance.

In each scenario treatments were ranked in order of increasing cost. Treatments that were more costly and less effective were excluded by simple dominance (e.g., ADAL-BSC compared with RTX-BSC). Treatments that had a higher *ICER* compared to a treatment lower down the ranking were excluded by extended dominance (e.g., INFL-BSC compared with RTX-BSC). The results show that if the cost-effectiveness threshold was €50 000 per QALY gained, then rituximab followed by infliximab followed by best supportive care would be cost-effective.

10.5.5 Net benefits

With all of the problems attached to *CER*s, it is not surprising that there have been challenges to their dominance. The most prominent of these is the net-benefit approach (Stinnett and Mullahy, 1998), which essentially restores the original concept of a cost–benefit analysis without the necessity of imposing a welfarist framework. Strangely, this was not mainly because of the theoretical problems of the *CER* but because of the undesirable mathematical and statistical properties referred to. The aim of this approach is to obtain a single number that is not a ratio. Recall that the *CER* is defined as $\Delta C / \Delta E$ where ΔC is measured in monetary terms and ΔE is not.

The net benefit of an activity is defined as $\Delta E - \Delta C$, where ΔC and ΔE are measured in the same units. In order to convert costs and effects to the same units, the net benefit approach relies on the use of the ceiling ratio (R_c) as an implicit value that is attached to a unit of effect. R_c can therefore be used as an exchange rate factor between costs and effects; it can be used to convert costs to the same units as effects, or effects to the same units as costs. If effects are converted, this results in *monetary net benefit* (*MNB*), defined as

$$MNB = (R_c)(\Delta E) - \Delta C \tag{10.2}$$

If costs are converted, this results in *health net benefit* (*HNB*), defined as

$$HNB = \Delta E - \Delta C / R_c \tag{10.3}$$

The decision rule is then straightforward. For *MNB*:

If $(R_c)(\Delta E) - \Delta C > 0$, the activity is cost-effective.
If $(R_c)(\Delta E) - \Delta C < 0$, the activity is not cost-effective.

For *HNB*:
If $\Delta E - \Delta C / R_c > 0$, the activity is cost-effective.
If $\Delta E - \Delta C / R_c < 0$, the activity is cost-effective.

The question is, however, which R_c should be used? If an organisation sets a specific value for this, then there is no problem. However, if we do not have such a value it is necessary to report the net benefit for each value of R_c. Figure 10.3 illustrates this for both *MNB* and *HNB*. The activity is cost-effective if R_c is above £10 000 per unit of effectiveness.

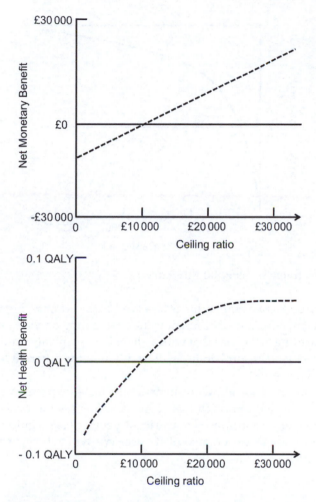

Figure 10.3 Net benefit curves

Of course, this gives exactly the same results as using *CER*s for a given level of R_c. It is also arguable that this is in effect CBA, although not of course of the full Paretian variety. On all of these grounds, the net benefit approach has considerable merits; further consideration of these in the context of statistical approaches to CEA will be discussed in Chapter 12.

10.5.6 Probabilistic approaches

Another response to the difficult properties of the *CER* is the cost-effectiveness acceptability curve (CEAC) (van Hout *et al.*, 1994). This again makes use of the cost-effectiveness threshold and the concept of acceptability described earlier. A full treatment of this is given in Chapter 12; here we note only the essentials with respect to decision rules. The *CER* is retained as the measure of cost-effectiveness and this is compared with a ceiling ratio. However, the

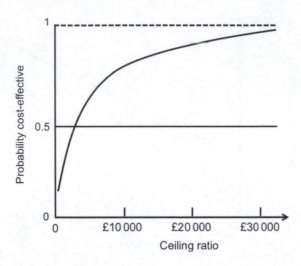

Figure 10.4 Cost-effectiveness acceptability curve

CER is no longer regarded as a number that is observed with certainty, but as a variable whose mean is observed. That mean can take different values depending on the sample of observations on which it is based, leading to the idea that with a given R_c we can only state the probability that the activity is cost-effective. This probability will be different for different levels of R_c. This can be represented as in Figure 10.4.

The CEAC has the merit of allowing uncertainty to be expressed while retaining the familiar concept of a *CER*. But although the CEAC is an interesting concept, it is difficult to know how decision makers are supposed to use it. As yet there is no guide to how to read and use a CEAC, and not enough experience of its use. We will return to this in Chapter 12, showing how in practice it is constructed.

10.6 Equity in economic evaluation

Despite the acceptance by most economists that the equity implications of decisions may be as important as efficiency issues, there is little in the way of formal evaluation of equity and nothing like the standardised quantitative routines that have been developed for efficiency measurement. However, there are some very important equity issues. The reason is that efficiency evaluations deal only with the amounts of resources used and the outputs achieved with them, not how these are distributed between different people, either individuals or groups in society. Most obviously, as was discussed in Chapter 9, a potential Pareto improvement may involve net gainers and net losers but does not require compensation to be paid from the first of these to the second. It also does not distinguish between programmes that redistribute benefits from the relatively poor to the relatively rich or from the rich to the poor, from the relatively sick to the relatively healthy or from the healthy to the sick, or that are neutral with respect to these groups. Even a Pareto improvement may require analysis of distributional effects if a goal in society is to change the distribution of costs and benefits in some way, for example to achieve greater equality in health at the expense of overall levels of health.

As an example of this in health care, the most commonly used practice in CUA is to use the QALY and moreover to assume that each QALY is worth the same irrespective of who gains it and by what route. This is utilitarian in practice if not by design. Similarly, CBA in practice focuses on sums of benefits compared to sums of costs, not on the distribution of these between people with different characteristics. It also does not usually take account of whether society places different weights on benefits experienced by different people; for example, there is evidence that many people would prefer health services to put a higher priority on improving the health of younger rather than older people (Tsuchiya *et al.*, 2003). Such distributional issues were discussed in Chapters 7 and 9 and will be considered in more detail in Chapter 13, including the issue of equity and QALYs.

Summary

1. Economic evaluation is a structured approach to help decision makers choose between alternative ways of using resources. It is largely concerned with measuring efficiency in areas where there is public involvement and there are no market-based measures available to judge this. The general term used for this in economics is cost–benefit analysis (CBA), which is used in investment appraisal.

2. Cost–benefit analysis involves constructing an inventory of all costs and benefits of an alternative, whatever they are and whoever incurs them; this forms a balance sheet in which they are weighed against each other. This is only possible if all costs and benefits are measured in the same unit; the obvious one is money as the measure of value most used in modern economies.

3. Cost-effectiveness analysis (CEA) is a partial form of cost–benefit analysis. The rationale for CEA is that while costs are usually measured in terms of money, it may be much more difficult to measure benefits that way. In health economics, cost-effectiveness analysis tries to identify where more health benefit can be produced at the same cost, or where a lower cost can be achieved for the same health benefit. A theoretical basis for this can be found in the theory of production efficiency.

4. Cost–utility analysis (CUA) is a form of economic evaluation in which health benefits are usually measured in terms of quality-adjusted life years (QALYs). These are a composite measure of gains in life expectancy and health-related quality of life.

5. In cost–benefit analysis the main decision rule is to undertake an activity if the sum of the benefits is greater than the sum of the costs or, equivalently, if the net benefit is positive. If only one activity with a positive net benefit can be undertaken (for example, if there are limited available funds), then the appropriate rule is to choose the activity with the highest net benefit.

6. In CEA (and CUA) a direct comparison between the value of effects and costs is not possible. The cost-effectiveness ratio (*CER*) measures the incremental cost of an activity relative to its best alternative divided by the incremental effect. The *CER* is used in decision making; it is compared to a ceiling ratio, which is a level of the *CER* that any intervention must meet if it is to be regarded as cost-effective.

7. *CER*s can be presented graphically on a cost-effectiveness plane, which shows the costs and the effects of an activity compared to some alternative, with costs on the north–south axis and effects on the east–west axis.

8. It is important to measure the *CER* correctly as a comparison with the best alternative rather than some other alternative. Because the costs and effects are incremental to the best alternative, it is often known as an incremental cost-effectiveness ratio (*ICER*).

9. *CER*s can be converted into monetary net benefit and health net benefit measures, using the ceiling ratio to convert incremental costs to incremental benefits or vice versa.

10. Cost-effectiveness acceptability curves account for statistical uncertainty in the *CER* and uncertainty in the ceiling ratio by presenting the probability that an intervention is cost-effective for different levels of the ceiling ratio.

11. Equity issues – the way in which health and health gains are distributed among peoples – are as important as efficiency concerns, yet theory and methods for addressing these within the practice of economic evaluation remain underdeveloped.

CHAPTER **11**

Measuring and valuing health care output

11.1 Introduction

In Chapter 3, we discussed how the output of health care can be defined either as the amount of care provided or the health that results from it. As before, we will regard both of these as valid concepts of output. Our focus in this chapter is how each type of output can be measured, with a particular focus on the use of these measures in economic evaluation. As mentioned in Chapter 10, we will also have a special interest in how output can be valued, rather than simply counted.

In most areas of economics, output measurement is relatively straightforward and valuing that output usually poses no real conceptual difficulties. For example, in the pharmaceutical manufacturing industry, output can be measured in physical terms, such as the quantity of drugs produced, and in value terms as the market value of drugs produced. But when a health professional uses these products to treat a particular illness, output measurement becomes more difficult. What is the measure of quantity? Is it numbers of treatments or improvements in health? How should improvements in health be measured? How are these to be valued? As discussed in Chapter 5, the economic conditions under which health care is usually traded are unusual and may mean that the market may not generate information from which measures of value can be calculated. A further difficulty is that health improvements cannot be directly sold in a market at all.

11.2 Monetary valuations of health care benefits

In Chapter 9, the concepts of *equivalent variation*, *compensating variation*, *willingness to pay* and *willingness to accept* were introduced as means of measuring welfare changes as a result of changes in resource allocation. These are the most usual means of measuring welfare changes in economics, and have money as their natural unit of value. They are the basis of the benefit side of cost–benefit analysis, providing estimates of changes in *consumer surplus*, the difference between what people pay and are willing to pay. In applying these theoretical concepts to the practical measurement of benefits, there are two broad approaches, known as *revealed preference* and *stated preference*.

11.2.1 Revealed preference

Revealed preference (RP) refers to valuations of goods and services that can be inferred from real choices that are made in the everyday world. It is based on the theory that the choices that people make arise from a comparison of the benefits of alternatives with their opportunity costs. People assess these benefits in accordance with their preferences. The choices that they make therefore reveal their preferences. For example, if we observe that someone will not purchase a dental check-up for £20 but will do so for £10, we can infer that the value they place upon a dental check-up lies between £10 and £20. If we were able to vary prices between these two limits and observe their choices, we would be able to make a more precise estimate of this value, their maximum willingness to pay for a check-up.

Usually, however, we are concerned with estimating the value of a good or service not to one person but to everyone who might consume it. We are more interested in what is demanded by all consumers at different prices. If patients attach different values to a dental check-up, then different numbers of them will choose to pay for one at different prices – which is, of course, the basis of the demand curve. Their average valuation of a dental check-up – their average willingness to pay – can be inferred from a market demand curve using the same reasoning as for individual consumers' demand curves.

One problem with using RP is that in cost–benefit analysis we are most often interested in markets where prices are not directly charged or do not reflect values. For example, health care is often free at the point of consumption or highly subsidised, which poses obvious difficulties for estimating a demand curve. Moreover, if we are interested in obtaining the value of health improvements, as opposed to the value of health services, then we cannot use RP directly as that commodity is not directly traded and has no market. However, there is another way of obtaining RP valuations, which is to search for other ways in which people make trade-offs between money and health care or health. Within this, there are two distinct methods, which have different justifications.

The first method is based on the observation that people may have to incur a number of different costs to obtain a good or service, not just its purchase price at the point of consumption. For example, even if a visit to a general practitioner is free, people may incur monetary outlays, such as the cost of travel to the surgery, and other opportunity costs, such as the cost of their time. If these user costs have an effect on demand similar to that we would observe with a purchase price, then it may be possible to derive a demand curve and to infer valuations from that.

The second method is based on the possibility that even if there is no direct market for a good or service, its benefits can be inferred from other markets in which those benefits are also assessed. If we are interested in measuring the value of changes in health as part of an assessment of the benefits of health care, it might be impossible to do that if health care is provided free. However, it may be possible to observe choices in markets where alterations in health are one of the outcomes, for example by observing wage differentials in labour markets between highly risky and less risky jobs (Viscusi, 2004), or by examining individual consumption decisions for goods that reduce the risk of ill health. The valuations of health that those choices reveal could then be used in an economic evaluation of health care. For example, suppose that we quantified a relationship between incomes and job characteristics like occupation and industry as well as the risk of death from a workplace accident. If we found that, all else being equal, an increase in the probability of death of 0.001 was associated with £5 000 higher incomes this indicates that the value of a life is £5 000/0.001 = £5 000 000.

11.2.2 Stated preference

Stated preference (SP) valuations are derived from surveys or experiments, which are often loosely known in health economics as willingness to pay (WTP) studies. These may simply ask people to give values directly, or infer them indirectly by, for example, offering people hypothetical choices and observing their responses. SP relies on the assumptions that the values that people state are really those that underlie their choices in the everyday world, and that the choices that they make within the survey are those that they would make if they were really faced with the alternatives offered. Unlike RP, the validity of which is based on economic reasoning, the main theoretical basis of SP is psychological and this makes SP controversial. An extreme view, associated with Austrian economics, is that only choices in the market have relevance to economic analysis; valuations derived from psychological experiments may be of interest but refer to an entirely different phenomenon from that which is relevant to economics. However, most economists seem to agree that it is acceptable to use SP techniques, as long as they are consistent with the aims of economic analysis.

Alternatives include surveys that are basically referendums on the issues. Others include simulated markets, in which the goods are actually provided under experimental conditions – for a health care example, see Bhatia and Fox-Rushby (2003). However, the most widely recognised technique is the *contingent valuation method* (CVM). This refers to the valuation of a good or service, the measurement of value being contingent on the description of the hypothetical market that is given to respondents.

In health economics, stated preference techniques have been used both for the measurement of the value of *health care* and for the valuation of *health*. Applications to health are considered separately below and here we concentrate on the application of contingent valuation to health *care*. Moreover, we will concentrate on contingent valuation studies in which respondents are asked for their *willingness to pay* for health care. In Section 11.8, we will discuss some alternatives to this in the context of valuations of health.

The most important issue in contingent valuation is ensuring that the values that are obtained from it are credible to those whose actions will be informed by any evaluation that uses them. The respondents must understand the market scenarios that are presented to them and find them plausible and meaningful. Otherwise, they will have no idea how to respond to the questions that are asked of them and may even not attempt to give serious answers to them. Among the elements regarded as essential are: descriptions, in sufficient detail to be understandable, plausible and meaningful, of the nature of the good or service that respondents would receive; how they would obtain it; and, how they would pay for it. The last of these, to be credible, must allow respondents to believe that they might actually be asked to do so. Other important features are to ensure that the sample used is representative of everyone who might be affected; that the exercise could be undertaken equally well by all of them; and that the purpose of the study is explained, again so that they provide serious and thoughtful responses. However, the information provided must be the minimum possible, to avoid respondents being overburdened, and must contain nothing irrelevant that might distract respondents.

SP techniques have been refined so that there are best practice guidelines available for conducting contingent valuation studies; for example, Pearce and Özdemiroglu (2002). Within health care, there are no universally accepted approaches to CVM studies, but Gafni (1991) has published a very strongly argued set of guidelines, which include the following elements.

- People cannot plan to consume health care, so their willingness to pay should be expressed as an insurance premium that must be paid so that the service is available if they need it. Furthermore, the scenario should state the probability that they will need it.
- Treatment effects should also be explained in probabilistic terms – the probability of success or failure.
- The willingness to pay of all members of the relevant population is required, so the survey should have a representative sample.

There are a number of well-known problems with contingent valuation studies that arise from the artificial nature of the choices that respondents have to make. We assume that in making choices in real life what matters to consumers is the trade-off between the benefits of the good being bought and its cost; their choice may of course be influenced by the environment in which they make the choice, but that is part of the market. In an experiment or survey, the respondent may still behave as a rational consumer, but the environment in which they make choices will not be a market; their choices may be influenced by utility derived from interactions with researchers rather than providers. In fact, we might expect rational consumers to behave in such a way, offering answers to questions that are strategic. For example, if they believe that they will be asked to pay for the good at some future time and that the study's results will be used to set prices, they have an incentive to state a lower WTP than they would really pay. Alternatively, if they believe that they will not be asked to pay and the study will simply be used to decide on whether or not the good or service should be provided free, they have an incentive to overstate their WTP.

Other problems may arise from respondents being unable to share the researchers' aims. For example, if they do not know or care about their WTP for something that they have never had to pay for or even encountered before, they may resort to a face-saving strategy that will please the researcher. For example, it may be embarrassing to reveal that they in fact know, understand or care little or nothing about something that is clearly of importance, and therefore guess at high WTP. They may seek guidance from interviewers, who must avoid giving any implied cues. Finally, there are a number of problems in making the market scenario realistic; for example, that if someone states that their WTP is £500, they understand that this will reduce their real income by that amount, and they will have £500 less to spend on other things.

Willingness to pay questions can be expressed in different ways, which may deal with some of these problems or possibly cause them! Box 11.1 shows two examples of how WTP questions have been asked, which illustrates some of the issues that researchers have to face.

These UK examples demonstrate well some of the problems that willingness to pay studies have and some ways of solving them. A particular problem in the UK is that researchers are not ethically allowed to imply that services that are currently free might in the future be charged for, which makes describing the context very difficult. Both examples attempt to explain what the task is about by describing it as a way of finding out how much people value things. The first example does try to describe the market context by reference to

---

BOX 11.1   Willingness to pay questions

Here are two examples of willingness to pay questions:

Example 1: Bone scans (Donaldson *et al.* 1997)

"We want to know how much women value the bone scan. A way of finding out the value of things, like the bone scan, is to ask what people would pay for it. Of course, the bone scan is free and will stay free. But imagine you lived in a country where you had to pay for the scan.

Before you answer, think about the scan you have just had. Also, remember the results of the scan will help you and your doctor to decide whether you need help to keep your bones in order.

What is the most that you would pay to have the scan?"

Example 2: *In Vitro* Fertilisation (IVF) (Ryan, 1997)

In this section I am concerned with how you **value** IVF treatment.

One way to do this is to find out what the maximum amount of money is that you would be willing to pay for each IVF attempt that you have. **You will not have to pay the amount you state. This is just a way of finding out how strongly you feel about IVF.**

Would you be willing to pay £2 000 for your **current** attempt at IVF? If you are not currently undergoing IVF, would you be willing to pay £2 000 for your next attempt at IVF?

Remember that any money that you spend on IVF will not be available for you to spend on other things.

another country, but this has to be qualified, making it clear that it is an entirely imaginary scenario, by emphasising that the current position is the real market. The second does not attempt to describe any market context in which payment would be made, and in fact uses boldface emphasis to make sure that the context is one of no payment.

The first example tries further to make the context real by asking respondents to think about the benefits that they will derive from the service. The second attempts to ensure that respondents treat the prices as if they were real, by reminding them that expenditure means a reduction in consumption of other goods and services.

There are four ways in which researchers ask respondents to record their answers to WTP questions, two of which are shown in Box 11.1. The most obvious is simply to let respondents choose whatever value they want, known as *open-ended* or *continuous* responses. The open-ended method has the merit of simplicity, but the problem with this is that this is far removed from the way that people are asked to behave in most markets: it would be unusual to find a market in which one would simply state a price and expect to receive the good or service whatever value was stated. Faced with such an unfamiliar task, people may give random or completely unrealistic responses. The second method is *closed-ended*, also known as *discrete choice* or *binary choice*, where respondents are given only a single value that they must choose to accept or reject. Different values are presented randomly to different people in a sample and WTP values are estimated from the average responses from the sample as a whole. The closed-ended scale is more easily recognisable as relevant to markets that have a fixed price for the good. The third method is a *payment scale*, where respondents are given a range of choices. This overcomes the problem of open-endedness, but at the cost of giving cues to the respondent on the size of WTP that will be considered sensible by the researchers. A variant of this, designed to make the task closer to the way that some markets operate, for example where haggling is permitted, is *iterative bidding*, which can really only be used in an interview. Respondents are given an initial price, and asked whether they would be willing to pay it or not. Depending on their choice, the price will be raised or lowered and their decision again recorded. This continues until they are unable to decide.

Box 11.2 gives an example of a WTP study.

BOX 11.2   Willingness to pay for child safety seats

Jarahi *et al.* (2011) examined parents' willingness to pay for child safety seats in Iran. Iran has one of the highest rates of road traffic crash deaths in the world and road traffic injuries are the leading cause of life years lost. Use of child safety seats is not mandatory. The authors interviewed in a pre-school setting 590 car-owner parents of children aged less than five years. Parents were shown pictures of the main types of safety seat, with evidence of their efficacy in reducing deaths and information on the incidence of child car passenger deaths in Iran. Using a payment scale format, parents chose the amount of money they were willing to pay for a safety seat, from seven options ($0, $15, $45, $80, $120, $180, $250), all measured in 2009 US$. The mean and median amounts that respondents were willing to pay were calculated and analysed with respect to demographic and socioeconomic characteristics of respondents and their families, whether or not they had received previous advice about car safety seats and past history of road traffic accidents.

13 participants (2.2%) were not willing to own a safety seat even if it was free. The median WTP among those willing to have one was $15 (interquartile range $15–$45); mean $52, standard deviation $66. Eighty-two (14%) were only willing to have a car seat if it was free. Excluding these responses, the median and mean WTP increased to $45 and $60, respectively. Higher household income and parents' education were positively associated with the amount parents were willing to pay. Age and sex of the child, sex of the parent, receiving previous advice about car seats, past history of road traffic accidents and having another child under five were not associated with parents' WTP.

The authors noted that the median and mean WTP for car safety seats was much lower than the actual price of safety seats in Iran, which was around $100. They concluded that interventions to provide free subsidised car safety seats should be considered.

11.2.3 Discrete choice experiments

A stated preference technique that is increasingly used by health economists is discrete choice experiments (DCEs). DCEs are based on a theory of demand originally suggested by Lancaster (1971), which views goods and services as bundles of characteristics or *attributes*, and that it is people's preferences for those attributes that determine the overall preferences for a good. The most common use of the technique involves presenting people with choices of scenarios described in terms of attributes and their associated levels. For each choice respondents are asked to choose their preferred scenario. Respondents are asked to make a number of such choices and the responses are then modelled using regression analysis. This identifies whether or not a particular attribute is important, the relative importance of each attribute, the rate at which respondents are willing to trade between the attributes, and the overall utility score associated with each combination of attributes. If cost is included as one of the attributes, it is possible to estimate WTP for a good with a given set of attributes.

Ryan and Farrar (2000) describe the stages in undertaking a DCE: identifying the attributes; assigning levels to the attributes; choosing the scenarios to include; establishing preferences using, for example discrete choices; and using regression analysis to analyse the responses. DCEs have been used in many different types of intervention, for example measuring patient preferences for smoking cessation medications, management of pregnancy and labour, colorectal cancer screening strategies, and use of home video game console fitness programmes by older people. DCEs have also been used to assess the preferences of providers of care, for example of physicians for oral versus intravenous drugs for treating cancer, GPs for preventive osteoporotic drug treatment and antenatal clinic workers for different strategies to prevent malaria in pregnancy. An example of a DCE is in Box 11.3.

BOX 11.3   **Discrete choice experiment to assess patient preferences for early rehabilitation management after stroke**

Laver *et al.* (2011) studied the preferences of stroke patients for different models of rehabilitation in Australia in 2009 and 2010. They identified from a literature review the attributes of stroke rehabilitation that were important to patients, and that were capable of being influenced by policy makers. These were confirmed by patients in qualitative interviews, and developed into four attributes with three levels each. A fifth attribute, cost, was also included to allow estimation of WTP assigned to each level of each of the attributes presented. These attributes and their associated levels were: mode of therapy (group therapy, individual therapy, computer therapy); dose of therapy (30 minutes per day, three hours per day, six hours per day); team providing therapy (community-based doctor and physiotherapist visiting, same specialist team from admission to discharge, different specialist team for each phase); amount of recovery made (70%, 80%, 90%); and, cost of therapy programme (no cost, Aus$50 per week, Aus$100 per week).

Three levels for each of the five attributes resulted in 243 possible scenarios. This was reduced to 18 choice sets between two different scenarios. These were divided into three versions, each containing six binary choice sets. A small pilot study ensured that the questions were understandable and that the levels were capable of being traded. Fifty patients were included in the full study, each completing the experiment within one month of their stroke. In each choice set, patients stated which rehabilitation programme they preferred. An example is the choice between the following two rehabilitation programmes.

Programme 1	Programme 2
Individual therapy	Group therapy
30 minutes per day	Six hours per day
Aus$100 per week	No cost
Same specialist team from admission to discharge	Community-based doctor and physiotherapist visiting
80% recovery	90% recovery

The resulting data were analysed using conditional logistic regression analysis, to account for the repeated observations for each person. The dependent variable was a binary variable reflecting whether the respondent chose programme 1 or 2 from each choice set. The independent variables were the differences between the levels of each rehabilitation programme attribute for each programme. The regression results identified 90% recovery as the most desirable attribute and individual therapy as also desirable. Computer therapy was the most undesirable attribute, with six hours' therapy per day and a cost of Aus$100 per week also undesirable. Other attributes and levels were not statistically significant. WTP figures for attribute levels were also given.

11.3 The measurement of health outcomes

Although the measurement of benefits in terms of money has considerable advantages from an economic theory point of view, the measurement of benefits in terms of improved health has dominated economic evaluation. This has at least four sources. The first is a recognition that plausible RP measures are rare in the health care market, along with a distrust of SP techniques, which has led to the rejection on practical grounds of money measures. The second is a belief that health care is a special good in which there is widespread rejection of willingness to pay as a criterion for resource allocation, and therefore an objection in principle to the use of monetary measures. The third is a belief that cost–benefit analysis is not a practical tool for analysis but cost-effectiveness analysis is, so that health is a more appropriate measure than money anyway. The fourth is that health measurement is a widespread activity in many social and biomedical disciplines and in particular in evaluations by health care professionals; economic analysis can therefore draw upon many existing sources of data and ideas, have a discourse with other disciplines, and in particular talk a common language with the dominant professional groups in health care.

Health was for many years appropriately measured by extreme health indicators – changes in survival, mortality and life expectancy. These are relatively easy to measure and where health problems are dominated by deadly diseases and premature death it is reasonable to concentrate on them. Moreover, at an aggregate level they are often strongly correlated with general levels of disease. However, as health has improved and health care has become more sophisticated, premature death has become relatively less important than other aspects of ill health. Clinical indicators of health based on biological markers or other signs and symptoms have become more important, for example changes in blood pressure or the chemical composition of body fluids. Recognition that these indicate only that there is disease, but not necessarily that the disease is having any impact on the patient, leads to interest in patient-oriented indicators. Originally, these were concerned mainly with 'function' – how well the patient was able to undertake activities of various sorts. Such functional indicators have the advantage that they are in principle straightforward to measure, either by observation of a patient or by questionnaire.

However, it was again recognised that this is a narrow view of the impact of disease on humans and that led to a widely accepted more general concept, that health can be measured by its impact on *quality of life* (QOL). This is a very useful concept, although it suffers from many conceptual difficulties and in particular is much less easy to measure than any of the indicators discussed above.

One of the major conceptual problems with QOL is that it is in principle all-encompassing, and this covers aspects of life not normally considered to be related to health. It is arguable that this is not really a problem in assessing the benefits of health care, since economic evaluation actively seeks to measure all benefits, whatever they are; also, as we noted in Chapter 9, some health-based interventions aim to improve not just health but also other factors affecting welfare. However, those who develop and use health indicators prefer to restrict the scope of their measures to those that they believe are related to health, not simply those that health care affects – often for the pragmatic reason that it is difficult enough to measure a complex concept like health and attempting to measure general QOL is a step too far beyond that. This has led to the concept which dominates health indicators of the kind used in economic evaluation – *health-related quality of life* (HRQOL).

HRQOL sounds like a good solution to conceptual problems, but of course it demands a criterion that will enable us to define what is health-related and what is not. This can only reasonably be done by invoking a theory of what health is, and underlying most HRQOL indicators is such a theory, even if it is not explicitly stated. Although open to dispute, the following definition offers an excellent example of what is required if an HRQOL measure is to avoid being merely *ad hoc*. Patrick and Erickson (1993) defined HRQOL as:

> [T]he value assigned to duration of life as modified by the impairments, functional status, perceptions and social opportunities that are influenced by disease, injury, treatment or policy.

The merits of this definition lie in its clear statement about what is to be counted as health and the reasons for doing that – which, in this case, is to measure *values* and to make sure that these are those that can be changed by health care. In other words, it is an ideal conceptual definition on which to base assessment of the benefits of health care in the context of economic evaluation. In the next section we will consider this issue in more detail.

This concern with QOL, and in particular with overall QOL, prompts a suggestion that to economists is obvious – do we not already have a measure of this, which we call utility, and is this not the concept that we should be using in economic analyses? This observation has led to some distinctive economics-based contributions to the HRQOL industry, but also to some disputes and confusion, as we shall see.

11.4 Making health status indicators fit for purpose

In Chapter 10, we discussed the origins of economic evaluation of health care as in part deriving from a more general, non-economic, set of evaluative techniques. This is nowhere more obvious than in the measurement of health status. As suggested, health status measurement is a very large topic deriving from a number of different disciplines, including both social and biomedical science. The different approaches that these bring may result in quite different and equally valid health indicators; health is a complex entity and it is unlikely that one approach is superior to any other. Moreover, health indicators are intended for a wide variety of uses, all of which may require a different type of indicator. To give only a few examples, they might be used for research into the causes and consequences of ill health at either the individual or collective level, monitoring the effect of economic and social phenomena or of government health policies on health or planning health services. An important point in thinking about which health indicator should be used in a particular circumstance is that there is a link between the *purpose* for which the indicator is required and the *way* in which it is measured. As we shall see, the purpose for which health state indicators are used in economic evaluation is quite specific, so it is very straightforward to define the specific requirements for its measurement.

Health indicators are derived from many different sources, using many different measures. For example, measures of mortality in a population may be derived from death certificates, and measures of morbidity from records compiled by health professionals or health care facilities. However, we are mainly concerned here with HRQOL indicators that are based on questionnaires or interview schedules, which we will call *instruments*, that are used with patients or members of the general population, whom we will call *respondents*.

There are some general criteria for judging how good an HRQOL instrument is, mainly based on its *psychometric* properties. (Psychometrics is the branch of psychology that is concerned with measurement of psychological phenomena, in the same way as econometrics concerns the measurement of economic phenomena.) The main criteria are reliability, validity, responsiveness and feasibility. *Reliability* means that the HRQOL instrument produces consistent measurements. A particularly important reliability issue is *test–retest* reliability, where the same instrument applied repeatedly to the same respondent under the same conditions produces the same results. *Validity* means that the instrument measures what it is supposed to measure. Validity can be defined in a number of different ways, including *criterion validity*, which is the extent to which the instrument's results correlate with other measures that are known to be valid; *construct validity*, which is how the instrument's results relate to other variables that are suggested by theory; and *content* or *face validity*, which is simply whether the instrument appears to contain and cover the concept that it is measuring. Validity and reliability are related: an instrument cannot be valid unless it is reliable, but a reliable measure need not be valid. *Responsiveness* is a more general social research criterion and in this context it usually means how sensitive the results from the HRQOL instrument are to changes in health. If people who have a serious illness have the same HRQOL scores as healthy people, we might suspect that the instrument is not very sensitive. *Feasibility* simply means whether or not it is possible to use the instrument. A particularly important issue is how acceptable it is to respondents, since if they cannot or will not complete it there will be many missing data.

These general criteria apply equally to an HRQOL indicator that is to be used for economic evaluation, but what are its special requirements? These derive directly from the need for a quantified measure of the benefits of activities that change health, such as health care and government health policies. This suggests that the following three properties are desirable.

First, it should provide an *unambiguous* measure of benefit. This means that we should be able to tell whether a treatment or policy has made health better or worse, or not affected it at all. Without this property, there is no way to judge how efficiency or equity will change, which is of course the point of economic evaluation. The obvious requirement is therefore for a *single number* that summarises the health change. This is sometimes regarded by critics as resulting from a geeky desire by economists to reduce everything to numbers, but it should be emphasised that it is derived from what economists want to do, rather than being wanted for its own sake.

The second desirable property is that it should be capable of comparing different possible uses of scarce resources. Again, this is because we are interested in the efficient and equitable use of those resources, and economic evaluation is about deciding which possible uses of them are better than others. This implies that it should be applicable to all kinds of possible treatments and policies and, moreover, should be applicable to all kinds of possible health problems.

The third is that it should be capable of being interpreted in terms of values. This is because the health benefits are to be compared with costs. Costs are essentially a measure of the value that we place on the resources used as inputs, so it is logical that the benefits should be measured as the value of outputs. Of course, not all kinds of economic evaluation require this – in particular cost-effectiveness analysis does not have such a requirement – but it is nevertheless desirable. At the very least, it should be able to say that more is preferred to less.

11.4.1 Generic and specific measures

Generic health state instruments are intended to be independent of particular health conditions and interventions and therefore applicable in all circumstances. They therefore in effect deal with the entire concept of what health is, and different generic measures reflect different ways in which health is regarded – that is, particular 'constructs' of health deriving from a particular theory of what health is. For example, we may believe that there are two dominant aspects of ill health, pain and disability, and these are quite separate. The instrument should therefore cover these two aspects separately. An entirely different instrument would be appropriate if, for example, our theory of health was based on a holistic view in which pain and disability are simply two different manifestations of ill health, or we believed in the ancient Greek theory of humours. Because of their intended wide applicability, generic instruments may contain elements irrelevant to particular conditions – for example, including pain when a particular condition is not painful. These measures are sometimes intended to be an all-encompassing measure that tells you all you need to know in every circumstance, and sometimes a common minimum data set to be collected with other measures, so that at least some key part can be compared across different illnesses and interventions.

The alternative is a *disease-*, *condition-*, *treatment-* or *domain-specific* health state instrument. By disease- or condition-specific, we mean that the measure is intended only for a specific illness; by treatment-specific that it is for a particular type of treatment; and by a domain we mean a particular aspect of health, for example pain. Rather than being derived from a theory of health, as generic measures are, they usually reflect the experience of particular conditions, domains or treatments by patients and health professionals. The advantages of specific questionnaires are said to be that they may have greater acceptability to those who complete them, because people are more interested in their own health. It is also alleged that the indicators derived from them may be more sensitive than generic measures, but the evidence in favour of this is not clear cut.

It follows from our earlier argument that for economic evaluation we will mainly be interested in generic measures. There are many different generic measures, based on standard questionnaires that have been developed by different groups of researchers. In this chapter we will examine in more detail one of these, the EQ-5D (Brooks, 1996), mainly because of its relative simplicity compared with many other instruments. The EQ-5D derives its name from the European group (EuroQol) that originally derived it, but it is now used worldwide. The Health Utilities Index (HUI) originated in Canada but is also used worldwide (Horsman *et al.*, 2003). The Finnish 15D instrument – named for the fact that it has 15 dimensions – is at present mostly used locally but it is widely regarded by researchers as having some desirable properties, though also some problems, one of which will be discussed below (Sintonen, 1981). Similarly of mainly local interest is the Australian Assessment of Quality of Life (AQOL), which is of particular interest because its development was very closely guided by theory; other indicators have used theory as a guide, but have been very heavily influenced by accumulated empirical experience of good practice in health measurement derived from a number of different sources (Hawthorne *et al.*, 1999). Lastly, there is a very widely used instrument, developed in the USA, that has a number of different variants and names given to it but is most widely known as the SF-36, an acronym which means that it is made up of 36 items and is a short form of a larger instrument (Brook *et al.*, 1979). In that form it is also known as the MOS SF-36, referring to the Medical Outcomes Survey that developed it, and the RAND-36, from one of its developers. Of particular importance for economic evaluation – because they have been used to derive health state valuations – are even shorter versions of it, the SF-12 and the SF-6, containing 12 and 6 items each.

Many condition-specific measures are designed only for a specific purpose and are stand-alone, for example the Asthma Quality of Life Questionnaire (AQLQ) (Juniper *et al.*, 1993). Others are actually enhanced generic measures, which have add-on questions specific to the condition, for example the MS-QOL54, which is the SF-36 plus 18 specific questions on issues of particular importance in multiple sclerosis (Vickrey *et al.*, 1995). Several thousand condition-specific and generic instruments currently exist for measuring health; a useful searchable data base of these instruments and the associated research literature is available from Oxford University (http://phi.uhce.ox.ac.uk/).

11.4.2 Profiles and indices

Earlier, we noted that health is a complex concept and that a key element of that is that most theories of health regard health as *multidimensional,* involving many different dimensions such as pain and disability. Any health state can be described as a combination of different levels of these different dimensions. If the health state measure simply consists of a set of dimensions that have different levels, it is known as a *profile*.

As an illustrative example, suppose that we have a health measure that only involves pain and disability. We might define these dimensions so that pain has five levels (none, slight, moderate, strong, severe) and disability has four (none, minor, major, complete). Within each dimension the levels are ranked, so that we can assume that, for example, severe pain – which is defined to be as bad as pain can be – is worse than strong pain, which is worse than moderate pain, which is worse than slight pain. Any particular health state will involve one level of each dimension, for example slight pain and minor disability or moderate pain and no disability. In this particular example, there are $5 \times 4 = 20$ possible health states.

Profile measures of health attempt to give an overall picture of health at a particular time, and although levels of health within any dimension can be compared, profiles do not make any comparisons between different dimensions. Important examples of measures that are mainly intended as profiles are the Sickness Impact Profile (Bergner *et al.*, 1981) and the SF-36 mentioned above. In these measures, the measurement within levels goes beyond ranking, assigning a score to each dimension; however, the scores are not comparable between dimensions. Another example is the EQ-5D, which is described in Box 11.4.

Profiles may have strong descriptive value, but the problem from the point of view of economic analysis is that a profile may not be able to identify whether one health state is better than another. Without additional information, we therefore may not be able to say whether a change in health state means that health has got better or worse or remained the same. For example, if someone has EQ-5D state 21111, they have some difficulties with mobility but otherwise no problems. We can say that this is better than, say, 22111, because that means that

---

BOX 11.4   The EQ-5D health-related quality of life classification

The EQ-5D contains five dimensions that describe health-related quality of life, with three levels in each dimension:

Mobility

1. No problems in walking about
2. Some problems in walking about
3. Confined to bed

Self-care

1. No problems with self-care
2. Some problems washing or dressing self
3. Unable to wash or dress self

Usual activities

1. No problems with performing usual activities (e.g. work, study, housework)
2. Some problems with performing usual activities
3. Unable to perform usual activities

Pain and discomfort

1. No pain or discomfort
2. Moderate pain or discomfort
3. Extreme pain or discomfort

Anxiety and depression

1. Not anxious or depressed
2. Moderately anxious or depressed
3. Extremely anxious or depressed

The EQ-5D classification therefore provides a profile of a person's health state. Each of the 243 possible health states can be uniquely identified by a five-digit number, for example '12212' would mean:

No problems in walking about
Some problems washing or dressing self
Some problems with performing usual activities
No pain or discomfort
Moderately anxious or depressed

The EuroQol Group (www.euroqol.org) has developed a new version, the EQ-5D-5L, which has the same dimensions as the original (now sometimes referred to as the EQ-5D-3L), but each has five levels (no, slight, moderate, severe, and extreme problems). This has $5^5 = 3\,125$ health states.

they also have some problems with self-care; however, we cannot say whether this is better than 12111 because they have self-care difficulties *instead of* mobility difficulties. We would only be able to say whether a change from 21111 to 12111 was an improvement or not if we knew how people rated mobility in comparison with self-care.

What is required is an *index*, which is a single number representing the overall level of health. This will allow an unambiguous judgement to be made about whether one state of health is better or worse than another and from an economics point of view this is an essential requirement. As will be discussed below, the numbers may have to have rather stronger properties than simply representing a ranking, because we will want to compare not just health state levels but *changes* in health states. The major disadvantage of an index is that if it is used as the only measure of health it may not provide or may mask important details of health state changes.

An index can be derived as a direct measurement of overall health or can be derived from a profile. The EQ-5D again provides a useful example, as it can be used to provide both types of index, as shown in Box 11.5.

BOX 11.5 **Health state indexes and the EQ-5D**

One way to obtain a single number representing a health state is simply to ask for it in that way! The EQ-5D instrument, shown here, provides a way to do this using a visual analogue scale known as the EQ-VAS.

The status of numbers collected in this way is disputed. It is reasonable to regard them as representing a ranking, but it is unclear that someone who rates their health state at one time as 25 and another as 50 is twice as healthy on the second occasion, or even that a change from 0 to 25 is valued the same as 25 to 50. However, this index has very

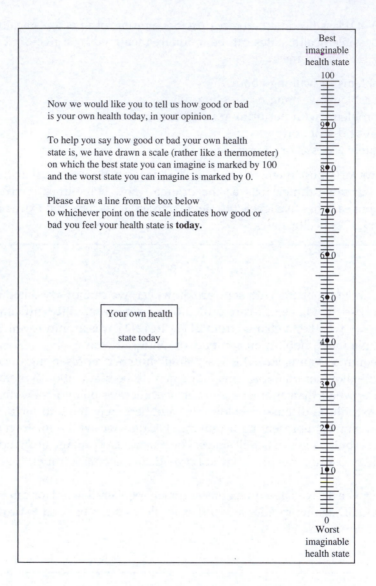

Now we would like you to tell us how good or bad
is your own health today, in your opinion.

To help you say how good or bad your own health
state is, we have drawn a scale (rather like a thermometer)
on which the best state you can imagine is marked by 100
and the worst state you can imagine is marked by 0.

Please draw a line from the box below
to whichever point on the scale indicates how good or
bad you feel your health state is **today.**

Your own health

state today

good properties in terms of reliability, and can be used in time series to show fluctuations in health.

An alternative is to convert a profile into an index. The York MVH project used a model derived from data from 2 997 people who completed a TTO exercise on 43 EQ-5D health states. Each state was regarded as a combination of attributes, and a regression model was estimated using levels 2 and 3 in each EQ-5D dimension as dummy variables, taking the value 1 if they exist and 0 otherwise. The resulting model was an additive multi-attribute utility function, with two complications: a constant term representing any deviation from full health, and a term representing very poor health, evidenced by level 3 in any dimension. The resulting equation was:

$U = 0.97 - 0.066 \times$ Mobility level $2 - 0.271 \times$ Mobility level $3 - 0.029 \times$ Self care level $2 - 0.097 \times$ Self care level $3 - 0.127 \times$ Usual activities level $2 - 0.224 \times$ Usual activities level $3 - 0.144 \times$ Pain & discomfort level $2 - 0.376 \times$ Pain & discomfort level $3 - 0.114 \times$ Anxiety & depression level $2 - 0.259 \times$ Anxiety & depression level $3 - 0.305 \times$ Any level 3

The index takes values from 0 to 1. Health state 12122, for example is valued at $0.97 - 0.029 - 0.144 - 0.114 = 0.683$, while health state 32111 is valued at $0.97 - 0.271 - 0.029 - 0.305 = 0.365$.

For a review of this and other EQ-5D valuation research, see Szende *et al.* (2007).

11.4.3 Measuring health-related quality of life: an indifference curve approach

We can draw together the economics issues involved in constructing an HRQOL indicator using an indifference curve approach, following Culyer, Williams and Lavers (1971). We will use the simple example of the pain and disability profile described above. In Figure 11.1 the five levels on the pain dimension are labelled P_0–P_4 and the four levels on the disability dimension are labelled D_0–D_3. Pain and disability both increase as they move from the origin. Each point X is a health profile describing a unique health state, in terms of a particular combination of pain and disability. The 20 points together describe every possible health state given this classification system.

In a strict profile measure of health, we cannot compare dimensions, but this does not mean that we cannot compare health states. In discussing how health profiles might be compared, Devlin, Parkin and Browne (2010) drew an analogy with the Pareto principle, that

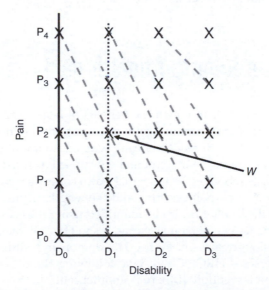

Figure 11.1 Measuring health-related quality of life: profile of ill-health, relative ranking and absolute values

there is an improvement if at least one person is made better off and no-one is made worse off. This suggests that:

- A health profile is better than another if it is better in at least one dimension, and is no worse in any other dimension.
- A health profile is worse than another if it is worse in at least one dimension, and is no better in any other dimension.

For example the point marked W is worse than any other point in the quadrant to the south-west of it, including those on the dotted lines, which are better in only one dimension. Similarly, point W is better than any point in the quadrant to the north-east of it, including those on the dotted lines. However, we cannot, without extra information, rank point W compared to any points inside the other two quadrants, north-west or south-east. In those quadrants, health is always worse in one dimension and better in another. Since dimensions are not compared, we cannot make an overall judgement. In other words, a profile cannot compare and rank every possible health state.

What is required is an explicit ranking of health states, which can be thought of as deriving from indifference curves that embody the relative weight given to different dimensions and to different levels within dimensions. As a first step, we might regard the dashed lines as representing equal rankings for the points on them. However, from an economics point of view it will be important to attach a number or weight to each line, which quantifies the relative value attached to each point. These weights incorporate relative values both for dimensions and for scale points within dimensions. If we maintain the indifference curve analogy, then these can be thought of as utilities, though in this case only utility derived from aspects of HRQOL and not any other aspect of life.

11.5 The measurement of health gain

Another way to describe the way in which the benefits of health care are best measured for economic evaluation is that the impact of health interventions should be measured as *health gain*, which is calculated as the difference in health with and without the intervention. This is consistent with the calculation of the incremental effect used as the denominator of the cost-effectiveness ratio (*CER*), as shown in Chapter 10. Health comprises two dimensions: the level of health experienced at a given point in time and the length of time for which that level of health is experienced. If the level of health is quantified using the concept of HRQOL, we can analyse the health experience of a person as variations in HRQOL over time, representing the prognoses with and without treatment. Figure 11.2 demonstrates this. The lower line represents the path that a person's HRQOL will take following the onset of a particular illness without any health care intervention. If there is an intervention, then the patient's prognosis will alter, and HRQOL will follow the path of the upper dashed line that starts at that point of intervention.

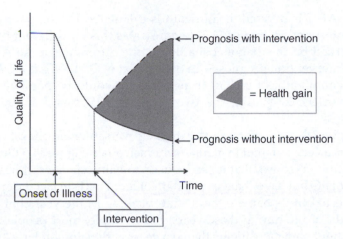

Figure 11.2 Measuring the health gain from interventions

The quantity on the vertical axis is a single number representing HRQOL at a point in time – the ways in which this can be derived are discussed in some detail below. It takes the value 1 for 'full health' – the implication being that this value is as good health as that person can experience. The value 0 is more complicated, as it represents the strange concept of 'no health'. Such a state most obviously exists when there is the absence of life, but it can also be experienced while alive if the health state is very poor. It is not the lowest value that health states can take, however, as it is possible to conceive of health states that are worse than being dead. In fact, there is in principle no lower bound to negative values for health.

The next step is to consider how this can be used to create an overall indicator of health and changes in health. In general, health is regarded as the product of the level of health and the length of time that it is experienced, in other words a measure of fully healthy time. For example, if we have an HRQOL of 0.5 and this is experienced for six days, we have experienced the equivalent of three days of full health. Given curves of the kind shown in Figure 11.2 representing prognosis, the total amount of health experienced with this prognosis will be measured by the area under the curve (AUC). The incremental effect of the intervention is the difference in the AUC with and without the intervention. This is shown by the shaded area in the figure.

Although this way of viewing the benefits of health changes as the AUC is widely accepted, there is less agreement about the way in which it should actually be calculated. The most commonly used measure is *quality-adjusted life years* (QALYs). These are calculated, in a similar way to the example above, by multiplying the amount of time in a particular health state by the quality of life during that time, summing over all time periods and standardising to a year. An example of how this is done is given in Chapter 12.

An alternative is *healthy year equivalents* (HYEs) (Mehrez and Gafni, 1989). One important critique of QALYs is the implied assumption that quality of life is valued independently of length of life; another is that it does not incorporate uncertainty. For these and other reasons, HYEs were devised to calculate directly the AUC. The precise way in which this is done is also shown in Chapter 12.

However the AUC is derived, health gain is calculated by comparing the AUC with and without the intervention. Figure 11.3 demonstrates this for different types of intervention. The area marked by the diagonal shading is the difference in the AUCs of the non-intervention and intervention prognoses. In the context of QALYs, it is a QALY gain, which could form the denominator of a *CER*. In principle it would be possible to estimate this directly rather than by estimating the two separate AUCs and subtracting one from the other.

The resulting health gain measure is extremely versatile, enabling the comparison of health effects that are very different in nature from each other. Figure 11.3 illustrates the range of possibilities. Graph (a) shows that it can be used to value changes in health that have no impact on quality of life but have changes in length of life. This is in fact the original concept of a QALY, best reflected in its name – there is an increase in life years but these should be weighted by quality of life during those years. For example, most people would value ten years' survival without pain more highly than ten years with pain; similarly, they would value

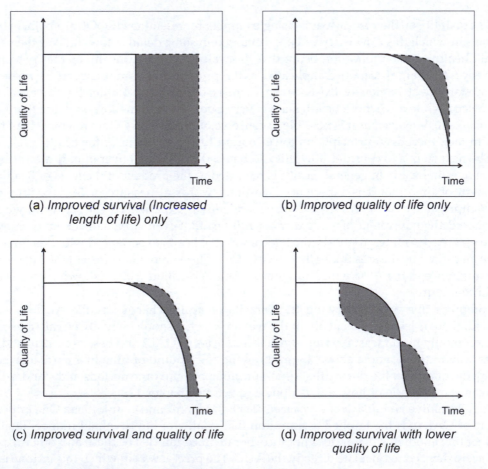

(a) *Improved survival (Increased length of life) only*

(b) *Improved quality of life only*

(c) *Improved survival and quality of life*

(d) *Improved survival with lower quality of life*

Figure 11.3 Measuring gains from different types of intervention

survival for ten years in whatever health state – assuming that it was not so bad that being dead was preferable – to five years in that state.

Graph (b) shows that the AUC measure can be used where there is no change at all in survival but a change in HRQOL during the person's remaining life.

Graph (c) shows another scenario, where both survival and HRQOL are changed. In this case not only is quality of life increased for the time that the person would live without the intervention, survival continues beyond that time.

Graph (d) is a more complex example illustrating further the versatility of the measure. This example might represent a radical treatment which reduces a person's quality of life but enables them to live longer. In this case, there is a positive health gain deriving from increased survival, measured as an increment of quality of life over the increased length of life, but this must be weighed against the decrement of HRQOL over the time that they would live without the intervention. A simple way to evaluate this would be to calculate a net benefit – does the positive area outweigh the negative?

That the AUC measure of health gain can measure very diverse types of effect, and therefore in principle all health care interventions that affect health, is a powerful one which many regard as its chief advantage. However, there is an opposing view, that this demonstrates a fatal weakness in the whole concept because changes in quality of life and in length of life can never be valued on the same scale. In this view, an improvement of 5% in quality of life for 20 years cannot really be equated to one year of extra life; the two cannot even be compared.

A third measure of this type is *disability-adjusted life years* (DALYs) (Fox-Rushby, 2002). DALYs are rather different in that they measure ill-health rather than health. QALYs and HYEs weight years by health, so that the more there are of them the better and the benefits of a health intervention are that QALYs or HYEs are gained. DALYs weight years by ill health, as measured by disability, so that the fewer there are the better, and a health intervention would be evaluated using reductions in DALYs. DALYs have been heavily promoted by the World Health Organization and the World Bank for use in developing countries, and their use in the Global Burden of Disease Project is discussed in Chapter 13. Details of how they are calculated are given below.

11.6 Non-monetary valuation of health states

We now have a health state indicator that meets almost all of the requirements that we stated earlier. All that remains is to ensure that it implies values. But what does this mean? Value is a quite general term that does have some specific meanings in economics – and in other social sciences – and it is not clear which should have primacy. We are here concerned with non-monetary values, and as suggested earlier, this usually means utilities. But utility itself is not a concept that has a single meaning, and moreover there is no well-defined way of measuring it. Hence there are controversies and disputes about how non-monetary values should be measured and there is no real consensus on the best approach.

It is therefore no surprise that there are several alternative techniques available and in widespread use. What is common to valuation methods is that they are usually based on interviews or questionnaires in which respondents are presented with 'scenarios' that describe a health state. Sometimes these are stylised descriptions based on the way that specific illnesses are experienced by patients; very often they are descriptions of particular health states according to a profile measure, such as the EQ-5D. Using a particular technique, respondents are asked to place a value on one or more health state.

Many of the techniques used to derive index numbers for health states originate from psychometrics, and indeed most were originally developed as part of psychophysics, the study of how people respond to physical stimuli. Techniques include *magnitude estimation*, where people are asked simply to give a direct estimate of size; *paired comparisons*, where people are asked to state which of two alternatives is preferred; and *rating scales*, which are discussed below. Other techniques have more economics-based origins, including the *standard gamble* and *time trade-off*, which are discussed below, and the *person trade-off* or *equivalence* method, where people are asked to judge the relative importance of health states in terms of equivalence – the number of people they would like to see cured of them. The following are the most commonly used methods.

11.6.1 Rating scales, category scales and visual analogue scales

These form a distinctive class of health measurement instruments that again originated in psychometric research. Although similar, they have some important distinctions, the labels that are applied to them are not always consistent and there are a number of important variants within them. What is similar about them is that they are a single scale on which respondents mark a point which they believe best represents a health state, either one that is or has been experienced or one that they are asked to imagine. We will not discuss the difference between rating and category scales as they are unclear and not important for our needs. Currently of most importance in economic evaluation is the *visual analogue scale* (VAS), although its role is controversial (Parkin and Devlin, 2006). This usually consists of a single line with verbal and numerical descriptors at each end. Scale markers are often added to the line, and these are sometimes also numbered. Respondents are presented with a set of health states and are asked to rate the desirability of each by placing it at some point on the line on or between the two endpoints. An example of a visual analogue scale is the EQ-VAS described earlier. The instrument described in Box 11.5, however, was intended for recording a respondent's current health state. There is a variant of this, the EQ-5D VAS, which has a similar design but records respondent's valuations of health state scenarios defined according to the EQ-5D classification system.

11.6.2 The standard gamble

The standard gamble (SG) was invented specifically to measure von Neumann–Morgenstern (vNM) utility. In its application to health, illustrated in the upper part of Figure 11.4,

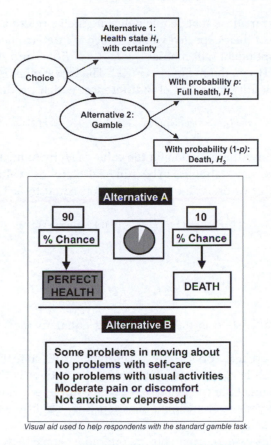

Visual aid used to help respondents with the standard gamble task

Figure 11.4 The standard gamble method for a chronic health state preferred to death

respondents are given a choice between two alternatives; one (Alternative 1; A_1) is a health state with certainty, (H_1) and the other (Alternative 2; A_2) is a gamble that has two possible outcomes that involve different states of health, H_2 and H_3, with particular probabilities attached to them, $p(H_2)$ and $p(H_3)$. The method relies on the fact that vNM utilities have the property that the expected value of a choice is the value multiplied by its probability. (In fact, vNM utilities can be defined as utilities to which these kind of mathematical manipulations apply.) Since H_1 is offered with certainty, its probability is equal to 1, so its expected value, $E(A_1)$, is equal to its value, $v(H_1)$. Therefore the choice is between

$$E(A_1) = v(H_1) \tag{11.1}$$

and

$$E(A_2) = v(H_2)p(H_2) + v(H_3)p(H_3) \tag{11.2}$$

Since there are only two alternatives, $p(H_2) + p(H_3) = 1$, which may be equivalently stated as $p(H_3) = 1 - p(H_2)$.

The key assumption made is that people will state their preferences for A_1 and A_2 on the basis of the relative size of their expected values, which are determined by different values of $p(H_3)$ and $p(H_2)$. The respondent will choose A_1 if $E(A_1) > E(A_2)$ and A_2 if $E(A_2) > E(A_1)$; and if they are indifferent between them, $E(A_1) = E(A_2)$. The experiment is intended to vary $p(H_3)$ and $p(H_2)$ in order to identify the point of indifference, which produces a simple equation:

$$v(H_1) = v(H_2)p(H_2) + v(H_3)(1 - p(H_2)) \tag{11.3}$$

The final step is to solve this equation for the value of H_1 by fixing the values of H_2 and H_3. The usual way to do this is by stating H_2 to be 'full health', whose value is by definition equal to 1, and H_3 to be 'death', whose value is by definition equal to 0. This produces

$$v(H_1) = (1)p(H_2) + (0)(1 - p(H_2)) \tag{11.4}$$

and therefore

$$v(H_1) = p(H_2) \tag{11.5}$$

The value of a health state is therefore simply equal to the probability accorded to obtaining full health.

The method described here applies only to a chronic health state that is preferred to death. The reason for this is slightly complicated. One of the alternatives within the gamble is death, which is of course permanent but can be viewed as the complete removal of HRQOL for what would otherwise be the person's remaining life span. So, a slightly different set of options is offered for a *temporary* health state in which the worst option can be related to a similar period as that health state. In this case, respondents are offered a choice between a temporary health state H_1 with certainty and a gamble with the possible outcomes of full health with probability p and the worst possible state H_2 with probability $(1 - p)$. If they are indifferent between these, the value of health state H_1 is $p + (1 - p)H_2$.

The lower part of Figure 11.4 is a stylised version of the kind of visual aids, or 'props', that are used by interviewers to assist respondents to give answers in an SG survey. These are necessary because what respondents are asked to do is likely to be an unfamiliar task for which they might require different types of explanation as to what they are supposed to do. A particular feature of this is the probability 'wheel' which seeks to demonstrate to respondents the meaning of probability, since that may be particularly difficult for some people to handle. As may be seen, in this stylised example we have presented a health state scenario in terms of an EQ-5D profile.

11.6.3 Time trade-off

The time trade-off (TTO) method was originally invented as a way of obtaining vNM utilities that were easier to use than the standard gamble. There are a number of different ways in which the TTO could be applied, but the most common is as follows. Respondents are given a choice between two health profiles: a particular health state for a given number of years and full health for a shorter period of time. In effect they are asked to trade between quality of life and length of life. The method tries to establish where they are indifferent between the two by varying the amount of time spent in full health. The assumption is that, other things being equal, people will choose the option that produces the highest QALY value, which is simply defined as the product of length of life (LOL) and quality of life (HRQOL). So, for profile i the QALYs are $QALY_i = (LOL_i)(HRQOL_i)$.

Figure 11.5(a) demonstrates this. If the respondent is indifferent between two health profiles, A and B, then $QALY_A = QALY_B$, or $(LOL_A)(HRQOL_A) = (LOL_B)(HRQOL_B)$. If B is the health state that we wish to value, we can calculate QOL_B by fixing LOL_B to be a particular number of years and by defining A as full health, thereby fixing the value of $HRQOL_A$ as 1. Therefore, $HRQOL_B = LOL_A/LOL_B$. For example, suppose that one of the alternatives is a particular state of health for 5 years and the respondent states that this is equivalent to 4 years in full health. The value of that health state is $4/5 = 0.8$.

Strictly speaking, this method applies only to a chronic health state preferred to death. For a chronic health state *worse* than death, the following method is often used, as illustrated in Figure 11.5(b). The respondent is offered a choice between (1) LOL_A years of full health plus

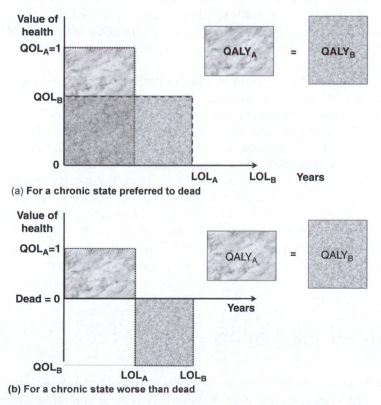

(a) **For a chronic state preferred to dead**

(b) **For a chronic state worse than dead**

Figure 11.5 The time trade-off method

(LOL$_B$ – LOL$_A$) years at health state HRQOL$_B$, which is worse than being dead, and (2) immediate death. If the respondent is indifferent between these, then the value of HRQOL$_B$ is LOL$_A$/(LOL$_A$ – LOL$_B$), which is a negative number. This is because the first alternative is valued as the sum of the positive and negative areas and the other alternative is valued as 0. If the respondent is indifferent between options, then their total values are equal, so $0 = (1)(LOL_A) – (QOL_B)(LOL_B – LOL_A)$.

11.6.4 How do we choose between these methods?

It is sometimes asserted that the so-called 'choice-based' measurement techniques, such as SG and TTO, are preferable for economic evaluation studies. Various reasons are given for this, mainly that people will not reveal their true preferences if they are not constrained to behave as they do in real life when expressing them, which is by choosing. However, these theoretical arguments are not as compelling as they might appear. All of the techniques – whether 'choice-based' or not – are experimental or survey-based and, while there are good reasons for applying economic behaviour reasoning to revealed preferences, there is less to applying it to stated preference experiments. This is particularly the case in measuring health values or utilities, since there is no real-world trading in them and therefore no plausible experimental replication of a market in which trading takes place. In addition, the use of SG and TTO requires careful consideration. For example, SG results are likely to be affected by the attitude to risk of the respondent (see Chapter 6) and TTO results are likely to be affected by their time preference (see Chapter 12).

Moreover, it will be obvious from our earlier definitions of stated preference (SP) and revealed preference (RP) that all of these techniques are based on SP. However, it is sometimes claimed (by for example Drummond *et al.*, 2005) that methods that *indirectly* provide values, such as SG and TTO, are RP and those that provide them *directly*, such as Magnitude Estimation and VAS, are SP. However, it is clear that this is simply an analogy, since in every case preferences are stated, and the theoretical superiority of RP in terms of having a basis in economic theory simply does not apply to indirect measures of values.

It is therefore sometimes argued that theoretical issues are of less importance than practical ones. The latter are largely based on the desirable psychometric properties, discussed earlier, that the data that result may have, plus the efficiency of their collection in terms of the cost of obtaining a sample of a particular size. In these terms, VAS measures are argued to have some advantages over others; however, the TTO is more widely used.

11.7 Multi-attribute utility measures

We have noted that economists have been particularly interested in health indicators that can be interpreted as utilities, since that is the standard concept for analysing issues of well-being and quality of life. A particularly important type of indicator, therefore, is one based on what is known as a *multi-attribute utility* (MAU) *function*. Sometimes such indicators are given this title explicitly; in other cases they can rather be interpreted as MAU-based indicators. Some of the measures described earlier fall into this class.

MAU theory is also derived from the Lancaster characteristics theory discussed earlier, in which the good is not health care but health. In a MAU model, utility is derived from health state *attributes*, a_i, which may be thought of as similar to the health state dimensions referred to earlier. The utility function is therefore $U = U(a_i)$.

In measuring health states, we are interested in particular in two properties of the utility function. One is the conditional utility of each attribute, its effect on utility with the other attributes held constant, which is defined as $\delta U / \delta a_i$. The other is the interaction of each attribute with each other attribute, expressed as the term $a_i a_j$.

Although the functional form of the utility function can take any shape, a popular and easy assumption is that it is additive, which if there are no interaction terms can be expressed as

$$U = \sum_{i=1}^{n} w_i a_i \qquad (11.6)$$

In this case the conditional utilities, w_i, are sometimes referred to as *weights*. This additive function can be made more complex by including interaction terms, for example,

$$U = \sum_{i=1}^{n} w_i a_i + \sum_{i=1}^{n} \sum_{j=1}^{n} w_{ij} a_i a_j \qquad (11.7)$$

where w_{ij} is the weight for the interaction term $a_i a_j$. Another widely used function is the multiplicative utility function, usually expressed in log linear form as

$$\log U = \sum_{i=1}^{n} w_i \log a_i \qquad (11.8)$$

The EQ-5D can be used within a MAU framework, and some widely used sets of health state valuations have been derived empirically using regression techniques to estimate a MAU model. The best-known of these is the York MVH model, described in Box 11.5. The data on which this is based were obtained from a study in the UK whose protocol and methods have been used extensively in other countries. All of the instruments discussed earlier (EQ-5D, HUI, 15D, AQOL) have MAU theory-based valuations attached to them. The SF-36 does not have a MAU model attached to it, but its even shorter versions, the SF-12 and the SF-6, have.

An attraction of MAU-based instruments is that in undertaking an assessment of health benefits we do not have to undertake valuation tasks of the kind described in the previous section. All that is required is to ask respondents to record their health state, for example using the EQ-5D descriptive system, and use the pre-scored MAU model, for example the algorithm in Box 11.5, to compute the HRQOL score.

In developing a useful MAU-type instrument, there are trade-offs to be made between their complexity, their descriptive value, their precision and their practicality in actual use. An important issue is the trade-off between the extent to which they are descriptively rich – having many fine gradations of health derived from large numbers of dimensions and large numbers of possible levels within them – and are practical in terms of the ability to place values on the health states. Indicators with a small number of possible states may lack descriptive richness, but may make it plausible for all of them to be valued directly, or at least a large proportion. If there are a very large number of states, an alternative strategy must be used, for example sampling from some health states and extrapolating to others. The EQ-5D is a very simple instrument in these terms, with 245 states, including 'unconscious' and 'dead'; the HUI has around one million, the AQOL one billion and the 15D, which has great descriptive richness, 30 billion.

11.8 The valuation of health states: willingness to pay for health changes

We began this chapter by discussing monetary valuation of health care and explained that dissatisfaction with this led economists to non-monetary valuation methods that dealt not with health care itself but with health. However, a middle way between these has been suggested, in which monetary values are derived for health, and stated preference techniques can and have been used as alternatives to the techniques described above in the measurement of health itself.

One possible way to do this is to use a variant of the willingness to pay methods described earlier for valuing health care. Of course, these are strictly not contingent valuation methods since there is no market for health itself and hence no possible description of such a market. It would be possible to describe the health care market that is assumed, but there is no imperative to do so and in some cases that might be quite inappropriate. Otherwise, many of the problems and good practices that apply to surveys relating to health care also apply to those relating to health.

CV, EV, WTP and willingness to accept (WTA) are defined according to two possible exogenously determined changes in states of the world with respect to health: other things being equal, it will either deteriorate or remain the same. In each case, it is assumed that this state can be altered, so that deterioration can be prevented or an improvement brought about. The different dimensions of benefit using each of these measures are as follows:

- Compensating variation (CV) involves compensation for a health change. If a person experiences health improvement money is taken away in compensation. If the person experiences health deterioration money is given to them.
- Equivalent variation (EV) involves compensation for *no* health change. If the person experiences no health improvement money is given to them in compensation. If they experience no health deterioration money is taken away.

- Willingness to pay (WTP) involves the person paying money to obtain a health improvement or prevent a health deterioration.
- Willingness to accept (WTA) involves the person being given money to compensate them for no health improvement or a health deterioration.

   If we assume that the difference between two health states can equivalently be regarded as a decline from the better health state or an improvement from the worst health state, then we have four ways of measuring the value of the change in health.

CV/WTP

- *Money amount*: maximum amount that must be taken away from a person.
- *Effect of money transfer*: to leave them as well off as they were before an improvement in health.
- *Example question*: "Suppose that a particular health treatment or health policy would improve your health from A to B. What is the most that you would be willing to pay for this?"

EV/WTP

- *Money amount*: maximum amount that must be taken away from a person.
- *Effect of money transfer*: to make them as well off as they would have been after a deterioration in health.
- *Example question*: "Suppose that a particular health treatment or health policy would prevent your health deteriorating from B to A. What is the most that you would be willing to pay for this?"

CV/WTA

- *Money amount*: minimum amount that must be given to a person.
- *Effect of money transfer*: to leave them as well off as they were before a deterioration in health.
- *Example question*: "Suppose that a particular health treatment or health policy would prevent your health deteriorating from A to B. The government does not provide the treatment or undertake the policy, so your health deteriorates. What is the minimum compensation that you would need to be as well off as if your health had not deteriorated?"

EV/WTA

- *Money amount*: minimum amount that must be given to a person.
- *Effect of money transfer*: to make them as well off as they would have been after an improvement in health.
- *Example question*: "Suppose that a particular health treatment or health policy would improve your health from A to B. The government does not provide the treatment or undertake the policy, so your health does not improve. What is the minimum compensation that you would need to be as well off as if your health had improved?"

   As an example, a respondent has an income of $£Y_1$ and health H_1, which produces a utility of U_1. Other things remaining the same, their health would deteriorate to H_2 but their income would remain at £Y_1, which would produce a lower utility of U_2. They are asked how much they would be willing to pay to prevent deterioration of their health to H_2. Strictly speaking, they should be asked to identify the point at which they are exactly compensated by the increase in their health for the loss of income brought about by the payment. Suppose that they were willing to pay £X_A; that would reduce their income to £$(Y_1 - X_A)$. This implies that the utility that they derive from £Y_1 and H_2 is the same as from £$(Y_1 - X_A)$ and H_1; that is, U_2. However, they could equally be asked what they would be willing to accept as compensation for the deterioration in their health. Suppose that they were willing to accept £X_B, which would increase their income to £$(Y_1 + X_B)$. This implies that the utility that they derive from £$(Y_1 + X_B)$ and H_2 is the same as from £Y_1 and H_1; that is U_1. In summary:

- Utility U_1 is achieved from health H_2 plus income £$(Y_1 - X_B)$ and from health H_1 plus income £Y_1.
- Utility U_2 is achieved from health H_2 plus income £Y_1 and from health H_1 plus income £$(Y_1 + X_A)$.

The willingness to pay value £X_A is an equivalent variation measure, because it is evaluated with respect to the final utility level U_2, and the willingness to accept value £X_B is a compensating variation measure, because it is evaluated with respect to the initial level of utility. There is no reason why these should be the same, even though they are equally valid measures of the value of the difference between H_1 and H_2. But what of the other two possibilities?

To evaluate these, we must reverse the scenario so that the initial health state is H_2 and the initial income is £Y_1 and then ask what they would be willing to pay to improve their health to H_1 or what they would be willing to accept as compensation for remaining at H_2. According to the above, this would mean that the initial utility was U_2 and therefore that the compensating variation – measured according to the initial utility – must be X_A. This implies that this would be the amount that they would be willing to accept as compensation for remaining at H_2. Using similar reasoning, the equivalent variation, which is the willingness to pay to improve their health to H_1, should be X_B.

In theory therefore, EV/WTP = CV/WTP and CV/WTA = EV/WTA. If a monetary evaluation study is carried out, EV and CV should produce the same value if the same method – WTP or WTA – is used, but it is not necessarily the case that EV measures produced under WTP and WTA will give the same value, and the same is true for CV measures. Looked at another way, although there is no reason why a WTP study should produce the same result as a WTA study, we would expect the values derived from a WTA study to be the same irrespective of whether a CV or EV measure is used, and the same to be true for a WTP study.

Can we say any more about the WTP and WTA values except that they may be different? With a typical good or service, the assumption is that it will form a small element of total consumption, with many other goods that could substitute for it. So, the good or service and income are perfect substitutes, with linear indifference curves, as in Figure 11.6(a). The change from H_1 to H_2, evaluated keeping U_1 constant, is X_B and keeping U_2 constant it is X_A. As you

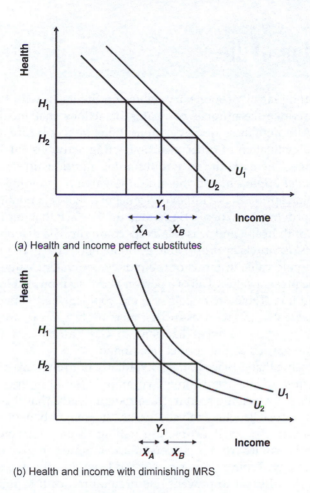

(a) Health and income perfect substitutes

(b) Health and income with diminishing MRS

Figure 11.6 Willingness to pay and willingness to accept

can verify from the figure, $X_B = X_A$, in other words WTA and WTP should be equal. However, in the case of health, it is arguable that health and wealth are not perfect substitutes; if we then make the usual assumption about the shape of indifference curves, that there is a diminishing marginal rate of substitution, then the indifference curves U_1 and U_2 will be as in Figure 11.6(b). As you may again verify, X_B should be greater than X_A – in other words, WTA should be greater than WTP.

In practice, it is usually found that WTA is greater than WTP for a wide range of goods and services, and it is often observed that the discrepancy is greater than can be explained by the existence of substitution effects. An explanation for this is *loss aversion* – people attach a greater value to something that they already have than to something that they can obtain. A bird in the hand is worth two in the bush even if it is certain that the birds in the bush will both end up in the hand!

11.9 The value of life

Finally, we look at the placing of monetary values on life itself, with the aim of evaluating either actions that reduce the number of deaths or actions that incidentally increase the number of deaths. Although these do have applications in health care, they are rather more widely found in the evaluation of other health-affecting activities, such as road safety and environmental change. There are in fact two different traditions in this, one which may be called the *human capital* approach, and the other the value of avoiding premature death.

The human capital approach is a rather old concept of how economics might measure the value of health improving activities, originating in the fact that mortality was the most important outcome of ill health and was relatively common. The evaluation of public health measures was therefore entirely appropriately evaluated in terms of reductions in numbers of deaths, and its economic value in terms of the money-equivalent value of those lives. In its crudest form, it is the present value of all of a person's contributions to Gross National Product (GNP) over their lifetime. There are of course more sophisticated versions of this, but in its essentials that is what it attempts to measure. It is an entirely appropriate measure to use if the evaluation is solely in terms of what happens to GNP and has a wider justification if maximising GNP is regarded as the correct maximand.

Measuring the value that is placed on the avoidance of premature death was often called in the past the *statistical value of life*. It is more commonly found in the evaluation of projects such as road building, in which the road traffic accident deaths that this will avert should be counted as part of a cost–benefit analysis, or as the major benefit of safety-improving measures. Essentially, it asks what people are willing to pay to avoid a reduction in the *risk* of death. The WTP values from each person are summed to give a value that they are collectively willing to pay. Typical figures calculated from this give the collective WTP value for a reduction in risk sufficient to prevent one premature death in millions of pounds.

Summary

1. Economic evaluation is concerned in part with how the output of health care can be defined, measured and valued.
2. Monetary valuation of health care benefits can be undertaken using revealed preference (RP) and stated preference (SP) approaches. RP refers to valuations of goods and services that can be inferred from real choices that are made in the everyday world. SP valuations are derived from surveys or experiments, which are often loosely known in health economics as willingness-to-pay (WTP) studies. The most widely recognised SP technique is the contingent valuation method. This refers to the valuation of a good or service, the measurement of value being contingent on the description of the hypothetical market that is given to respondents.

3. A recent addition to techniques of SP are discrete choice experiments, which view goods and services as bundles of characteristics or attributes, and it is people's preferences for those attributes that determine the overall preferences for a good.

4. The measurement of benefits in terms of improved health is common in economic evaluation. In particular, the concept of health-related quality of life (HRQOL) has dominated health indicators of the kind used in economic evaluation.

5. Indicators for measuring benefits that are based on questionnaires or interview schedules are called instruments. There are some general criteria for judging how good an instrument is, based on its reliability, validity, responsiveness and feasibility.

6. Instruments can be generic or disease-, condition-, treatment- or domain-specific.

7. If the instrument consists of a set of dimensions that have different levels, it is known as a profile. If the instrument is an index, then it can produce a single number representing the overall level of health.

8. Health can be regarded as the product of the level of health and the length of time that it is experienced, in other words a measure of fully healthy time. If the level of health is quantified using the concept of HRQOL, we can analyse the health experience of a person as variations in HRQOL over time, representing the prognoses with and without treatment.

9. The most commonly used measure that follows this approach is quality-adjusted life years (QALYs). This is calculated by multiplying the amount of time in a particular health state by the quality of life during that time, summing over all time periods and standardising to a year. Alternatives to QALYs are healthy year equivalents (HYEs) and disability-adjusted life years (DALYs).

10. Non-monetary valuation of health states can be undertaken with a variety of means, including rating scales, category scales and visual analogue scales, the standard gamble and the time trade-off.

11. Multi-attribute utility (MAU) measures can be used to compute the utility associated with different health states. In a MAU model, utility is derived from health state attributes. When estimating MAU models we are interested in the conditional utility of each attribute, which is quantified by the weights given to each attribute and their interactions.

12. An alternative to monetary valuation of health care benefits and the measurement of benefits in terms of improved health is to value the willingness to pay for health changes. This utilises the concepts of compensating and equivalent variation and of willingness to pay and to accept.

13. It is possible to place monetary values on life itself using a human capital approach or using avoidance of premature death studies.

CHAPTER 12

Economic evaluation methods

12.1 Introduction

This chapter provides an overview of the way economic evaluation methods are used in the health sector to assess value for money. Whereas Chapters 9 and 10 examined the theory and principles underpinning economic evaluation, our focus here is on the *practice* of economic evaluation – although clearly the theory and principles of economics informs both the evaluator's methodological tool kit and the way results are interpreted in order to draw conclusions about resource allocation.

One way to view economic evaluation is that it is a balance sheet, in which the costs and benefits of the outcomes of decisions are weighed together. It might be thought that the economist's task is simply to fill in that balance sheet and produce summaries of the results, but in practice economic evaluation is much more complicated. An obvious example is that we are usually evaluating non-marketed goods, and because information on costs and benefits are not automatically generated by a market these data must be specially collected or generated. Moreover, the vision of a balance sheet does not reflect the complexity of real-world decision making, in which there is considerable uncertainty about the actual numerical values that should be attached to costs and benefits. This chapter is about how in practice we obtain and use the data that economic evaluation requires.

12.2 Selecting the viewpoint

The motivation for any economic evaluation is a practical question asked in a specific context: Should we fund drugs for all patients with Alzheimer's disease, or only for those with moderate to severe forms of that condition? How frequently should mammography screening be done, and for women of what ages? Which is better: an expensive hip prosthesis that lasts longer, or a cheaper version with a greater probability of revision in the future? These are all examples of quite different sorts of questions confronting policy makers and which economic evaluation can inform.

Which method is to be used, even what constitutes a benefit and a cost, and how these are to be valued, depends on *who* is asking these questions, and *why*. Is it patients, lobbying for better health services? A health care provider, for example a hospital, trying to improve its efficiency? A third-party funder, trying to ensure that health care budgets are being used wisely? Or a medical devices company, wanting to market its products? The purpose of the economic evaluation will have a fundamental impact on the viewpoint from which the evaluation is to be performed; and the viewpoint chosen can occasionally have an important effect on the judgement whether something is or is not good value for money. Consider the pairs of options compared in Table 12.1. The characteristics of these options, their impacts, and the way in which different sorts of costs and benefits are spread between different parties, mean that in each case the choice about what viewpoint to adopt is likely to have an important influence on the results and conclusions of an economic evaluation.

There is a connection between the choice about perspective and the choice about the preferred method of economic evaluation. For example, cost–benefit analysis (CBA) generally adopts a societal perspective (Mishan, 1971; Dasgupta and Pearce, 1972), in keeping with its foundations in welfare economics, as detailed in Chapter 9. However, in practice CBA is rarely used in the health care sector. The question of perspective is somewhat more complicated in the more common case where cost-effectiveness analysis (CEA) or cost–utility analysis (CUA) are to be used, since benefits and costs are not measured in the same units and how any given perspective is interpreted may be different for the numerator and the denominator of the cost-effectiveness ratio (*CER*). Gold *et al.* (1996), reporting on the US Washington Panel on CEA, advocated taking a societal perspective on costs. However, they suggested that changes in productivity as a result of improved health – which have a monetary value – should not be offset against health care costs in the denominator as that might result in 'double counting' if the value of improvements in productivity are already factored into the utilities used to calculate QALYs in the numerator. Drummond *et al.* (2005) are less directly prescriptive but suggest that, 'when in doubt, the analyst should always adopt the societal point of view, which is the broadest one and is always relevant'.

An important advantage of the societal perspective on costs in CEA is that it avoids the possibility of identifying as cost-effective options that appear so merely because they shift costs between sectors or groups. Gerard and Mooney (1993) argue that where benefits are considered in terms of health outcomes, as in CUA, the costs should be restricted to those that have opportunity costs in terms of health outcomes. Another way of thinking about this is that it reflects the decision makers' approach to evaluation and the extra-welfarist foundations of such techniques. That is, if the aim is to maximise health gain from a fixed budget, then arguably only costs that fall within that budget should be taken into account. Applying this argument to the evaluations undertaken by the National Institute for Health and Clinical Excellence (NICE) in the UK, Devlin, Appleby and Parkin (2003) noted that:

TABLE 12.1 Why does perspective matter?

Option 1	Characteristics	Option 2	Characteristics
A law making cycle helmets compulsory	Government enacts the legislation and incurs some law enforcement costs – but the vast majority of the costs are borne by cyclists who are compelled to purchase helmets. See Hansen and Scuffham (1995).	Routine addition of fluoride into reticulated water supplies	Taxpayers bear the cost; everyone benefits from reduced risk of dental illness, but especially those with lower incomes. See Griffin *et al.* (2001).
An effective treatment for back pain is discovered	Back pain impacts on the use of health services but has a substantial effect on the ability of sufferers to return to work. From a societal viewpoint, improvements in productivity are important, but any reductions in the payment of sickness benefits are merely transfers from one person to another, with no net gain or loss. Changes in benefit payments would therefore not be included, although from the point of view of taxpayers, the reduced costs would be seen as an important benefit. See Maniadakis and Gray (2000).	Screening for breast cancer	Mammography screening results in early detection and effective treatment of breast cancer; evidence suggests it is most effective in older women. It is generally shown to be cost-effective. The improvements in life expectancy and quality of life that are produced are dominated by those whose workforce participation is typically low; productivity gain is not an important benefit of this intervention. See Szeto and Devlin (1996).
At-home treatment or supportive care is substituted for in-hospital care facilitating early discharge	From the health service point of view, this might be cost-neutral, cost-saving or cost increasing overall. Similarly, transferring services out of hospitals may increase or decrease costs incurred by patients and their caregivers. Many conclusions about the cost effectiveness of early discharge restrict their perspective to that of the health service, ignoring the costs to families. See Dougherty *et al.* (1998) and Beech *et al.* (1999).	Inclusion of IVF in health insurance or health system funded cover	A difficulty in the economic evaluation of IVF is that, while it is a health service, the benefits are not improvements to *health-related* quality of life as such, so measures such as QALYs are not appropriate. This suggests CBA would be a more appropriate method; with benefits assessed using willingness to pay, and a social perspective on costs. The problem is that this evidence on value for money is not readily compared to that from other health services. See Devlin and Parkin (2003).

A wider perspective on costs would require NICE to extend its remit to optimising resource use in the public sector generally, not just health care, and indeed in the economy as a whole. In other words, an 'über-NICE' would be required to compare all possible uses of society's total resources. Decisions made from this broader perspective might maximise society's welfare but would not maximise health gain from the NHS budget.

Restricting the perspective on costs in CUA and CEA to health service costs is by far the most common practice in published papers. However, as Johannesson (1995) and Byford and Raftery (1998) point out, this approach would lead to an allocation of resources that is not allocatively efficient in the welfarist sense; indeed Johannesson (1995) argues that, taken to the extreme, it would imply that the only costs that should be included are health service costs arising in one fixed-budget period, for example ignoring changes in future costs and resource use.

Restricting the perspective to health service costs is often problematic in the case of public health interventions, where the majority of the costs and benefits can be borne by organisations outside the health service, including by firms and other public sector organisations. NICE, in its public health guidance, recommends that analyses should be based on a public sector perspective (NICE, 2009), but that sensitivity analysis should be used to explore the impact of different perspectives.

The issue of what perspective to adopt in economic evaluation also affects the way health benefits are to be measured and valued in CUA. Although the perspective commonly taken in assessing costs in CUA is that of the health service, a social perspective is commonly adopted in the valuation of health outcomes – QALYs are estimated using social values, rather than those of patients (Gold et al., 1996; NICE, 2004). Nevertheless, some guidelines for economic evaluation (for example those of Ramsey et al., 2005) recommend that analysts collect preference weights as part of clinical trials, so that patients' preferences can be incorporated into CUA. This remains controversial, partly because there is evidence of systematic differences between patients' and the general public's valuation of health, particularly for chronic states: those experiencing ill health appear to adjust to it and to attach less disutility to it than those asked to imagine being in those states (Brazier et al., 2005). There is also the question whether the preferences of those who pay rather than those who consume should be used. A further issue concerns whose health is measured: the health outcomes that are measured and valued in CUA are usually, but not always, restricted to the recipients of treatment, rather than directly incorporating spill-over effects on the health-related quality of life of others. We will discuss these issues in more detail in Section 12.3.

Given the contention over the issue of perspective, what practical guidance is available? Brouwer et al. (2006b) suggest adopting a two-perspective approach in all routine analyses, presenting one cost-effectiveness ratio based on the health care perspective and another based on the broader societal perspective. They argue that 'the health-care perspective may assist the health-care policymaker better in achieving health-care goals, while the societal perspective indicates whether the local rationality of the narrow health-care perspective is also in line with societal optimality'.

In health care systems where economic evaluation evidence is used as part of a systematic decision-making process, the perspective is, for all intents and purposes, dictated by the stated requirements issued by the government body charged with preparing or considering evidence (for example, NICE, 2004). Byford and Raftery (1998) conclude that 'at the very least, economic evaluations should be explicit about the perspective they adopt. The exclusion of items, whether for practical reasons or as a result of pre-trial assessments, must be made explicit, explained, and discussed in terms of their likely influence on the final results.'

The following sections detail the practical steps involved in identifying, quantifying and valuing resource use and benefits.

12.3 Estimating costs

As we emphasised in Chapter 1, resources are limited – with the implication that the devotion of resources to any existing or proposed health care intervention necessarily diverts resources from some alternative use. This notion of opportunity cost is fundamental to the way costing is undertaken in economic evaluation. Costs are, in essence, the value of the resources used. In CBA 'the analyst must be interested in the benefits to be derived from the expenditure in question compared to the benefits that would have been obtained if the money had been used elsewhere' (Dasgupta and Pearce, 1972). This concept, social opportunity cost, may also be relevant in CEA or CUA in cases where the analysis adopts a societal perspective (see previous section). In the more common case, where the more restrictive health service perspective is used, opportunity cost still provides the conceptual basis for valuing resource use, but what is forgone is interpreted in a more restricted way: the next best opportunity forgone within the health sector.

The basis of economic costing is therefore quite distinct from accounting or financial cost approaches. The process of costing involves three steps: (1) identify and describe the changes in resource use, both increases and decreases, that are associated with the options to be evaluated; (2) quantify those changes in resource use in physical units; and (3) value those resources.

Most of the relevant resources, for example disposable rubber gloves, are bought and sold in markets, and prices for these are readily observable. Providing that these markets are competitive, firms will adopt technically efficient production processes to minimise production costs, and competition between firms will ensure that prices reflect the opportunity cost of these items. This draws on the proof, in welfare economics, of the First Fundamental Theorem of Welfare Economics, which was discussed in Chapter 5: in competitive markets, equilibrium prices of a good exactly equal both the marginal cost of their production *and* the marginal value consumers attach to them. Under these circumstances, economic costing is relatively straightforward: costs equal the quantity of a resource used multiplied by its price.

In reality, many markets are not fully competitive. For example, the wages paid to doctors may be a reflection of the lobbying power of medical associations or restrictions to licensing, rather than the value of their skills – see Chapter 8. The prices of drugs may reflect the effect of government regulations on licensing, pricing and intellectual property. Deviations of price from opportunity cost may arise from factors such as imperfect competition created by the inherent characteristics of the marketplace, for example a natural monopoly, or from distortions to markets created by government interventions. Where these are known, prices should be adjusted so that they better reflect opportunity cost. In practice, such adjustments are difficult to make and would rely on good information on the underlying costs of production, which is often not available. Further, where the perspective is that of the health service, there is an argument for not adjusting prices, on the grounds that the prevailing prices, even if inefficient, are *those they must pay* and are relevant to their budget. For example, the fixed prices for Healthcare Related Groups (HRGs) for hospital procedures, set by the UK NHS, are highly unlikely to be a reflection of the marginal cost of every UK hospital. However, they are the prices which are used by those who commission services and are therefore relevant for use as a basis for costing hospital care from an NHS perspective.

Where prices are used, it is important to consider whether the option being evaluated will, if implemented, result in price changes. This may be particularly important when the option will result in large changes to market conditions. For example, the inclusion of varicella vaccine on the schedule for routine immunisation, compared to its being available for individual purchase, changes both supply and demand conditions. Demand will increase because of the resulting subsidy to consumers; this enables large-scale manufacture and distribution; but the government may effectively become a monopsonist with great power to negotiate prices centrally. Predicting the effects on market prices is extremely difficult, and is best dealt with by incorporating plausible ranges around existing prices in sensitivity analysis, which is considered further in Section 12.6.

Valuing resource use becomes still more difficult in cases where there are *no* markets. This includes the value of patients' time in seeking and receiving care or of caregivers' time in providing informal supportive care. The latter can be an important element of costs and, as we saw in Table 12.1, may be particularly important in the evaluation of health care options that rely on such inputs. Values can be assigned to these resources using the same principle – opportunity costs. A carer's time may be valued at the wage rate where work is forgone, or at the value of leisure forgone. The attribution of values to non-market activities, sometimes called 'shadow pricing', can require heroic assumptions, so evaluations for which these costs are important should undertake a sensitivity analysis of plausible alternative valuations for these resources.

Finally, although the emphasis in economic evaluation is on marginal changes in costs and benefits, the available data frequently relate to *average* costs across patients in a given setting, or across settings. Average cost data have the principal advantage that they are readily available and that they will give an indication of the changes in costs *on average* that will be experienced when results are generalised or transferred to other settings. There are two issues with using average cost data. First, the addition to or reduction in costs from increased or decreased resource use may be higher, lower or the same as the average cost. Unfortunately, knowing what the relationship is between average and marginal cost requires information on the latter – the absence of which is the reason average costs are used! Secondly, average cost data obscure potentially important issues with respect to the technical efficiency of providers. If average costs are derived in one setting, for example a hospital, this assumes that the hospital is using the optimal combination of inputs. If average costs are derived from multiple settings, they will include a variety of underlying production technologies and a variety of underlying levels of production efficiency. Average costs are therefore less than ideal, because they comprise a 'black box' of underlying cost and production decisions. Analysts can add considerable value to their analyses – and aid the transferability of results – by describing and analysing the production technologies that underlie aggregate cost data.

12.3.1 Methods and data used in estimating costs

Approaches to costing fall into two broad types: macro- or 'top-down' costing, and micro- or 'bottom-up' costing. These are distinguished largely on the basis of the level of disaggregation at which individual resources are measured and valued as separate components.

A top-down approach may involve using pre-existing data on total or average costs and apportioning these in some way to the options being evaluated. Costs are not decomposed into their constituent quantities and prices. In contrast, a bottom-up approach identifies, quantifies and values resources in a disaggregated way, so that each element of costs is estimated individually and they are summed up at the end. The latter provides a greater insight into the health care programme being evaluated and facilitates the reporting of costs as components of quantities and prices – which in turn is a considerable advantage for transferability of findings between settings. For example, it facilitates re-analysis for different sets of prices that might prevail in different health care settings. It is, however, more time consuming. Table 12.2 shows the types of resource use that might be included in a bottom-up costing, and the manner in which the quantities and values may be dealt with in each.

Costing exercises may draw on a wide range of sources of data. Top-down studies generally rely on secondary data sources, such as routine accounting or management data. At the other extreme, clinical trials can design costing into the research design, so that individual record data of health care resource or patient costs are collected alongside clinical data. These data are amenable to more sophisticated statistical analyses, as will be discussed below. The separation of top-down and bottom-up costing approaches is not always clear. For example, often top-down studies are used to calculate unit costs, which are then combined with resource use data in bottom-up studies.

Patient costs may be obtained via patient and caregiver surveys. These may rely on retrospective recall of costs, or may take the form of patient diaries.

12.3.2 Which costs should we include?

Any new health care programme can have a complex and wide-ranging effect on resource use. In addition to the costs of delivering a service, there are costs that might be offset elsewhere in the system, including knock-on effects for future resource use in the health service or elsewhere. The identification of changes in resources may reveal a very long list of resource implications 'rippling out' from a given programme. However, in practice, it may not be possible for all these costs to be measured and valued in an economic evaluation.

TABLE 12.2	**Categories of resource use in micro-costing**

Type of cost	Quantity of resource	Value of resources: prices, imputed prices, or unit costs
Health service		
Staff (by type of staff)	Time	Wages + on-costs
Consumables (e.g. food; medicines; syringes)	Number/amount	Price
Overheads (shared institutional costs)	Proportion of total (or an approximation, e.g. m² floor space for the programme)	Proportional allocation
Capital items	Number of uses/proportion of total lifetime uses	Market price/rental value/replacement value
Other services (For example, social services, ambulance services, voluntary agencies)	Amount (as above, for health services)	Price (as above, for health services)
Patients, families and carers		
Time	Hours	Wage rates/imputed values
Out of pocket costs	Amount	Price
Changes in production and earnings	Time	Wage rates

Indeed, in some cases the magnitude of resources involved may be quite minor, of little consequence for results, and not worth the analytical effort that would be involved in generating cost data.

Moreover, in economic evaluation we are usually interested in incremental costs. There may be little need to quantify costs that are incurred equally by the options being compared. In all these circumstances, 'a good case can be made for excluding particular effects if they are likely to have little impact on the overall results. Pre-trial literature reviews and modelling can help prioritise items of importance' (Knapp and Beecham, 1993). This 'reduced list' method has been demonstrated by Knapp and Beecham (1993) to capture most relevant costs in mental health service evaluations, with the top five most costly services accounting for 94% of the total cost and the next five for only 4%. Byford and Raftery (1998) suggest that caution is required, however, citing a study costing screening for colorectal cancer that found reduced list costing to be less successful (Whynes and Walker, 1995). However, all studies inevitably have to address the issue of where to draw the line in costing. The analyst has a responsibility to justify any subjective decisions about which types of resource use are to be included and which excluded.

12.3.3 Should future costs and cost savings be included?

Health care programmes can affect both length and quality of life; these in turn interact with both current and future health care use, relating both to the condition of interest and to other conditions. Weinstein and Stason (1977) argue that the cost of 'saving' life in one way should include the future costs to the health service of death from other causes. The basis for this argument is that preventing premature death yields a benefit, captured in the denominator of a *CER*, but also a cost of the health services that would otherwise not have been consumed. Potentially, this argument would also extend to other sorts of non-health care costs. Should a smoking cessation programme factor in the increased health, pension, residential care and other costs associated with extending the lives of smokers?

Moskowitz (1987) argues against this, suggesting that 'this argument is inexhaustible and philosophically difficult to justify. If carried to the extreme, it would lead us to abandon all medical care. This would be the ultimate cost effective strategy.' In practice, different analysts respond to this issue in different ways: examples may be found of economic evaluations of mammography screening that do (Gravelle *et al.*, 1982) and do not (Szeto and Devlin, 1996) incorporate future health care costs. Methodological differences of this sort reduce the ability to make valid comparisons between results. A cogent argument against the inclusion of future costs is that these relate to specific programmes or treatments which *in themselves* ought properly to be the subject of economic evaluation.

In practical terms, this issue is a matter of researcher discretion, similar to the wider issues already noted concerning the appropriate boundaries for costs to be considered in an evaluation. Pragmatically, costs in the distant future, once discounted, may tend not to exert much influence on results (see Section 12.5), in which case the issue is largely irrelevant.

12.3.4 What if cost data are from different time periods?

A common issue in evaluation is that some cost or price data pertain to one, recent period, and other costs or prices relate to other, earlier periods. It is important to ensure that, where cost data relate to different years, these are inflation-adjusted prior to analysis. This is because the purchasing power of a pound, or any currency, changes through time and therefore a pound in one year does not mean the same thing as a pound in another year. Even where this is not an issue, *all* studies should report the year and currency in which their results are reported (for example '2004 Australian dollars') as this facilitates the transferability of results from that setting to others.

In the rest of this chapter, we will assume that any costs are reported in comparable, inflation-adjusted currency units. In Section 12.5 we will discuss a completely separate issue: whether or not we should *value* future costs and benefits differently from those in the present.

12.4 The measurement of health gain

Chapter 11 described the theory and practice of the measurement of health, and described how in principle we can use the resulting data to measure the gains in health from health care interventions. Here we outline how in practice these health gains can be measured. The most widely used measure in economic evaluation is QALYs, but we also consider two other possible measures of health gain: one healthy year equivalents (HYEs), because of its theoretical interest and the other, disability-adjusted life years (DALYs), because it is very widely used for economic analysis in developing countries and may be of increasing importance in economic evaluation studies in such countries.

12.4.1 Measuring quality-adjusted life year (QALY) gains

In Chapter 10, we described QALYs as being an area under the curve (AUC) measure, and illustrated this as a continuous function relating HRQOL to time. In practice, health state measurement is not so precise as to allow the detail that such a function would require, and the ways in which illnesses progress are not as neat. The usual way in which QALYs are calculated is by means of assessment at discrete points over time. In the intervals between these points, HRQOL is sometimes assumed to be constant. Box 12.1 illustrates this with a hypothetical example.

It is in fact rare to find data such as those in Box 12.1 in the real world, as the natural history of diseases – that is, the details of how they progress over time in people – is a very complex topic, requiring data that are hard to collect and analyse. For many diseases, the natural history is not known with precision; details relevant to quality of life issues over time are rarely known; it is even rarer for time series information on quality of life itself to be known; and the time intervals at which data are recorded are rarely capable of capturing key points in disease progression but are instead determined by other factors, such as when patients consult a doctor.

For the calculations in Box 12.1 HRQOL is constant between measurement points. Other assumptions are also used, such as linear increases or decreases (where the area under the curve is estimated using the trapezium rule), or curve fitting estimators between two fixed points – see Figure 12.1 for some examples.

The simple QALY model in Box 12.1 incorporates some assumptions about the relationship between the value assigned to health at particular times and the time itself. First, although values may change over time owing to changes in underlying health, they do not change because of the length of time for which they are experienced. For example, if a health state is given a value of 0.96, then every month spent in it is assumed to be worth 0.08 QALYs and every year in that state is worth 0.96 QALYs. This assumption is known as *constant proportionality*. It is quite plausible, however, that time and value are not independent in this way; for example, strong pain may be tolerable for short periods, but not for very long – this is known as *maximum endurable time*. In theory it would be possible to obtain valuations for

BOX 12.1   **Measuring QALY gains**

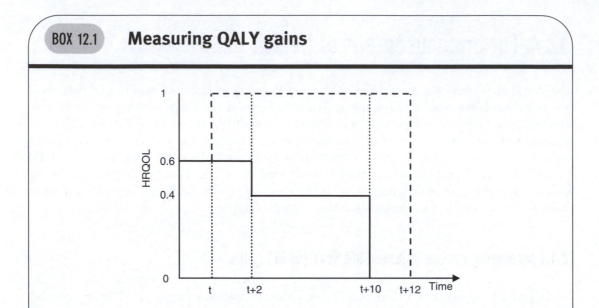

At time t, the patient has a health state valued at 0.6. If they have no treatment, their health will follow the solid line. It will deteriorate after 2 years (time t + 2) to 0.4 and remain at that level until death 8 years later (time t + 10). If they have treatment, shown by the dashed line, then their health state will immediately rise to full health, valued at 1.0, and remain at that level until death 12 years later (t + 12).

The QALY gain can be calculated in two equivalent ways. First, we can calculate total QALYs with and without the treatment and subtract the latter from the former. Without the treatment, the patient has 2 years at 0.6, which is 1.2 QALYs, plus 8 years at 0.4, which is 3.2 QALYs, making a total of 4.4 QALYs. With the treatment, the patient has 12 years at full health, which is 12 QALYs. The gain is therefore 7.6 QALYs. Alternatively, we can calculate the QALY gain directly. The first 2 years have a QOL improvement from 0.6 to 1, which is 0.4, giving a QALY gain of 0.8. The next 8 years have a QOL improvement from 0.4 to 1, which is 0.6, giving a QALY gain of 4.8. The final 2 years are additional years at full health, which is 2 QALYs gained. This gives a total of 7.6 QALYs gained, as before.

health states that relate to different durations, but this would require a lot of information that, to date, has not been practical to collect, so the assumption of constant proportionality is usually made on the grounds that it provides a reasonable approximation.

Secondly, the model assumes that QALYs are valued equally, whenever they are gained or lost, so that an improvement of 1 QALY spread over the next 5 years is valued equally to no improvement in the next 5 years but an improvement of 1 QALY spread over the following 5 years. Again, this may not be true, since in general people prefer to have benefits sooner rather than later, and in the context of QALY losses they may prefer to have them later rather

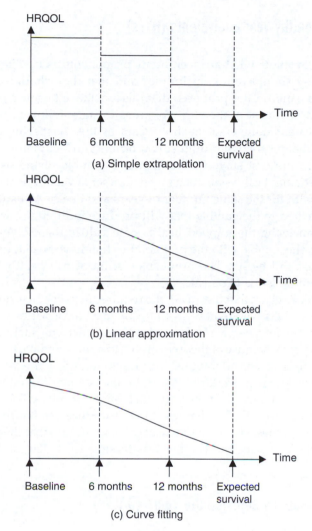

Figure 12.1 Estimating QALYs when HRQOL is measured at discrete points in time

than sooner. This can be, and is, dealt with by discounting, which is considered in more detail in Section 12.5, but as we will see it is controversial.

Finally, the periods of time in QALY estimates refer to periods of people's lives and therefore in effect also describe the progress of illness as their age changes. Any changes in underlying illness due to age can again easily be incorporated in this model, but it may also be that *values* are different at different ages. This makes matters far more complicated, though it can be taken into account by attaching different weights to different ages. But this is again controversial, especially since, as discussed in Chapter 7, it is sometimes asserted that values attached to older people's health should be lower. We will discuss it further in Chapter 13.

12.4.2 Measuring healthy year equivalents (HYEs)

HYEs attempt to incorporate what are seen by its proponents as two key features of health state values: that they should represent utilities and that they should place life-years and health within the same metric. It is proposed that this is achieved using a two-stage procedure involving an initial assessment of the utility of a health state, followed by conversion of the utility into an equivalent number of healthy years of life. A specific proposal is that an assumption is made that respondents' utilities conform to von Neumann–Morgenstern (vNM) axioms and therefore the first stage uses a standard gamble of the usual kind, in which alternatives are a particular health state for a given number of years, and a gamble in which the outcomes are full health for the same number of years and death. As usual, the aim is to find the probabilities attached to the gamble that will produce indifference with the health state. However, rather than using the implied health state values themselves, a second stage is undertaken in which the gamble with the probabilities that have been found is valued using a time trade-off against full health. The number of years of full health that is found to be equivalent to the gamble is the HYE value.

Proponents of HYEs claim that they meet the requirements for an economics measure that can be understood by others who require cost-effectiveness information, while QALYs do not (Gafni and Birch, 1993). However, HYEs have also been criticised (Buckingham, 1993; Culyer and Wagstaff, 1993), partly because of theoretical shortcomings and partly because of practical considerations. Theoretical considerations include that under the assumptions that are incorporated in the two-stage procedure the result must be identical to the results of a simple time trade-off, and any observed differences that might result will be due to the use of uncertainty and differences in the mechanics of the procedures, rather than reflecting a more accurate assessment of values. The main practical consideration is that the proposed method is very complex and there are doubts whether it is feasible to undertake large-scale research using it.

12.4.3 Measuring disability-adjusted life years (DALYs)

DALYs were developed by the World Health Organisation (WHO) and the World Bank as a health indicator that would be relatively easily measured in a wide variety of countries, especially those with lower incomes and therefore lower health care budgets and unsophisticated health information systems. They were seen as an improvement on using mortality alone and, by including disability, which was seen as being more easily measured than quality of life, they promoted the measurement of morbidity. Essentially, the DALY is a measure of population ill-health that combines information on the time that people live with a disability and the time that they lose to premature mortality. The aim is therefore to reduce DALYs.

Disability is measured with respect to functional status only, on a scale that ranges from 0, which is perfect functional health, to 1, which is as bad as disability can be. Mortality is measured by comparison to what is regarded as the maximum life expectancy that humans can expect to have – which currently is that of women in Japan. The standard procedure with DALYs is to map them to particular diseases. Discounting – see the next section – at a rate of

5% is standard. The values that are applied to health states are established by a person trade-off (PTO) valuation of health states by international experts in public health.

DALYs have been subject to severe criticism as part of a general critique of the WHO/World Bank Global Burden of Disease project. These are considered in Chapter 13.

12.5 Discounting

12.5.1 The rationale for discounting monetary costs and benefits

The options compared using economic evaluation may differ not only in how big costs and benefits are, but also when they occur. Consider the following options:

- A screening programme for the early detection of sexually transmitted disease, Chlamydia, incurs costs now, but the benefits in terms of the prevention of infertility will not be evident until some time in the future.
- Cataract surgery incurs costs now but also produces immediate benefits in terms of improved vision, which persist through time.
- Heart transplantation incurs costs now and produces immediate benefits, but requires a substantial annual cost for the remainder of the recipient's life, because of the drugs needed to prevent rejection of transplanted organs.

These interventions have very different time profiles of costs and benefits. This is relevant to economic evaluation because people are not indifferent to the timing of costs and benefits. We generally prefer to postpone costs and to enjoy benefits now. In other words, the value we attach to the benefit or cost reduces over time.

This phenomenon, known as positive *time preference*, is also argued to be relevant to social choices. Consider the following thought experiment. As a health care funder for your region, you are given an additional budget of £10 000 to spend on health care, which must be spent entirely on one of two government priorities, disease 1 and disease 2. With disease 1, the extra £10 000 incurred now will yield an extra 10 QALYs now. With disease 2, the same costs incurred now will yield an extra 10 QALYs *in 10 years' time*. The interventions are mutually exclusive and, if you do not spend the money, it will be clawed back by the government. Which would you choose?

Most people, it is argued, will prefer to spend the money on disease 1, since the payoff in terms of health gain is immediate. This suggests that there is positive *social time preference* and therefore it is argued that costs and outcomes that occur in the future should be given a lower weight compared to those that occur in the present. This is known as *discounting*; its precise use in evaluation is outlined below.

There are a number of reasons for people, individually and collectively, to have a positive time preference. One reason is that in a growing economy, where people will be better off in the future, the idea that people have a diminishing marginal utility of income implies that we will derive more satisfaction from an event now, when we have less income, than in the future, when we will be richer. A second is that people have a risk of death and other adverse events, so that we may wish to take account of the possibility that we will not be able to consume in the future. This is not an argument usually made at the societal level, however. A final reason is sometimes called short-sightedness, irrationality or impatience, but from an economics point of view it is a legitimate preference for anyone to have. It is less clear that it is an acceptable preference for society in general.

There is an alternative argument for discounting in public sector investment decisions, which is known as *social opportunity cost*. The resources invested in public projects, such as a particular health care programme, could have been invested in a private sector project, which would earn a rate of return on the investment. If there is no discounting in the public sector, the rate of return on society's scarce resources will be overvalued compared to their use in the private sector, which may lead to public sector projects being undertaken instead of more socially beneficial private sector projects. To avoid such inefficiency, it is necessary to ensure that public and private projects have a consistent discount rate, sometimes implicit in the private sector, but always explicit in the public sector.

A now-discredited argument is couched in terms of risk and uncertainty. The more distant in time a particular event, the less certain we are that it will occur and if it does how important it will be. We therefore place a higher value on the present, about which we are more certain, and the suggestion is that a *risk premium* should be added to the discount rate. This has long been recognised as a dubious approach (Sugden and Williams, 1978), but government agencies, such as the UK Treasury, have only recently recognised that risk is more appropriately addressed by calculating the *expected* value of future costs and benefits. Indeed, this was an important factor affecting the UK Treasury's revision downwards, in 2003, of the discount rate to be applied in public sector appraisal from 6% to 3.5% (HM Treasury, 2003).

12.5.2 The discounting formula

The use of discounting has the effect of giving less weight to future events. Economic evaluation weights future costs and benefits using a discount rate (r) according to the year in which they accrue, then adds them up and expresses them in present value (PV) terms. In effect, the discounting formula allows us to calculate, for any given monetary amount in the future (for example £100 in 2 years' time), the amount of money in the current time period (for example £90) such that someone would be indifferent between them. The discounting formula used is:

$$PV = FV\left(\frac{1}{(1+r)^t}\right) \qquad (12.1)$$

where PV = present value, FV = future value, r = discount rate, t = time period. The expression $1/(1+r)^t$ is known as the discount factor.

This discounting formula, which is the one conventionally used in economics, assumes a single, constant discount rate and an exponential functional form, as first proposed by Samuelson (1937). The discount rate that is chosen is applied to all time periods but, just as compound interest increases any initial amount invested exponentially, so discounting works to reduce the present value of future amounts.

An increasing body of research has used surveys to estimate peoples' discount rates for different health care programmes and has often found that people do not adhere to the exponential model. The emerging economics and psychology literature has given rise to alternative models of discounting, such as 'hyperbolic' (Henderson and Bateman, 1995), 'proportional' (Harvey, 1995) and 'slow' discounting (Weitzman, 1994, 1999). Under each of these schemes, the discount rate declines as impacts of the programme occur farther into the future. These alternative models suggest that time preference is better represented as decreasing impatience. For example, if offered the choice between £100 now and £120 in one year's time, most people will choose the immediate £100. However, given the choice between £100 in 5 years and £120 in 6 years most people will choose £120 in 6 years.

The impact on the present value of a project of using proportional instead of standard discounting procedures is quite dramatic: discounting with a constant discount rate of 10% per year values outcomes that occur now to be about 14 000 times more important than outcomes that will occur in 100 years. In contrast, proportional discounting, with an initial discount rate of 10%, values outcomes that occur now to be 11 times more important than outcomes that will occur in 100 years (Harvey, 1995). These alternative approaches remain contentious in economics, not least because the idea of a changing discount rate violates our usual economic assumptions about stability of preferences and gives rise to time inconsistencies. For that reason, the standard discounting formula continues to be used.

The application of discounting is straightforward using spreadsheets, but it is helpful to have a good intuitive understanding of the arithmetic, so a simple example is provided in Box 12.2.

It is usual for discounting to operate on an annual basis. This means that any costs that are incurred within one year from the introduction of a health care programme are classified as being in the present time period and are therefore not discounted. With regard to the discount formula, such costs are said to occur in year 0 and therefore have a discount factor of 1. The implication is that any health care option that has its incremental costs and effects within the current one year need not be discounted.

12.5.3 The choice of discount rate

The degree of time preference is represented by a discount rate, r. Clearly the choice of discount rate is important, because this will affect the magnitude of costs in an economic evaluation. The larger the value of r, the less weight is given to future events, so the present value of costs incurred in the future is smaller. Conversely, the smaller the value of r, the more weight is given to future events, so the present value of costs incurred in the future is greater.

BOX 12.2   **Discounting a future stream of costs**

Imagine a project which incurs costs of exactly £100 in the current year and for each of the following four years. To estimate the total costs of the programme, we need to add up these costs. But because they occur in different time periods, we must discount the future values to convert them into present value equivalents, before summing them. The profile of costs through time looks like this:

t_0	t_1	t_2	t_3	t_4
£100	£100	£100	£100	£100

't_0' effectively means 'now', or anything within the current one-year time horizon, since discounting is usually done on an annual basis. t_1 means next year, t_2 the year after that, and so on, to t_4.

We apply the discounting formula by giving values to 'r' and 't'. If the discount rate is 5%, then $r = 0.05$. 't' is the subscripted value for the time periods 0 (now), 1 (next year) and so on, as follows:

t_0	t_1	t_2	t_3	t_4
£100x1/$(1+0.05)^0$	£100x1/$(1+0.05)^1$	£100x1/$(1+0.05)^2$	£100x1/$(1+0.05)^3$	£100x1/$(1+0.05)^4$

At t_0, the discount factor $1/(1+0.05)^0$ is equal to 1, which means that £100 at t_0 has a present value of exactly £100. It is not discounted, because we are valuing all costs at their current value. At t_1, The discount factor is $1/(1+0.05)^1$ which equals 0.9524. We take the £100 in t_1 and multiply it by 0.9524, which gives £95.24. This is lower than £100, because we have discounted it, which gives a lower current value as future costs are less important to us. Extending this to all future years gives the following present values:

t_0	t_1	t_2	t_3	t_4
£100	£95.24	£90.70	£86.38	£82.27

Adding these up gives a total present value of £454, compared to the £500 that would be obtained by adding up the future amounts without discounting. Discounting places increasingly less importance on things that happen in the future. For example, if the stream of £100 continued until year 10, undiscounted costs would be £1 000, but discounted costs would be £810.

There is controversy surrounding the choice of discount rate to be used in economic evaluations. In practice, it is usually admissible to select a central best estimate and to vary this systematically in a sensitivity analysis to determine the impact of the choice on the conclusions of the study. The criteria to use in selecting the base-case value for the discount rate and the range of values for inclusion in sensitivity analysis are that they should be consistent with economic theory; should include any government recommended rates; and should include rates that have been used in other published studies to which the results may be compared or be consistent with current practice.

Further controversy arises from considering the possibility of a *negative* discount rate. Research in psychology has found that, in decisions involving health rather than money, choices are made that are inconsistent with positive discount rates. For example, if offered a choice between 10 days of illness now or in one year's time, people may prefer to have the illness now. They prefer to get it over with, so that they can enjoy future good health. Loewenstein and Prelec (1993) argued that this could give rise to negative discount rates for health, as people have preferences for the *ordering* not just their *timing*. Positive discount rates, by contrast, would suggest that people would prefer to delay illness until the future.

In general, the baseline discount rate adopted by most economic evaluations of health care programmes within the National Health Service in the UK, including by NICE, is that used by HM Treasury (2003) for appraising investment in public sector projects. At the present time, this discount rate is 3.5%. The database of guidelines on the International Society for Pharmacoeconomic Outcomes and Research (ISPOR) website shows that a variety of discount rates for costs are recommended across countries, ranging from 3% to 7% in the base case. Given the sensitivity of the results of an economic evaluation to the choice of discount rate, and the fact that the rate chosen will affect the cost ranking of different projects with different time profiles, it is good practice to calculate costs using a range of discount rates. There is no agreement regarding the best range of discount rates to use for this, though it would be normal to vary the discount rate between 0%, that is, no discounting, and 10%.

12.5.4 Discounting health effects

It is generally accepted that future costs should be discounted in an economic evaluation and, in CBA, it is also relatively non-controversial that benefits, in monetary terms, should also be discounted. In contrast, there is considerable debate surrounding the issue of whether to discount health outcomes such as QALYs, and what the appropriate discount rate is.

This debate has arisen for various reasons. A key feature, however, is that health outcomes are not usually expressed in monetary terms: it is generally accepted that a sum of money received in the present is worth more than that same sum of money received in the future, and this is why we discount costs expressed in monetary terms. However, it may be argued that health benefits are not 'tradable' in the same way because at an individual level one cannot 'give up a year of life' now, invest it, and obtain more than a year of life in the future.

The debate therefore concentrates on the issue of whether people have a time preference for receiving health benefits now rather than in the future in the same way that they might have a time preference for gaining monetary benefits now rather than later in life. Arguments both for and against this view are plausible, and the issue is currently unresolved.

Since it is usual for discounting to operate on an annual basis, health benefits that have an effect with a duration of less than one year would not normally be discounted anyway. Therefore, the issue of whether or not to discount health benefits only becomes important if the health care programme under consideration produces benefits that last for more than one year.

The effect of not discounting health benefits is to improve the cost-effectiveness of all health care programmes that have benefits beyond the current time period, because not discounting increases the magnitude of the health benefits. But as well as affecting the apparent cost-effectiveness of programmes relative to some benchmark or threshold, the choice of whether to discount will also affect the cost-effectiveness of different health care programmes relative to each other; that is, it may affect the *relative* cost-effectiveness of health care programmes. Discounting health benefits tends to make those health care programmes with benefits realised mostly in the future, such as prevention, less cost-effective relative to those with benefits realised mostly in the present, such as cure.

Most national guidelines for pharmacoeconomic research recommend that both costs and benefits should be discounted, and at the same rate. In 2004, NICE, for example, changed its recommended discount rate from 6% for costs and 1.5% for effects to 3.5% for both. But there remains considerable debate on this issue (see Brouwer *et al.*, 2006a). Theoretical arguments advanced in favour of discounting benefits, and for applying the same rate to both costs and effects, include the consistency argument (Weinstein and Stason, 1977) and the paralysing paradox (Keeler and Cretin, 1983), which we will consider below.

Table 12.3 describes a health care programme A which costs £10 000 now and yields 1 QALY in 40 years' time. Option B costs £10 000 now, and yields 1 QALY now. To argue that health outcomes should not be discounted is equivalent to saying that society is indifferent between A and B. However, because costs *are* discounted, this invokes a consistency problem. Consider A1–A3, each of which is a variant of programme A. In A1, the cost is £70 000 in 40 years' time, the present value of which, where $r = 5\%$, is £10 000 now, so both A and A1 have identical costs. Both have as their benefit 1 QALY in 40 years' time. So A and A1 are equally

---

TABLE 12.3   Weinstein and Stason's consistency argument

Programme	Cost	Benefit
A	$10 000 now	1 QALY in 40 years' time
A1	$70 000 in 40 years' time	1 QALY in 40 years' time
A2	$70 000 now	1 QALY now
A3	$10 000 now	1/7th of a QALY now
B	$10 000 now	1 QALY now

| TABLE 12.4 | Keeler and Cretin's paralysing paradox |

Programme	Time period		
	t_0	t_1	t_2
Option 1	Costs t_0/QALYS t_0		
Option 2		Costs t_1/QALYS t_0	
Option 3			Costs t_2/QALYs t_0

good value for money. Now consider A2: this is a programme that has £70 000 costs now and gains 1 QALY now. This programme is rather as if we could pull both the future costs and QALYs in A1 from 40 years' time into the current period. Because both costs and benefits are being transformed in this way, the *CER* in A2 is the same as in A1. So, in terms of a social ranking of programmes, A = A1 = A2. Now consider A3. Again, a transformation has been applied: both the benefits and the costs in A2 have been divided by 7, so the *CER* for A3 is identical to A2, and A = A1 = A2 = A3. Note that none of the options A1, A2 or A3 involves discounting QALYs, so the initial proposition that QALYs should not be discounted has been preserved in those variants of A. However, clearly A3 is *not* equal to B. Discounting costs and not discounting effects lead to a logical inconsistency.

A related argument is provided by Keeler and Cretin's (1983) paralysing paradox, illustrated in Table 12.4. Consider a health care programme, option 1, which is assessed in the current time period, t_0. The *CER* obtained by dividing the costs by the QALYs gained may well suggest that option 1 is good value for money. However, in a situation where costs are discounted but not health effects, it would be desirable for the decision maker to delay implementation of that programme until the following year (option 2). Considered from the current time period (t_0), option 2 has lower costs, but the same QALYs, and therefore a more favourable *CER*. The decision maker will prefer option 2 to option 1. However, delaying the programme for yet another year – option 3 – reduces costs, and the *CER*, still further. So option 3 > option 2 > option 1. Delaying the programme always improves cost-effectiveness, yielding the prediction that, where costs are discounted but QALYs are not, cost-effective interventions will always be delayed. Turning the proverb on its head: always leave to tomorrow what can be done today!

There have been some important challenges to these theoretical arguments. For example, the Keeler and Cretin finding relies on a set of assumptions that do not reflect reality. In practice, health care funders have time-limited budgets and do not defer decisions indefinitely (Parsonage and Neuberger, 1992). Van Hout (1998) has argued that the discount rate for health could be based on the expected growth in healthy life expectancy and the diminishing marginal utility related to such additional health, rather than the diminishing marginal value placed on income, as for costs. Gravelle and Smith (2001) argue that if the value of health grows over time, discount rates that are used for costs cannot directly be applied to effects, and should therefore be adjusted downwards.

12.6 Modelling-based economic evaluation

Earlier, we claimed that economic evaluation is much more complex than filling in and summarising a balance sheet. There are many calculations behind the estimates of costs and benefits, which are embodied in what is called an economic evaluation model. In practice, all economic evaluation in health care is now conducted in this way, and there are two reasons for this. One is that economic evaluations are usually based on different sources of data, which have to be linked together. The other is that there are many sources of uncertainty about the numerical information used in an economic evaluation, which will result in uncertainty about its results. In both cases, a formal model will help. We will first discuss the use of multiple data sources. Uncertainty is discussed in detail in Section 12.8, and here we discuss the modelling framework in which uncertainty is examined, called decision analysis.

12.6.1 Using multiple sources of data

It is very unlikely that all of the data that are required for an economic evaluation will be generated from a single source. Of course, it is in principle possible to design an experiment that would generate all of the data, but this is in fact rarely done. The reason for this is explained in Section 12.7, where we discuss the use of economic analysis as a part of a clinical trial. So, in practice the information on outcomes is obtained from multiple sources that need to be linked, sometimes in complicated ways, particularly because it is possible that they will not be entirely consistent.

Figure 12.2 illustrates how a simple economic model links data from different sources. It describes a hypothetical CUA of a new treatment for a chronic disease, the objective of which is to obtain an estimate of the treatment's *CER* compared to the alternative, which is the way in which the disease is currently managed by the health care team. This *CER* is located in the box to the far right of the diagram. A simple balance sheet that would enable us to calculate this would contain the data in the two boxes to the left of that – the estimated costs with and without treatment and the estimated utilities with and without the new treatment. However, these data are not observed directly, but must be obtained by calculation from other sources. The data that we actually have are contained in the boxes with straight line borders, and data calculated from them are contained in boxes with wavy borders.

A critical piece of information is a numerical value for the difference that the new treatment makes to costs and benefits. In this case, the source of this information is a clinical trial that compared the alternatives of the new treatment and existing disease management. This produced an estimate of the treatment effect, the effectiveness of the new treatment compared to existing disease management, contained in the box labelled 'Trial Data'. This information can be applied to data on the cost and benefit outcomes of current management to estimate the costs and benefits of the new treatment, which is what we need to calculate the *CER*.

Unfortunately, we also do not have data on the costs and benefits of existing management, because this would require a study that measured all of the outcomes over the whole

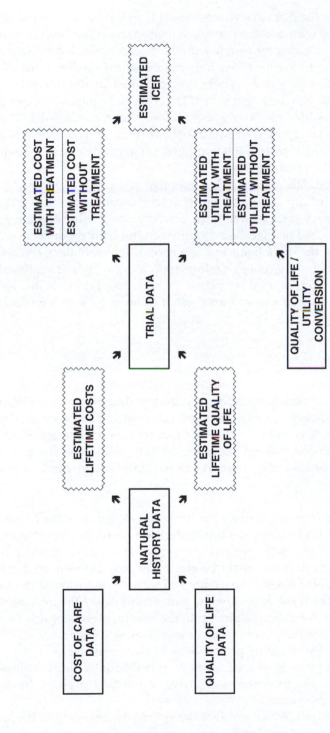

Figure 12.2 Economic evaluation model

time that the patient has the disease – which since it is a chronic disease means the patient's whole lifetime. However we are able to calculate them using other sources of data. We have information on the cost of caring for people with the disease, collected by a survey of a cross-sectional sample of patients. We also have information on the quality of life of patients with the disease, from a different survey. These are contained in the boxes to the far left of Figure 12.2. But they will only be a snapshot of the costs and quality of life of patients, not a profile over the patient's lifetime. So, we use another study, contained in the box labelled 'Natural History Data', that reported on how the disease evolves over time in people, and their life expectancy. This detailed information is applied to the yearly cost and quality of life data to give us the lifetime data that we need.

There is a final issue. The quality of life data that were published used a health status instrument in the form of a profile, and we wish to measure benefits in terms of utilities. Fortunately, another survey calculated utilities for every possible health state defined by that instrument, contained in the box labelled 'Quality of Life/Utility Conversion'.

We now have all of the ingredients that are needed to create the *CER*, and a recipe for combining them. But do we have enough information to make a decision based on the *CER*? That may depend on the degree of certainty that we have about the data that have been used. To examine this issue, we need a more formal set of techniques, which go under the general title of *decision analysis*.

12.6.2 Decision analysis

The main purpose of economic evaluation is to inform decisions about alternative uses of scarce resources. This involves using uncertain information; in practice, although uncertainty can be reduced, it is unlikely that we can remove it entirely. Decision analysis specifically looks at decision making under uncertainty, using theories of probability and of expected utility. It has a set of quantitative techniques that are applied in the following five steps.

1. Structure the problem by constructing a mathematical model of decision making as a series of connected events. This involves identifying decision alternatives, or strategies, listing the possible outcomes of each alternative and specifying the sequence in which the events take place. For example, the decision might be about choosing between medical and surgical treatment for a particular illness. The events will include provision of the treatments and the outcomes will include the impact on the patient's health of the treatment. Some of the events will be certain, for example providing the treatment; others will be uncertain, for example whether or not the patient's health improves as a result.
2. Quantify uncertainty by assigning probabilities to chance events.
3. Quantify preferences by assigning values to all possible outcomes of chance events.
4. Combine uncertainty and preferences to arrive at the best decision by calculating the expected value of each strategy.
5. Perform *sensitivity analysis*, which involves the systematic changing of the assumptions in steps 1–3 to see the impact on step 4.

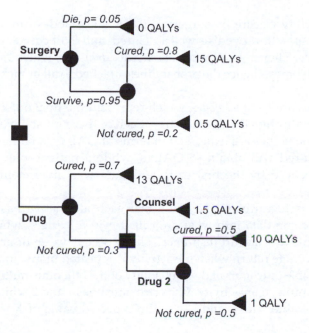

Die, p= 0.05
0 QALYs
Surgery
Cured, p =0.8
15 QALYs
Survive, p=0.95
0.5 QALYs
Not cured, p =0.2
Cured, p =0.7
13 QALYs
Counsel
1.5 QALYs
Drug
Cured, p =0.5
10 QALYs
Not cured, p =0.3
Drug 2
1 QALY
Not cured, p =0.5

Figure 12.3 Decision tree

Although not the only decision analysis technique, the most common involves use of a *decision tree*, which is a useful way of envisioning a decision analysis model. Figure 12.3 illustrates a decision tree for a hypothetical example. The tree is made up of *nodes*, which represent events and *branches*, which connect the nodes.

Square nodes are *decision nodes*, which represent decision points controlled by the decision maker. In our example, the initial decision is between medical treatment, leading to a branch labelled 'Drug', and surgical treatment, with a branch labelled 'Surgery'. There is also a second decision, which is contingent on whether or not the first drug provides a cure. If it does not, there is a decision between a second-line drug and counselling to help the patient cope with the decision not to try further treatment. A decision node can have more than two alternatives, for example, physiotherapy as well as surgery and the drug, but these must be *mutually exclusive* – the patient cannot have two of these therapies at the same time or all three. If it *is* possible to have more than one, then there should be an explicit alternative – in our example, that would require a third branch, labelled 'Drug and Surgery'.

Circular nodes are *chance nodes* or *probability nodes*, which represent chance occurrences that are not under the control of the decision maker. In our example, there are four chance nodes. The surgery branch has an initial chance node representing the probability that the patient survives the operation. There is then a second-chance node for those patients who do survive, which shows the probability that they are cured or not. The drug branch has an initial chance node showing the probability of cure with the first-line drug, and a second-chance node for those patients who have not been cured by this and have been offered the second-line drug. Each branch leading from a chance node must have a probability attached to it – for example, the probability of cure by surgery is 0.8. Chance nodes can also have more than alternatives, for example 'Improved' as well as 'Cured' and 'Not cured', but again these must be mutually exclusive. They must also be *collectively exhaustive*, which means that they must cover all possible outcomes – hence the probabilities attached to all branches from a node must sum to exactly 1.

Triangular nodes are *terminal nodes*, which represent the final outcome associated with a particular pathway through the decision tree. Each of these must have a value assigned to it. In our example, the values are expressed in terms of QALYs; a patient who has survived surgery and been cured will obtain 15 QALYs, while a patient who was given medical treatment, was not cured by the first drug and then was given counselling will obtain 1.5 QALYs.

The next stage is to calculate the value that each alternative has, by combining the uncertainty and outcome data into what are called *expected values*, which we discussed in Chapter 6 in the context of health insurance. The expected value of an activity which has known risks is the average return when the activity is repeated many times. It is calculated as the sum over all possible outcomes of the probability of the outcome multiplied by the value of the outcome. For example, if an activity X has two outcomes 1 and 2 which have probabilities $p(X_1)$ and $p(X_2)$ and values $U(X_1)$ and $U(X_2)$, the expected value of X is

$$E(X) = p(X_1)U(X_1) + p(X_2)U(X_2) \tag{12.2}$$

More generally:

$$E(X) = \sum_{i=1}^{n} p(X_i)U(X_i) \tag{12.3}$$

A way in which this is often done is *folding back* or *pruning* the decision tree, so that separate expected values for all events are revealed. This procedure is undertaken from right to left, working back from the final outcomes, pruning branches of the tree at the decision nodes, and finishing with the original choice. In our example, the first expected value to be calculated is for those who survive surgery; it combines the probability of cure and the QALYs obtained by those who are cured and those who are not cured, and is given by $0.8 \times 15 + 0.2 \times 0.5 = 12.1$. Similarly, the expected value for those who have the second drug is $0.5 \times 10 + 0.5 \times 1 = 5.5$. This expected value enables us to make our first decision. The expected value of Drug 2 is greater than the value of counselling. So, we would choose Drug 2 if the patient was not cured by Drug 1.

The next step is to calculate the expected value of surgery. One of the values to be incorporated is no QALYs for those who do not survive, which is one of the final outcomes. However, the other value, for those who do survive, is not a final outcome but is the expected value for those who survive surgery, calculated above. So the expected value of surgery is $0.05 \times 0 + 0.95 \times 12.1 = 11.495$. Similarly, the expected value of medical therapy is made up of a final outcome, if the patient is cured, and an expected value, if the patient is not cured and has the second line drug. The calculation is $0.7 \times 13 + 0.3 \times 5.5 = 10.75$. We now have all of the information required to compare the alternative strategies. The expected value of surgical treatment is greater than that of medical treatment, and if the decision-making criterion is to choose the most beneficial option, then it should be surgery. We are also able to quantify the advantage of surgical treatment, which is $11.495 - 10.75 = 0.745$ QALYs.

12.6.3 Markov models

The decision analysis model that we have looked at describes a process in which a fixed sequence of events leads to an outcome and, except that they are sequential, does not involve as an important feature a time dimension. But many real-world processes are dynamic – patients are not usually simply cured or not as a result of treatment, they may initially get worse, then improve, perhaps relapse and improve again before they are finally thought of as cured. *Markov models* are a way in which these processes can be structured and analysed.

In health care evaluation, the most common use of Markov models is in analysing the evolution of health states over time for a particular illness. The models assume that patients at any time are in one of a specific number of *Markov states*, in this case health states. Over specific time periods, called *cycles*, they either stay in the same state or move to one of the other states, with a given probability of moving known as a *transition probability*. Figure 12.4 shows a simple example in which there are three possible states: well, sick and dead. There will be an initial distribution of a population between these states; if this is a patient population, all will be in the state 'sick'. During the first cycle, some will become well, some will die and others will remain sick, giving a new distribution. This will be repeated for the second cycle, but there are

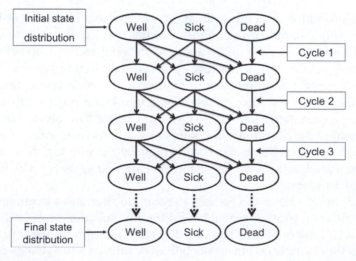

Figure 12.4 Markov states

now two other states that have to be taken into account: if the patients are well, they may remain well, become sick or even die; but those who died during the first cycle cannot of course move from that state – which is known as an *absorbing state*. This can be repeated as many times as required, although in this particular model eventually everyone will end up in the absorbing state, demonstrating Keynes' assertion that in the long run we are all dead.

How the distribution changes over time and how quickly it converges to a final state depends on the size of the probabilities, which are often expressed in the form of a *transition matrix*, such as:

| | | Finishing state | |
	Well	Sick	Dead
Well	0.5	0.4	0.1
Starting state **Sick**	0.2	0.5	0.3
Dead	0	0	1

If we consider a group of 1 000 sick patients, in the first cycle, 500 will remain sick, 200 will become well and 300 will die. In the second cycle, of the 500 who are sick, 250 will remain sick, 100 will become well and 150 will die. Of the 200 who are well, 100 will remain well, giving a total of 200 well people; 80 will become sick, giving a total of 330 sick people; and 20 will die, making 170 total deaths and therefore a total of 470 dead people. This will continue for as many cycles as are required. Table 12.5 shows the distributions for the first 20 cycles. Note that the total always remains the same. In this model, everyone is dead by the 30th cycle.

To make this useful for economic evaluation, we have to add in costs or benefits or both; we will give an example of measuring utilities. For this, we require a utility value for each of the health states. Suppose that the utility assigned to being well is 1, to being dead is 0 and to being sick is 0.6. At the end of the first cycle we will accumulate for that time period $500 \times 0.6 + 200 \times 1 = 500$ utility units; let us assume that a cycle is one year, so that means 500 QALYs. At the end of the second cycle we accumulate a further $330 \times 0.6 + 200 \times 1 = 398$ QALYs, giving a cumulative total of 898 QALYs. The last two columns of Table 12.5 show how QALYs accumulate over time; for simplicity we have ignored the effect of time preference, though this could be taken into account by discounting. Note that most of the QALYs are accumulated in the early years; the total after 30 years is 2 340, but 90% of this is gained in the first 10 years.

A simple way in which this can be used to compare alternative treatments is to make an assumption that different treatments will have different transition probabilities and therefore generate different utilities or costs. There are different assumptions that can be made within Markov models – for example that the probabilities or utility values change over cycles – and states and the transitions between them can be made much more sophisticated.

TABLE 12.5		**Markov process**				
Cycle	Well	Sick	Dead	Total	Total Utility	Cumulative Utility
0	0	1 000	0	1 000		
1	200	500	300	1 000	500	500
2	200	330	470	1 000	398	898
3	166	245	589	1 000	313	1 211
4	132	189	679	1 000	245	1 456
5	104	147	749	1 000	192	1 648
6	81	115	804	1 000	150	1 799
7	64	90	846	1 000	118	1 917
8	50	71	880	1 000	92	2 009
9	39	55	906	1 000	72	2 081
10	31	43	926	1 000	56	2 138
11	24	34	942	1 000	44	2 182
12	19	26	955	1 000	35	2 216
13	15	21	965	1 000	27	2 243
14	11	16	972	1 000	21	2 265
15	9	13	978	1 000	17	2 281
16	7	10	983	1 000	13	2 294
17	6	8	987	1 000	10	2 304
18	4	6	990	1 000	8	2 312
19	3	5	992	1 000	6	2 319
20	3	4	994	1 000	5	2 324

12.7 Trial-based economic evaluation

Although from an economics point of view, economic evaluation in health care is just an application of more general cost–benefit techniques, from a health care point of view, cost–benefit and cost-effectiveness analyses are just special kinds of more general health care evaluation. The dominant technique in general health care evaluation is the clinical trial, in which an experiment is carried out under controlled conditions to determine in a scientific way which of a number of possibilities is best. This is promoted for good reason, because its focus is on the *efficacy* or *effectiveness* of health care interventions. Other methods of determining effectiveness, such as case records and uncontrolled experiments, are open to bias and the consequences of carrying out ineffective, or even harmful, procedures may be great, as will the consequences of not carrying out effective procedures.

As a result, there have been considerable efforts to include economic analysis within trials. In theory, this is reasonable and indeed desirable, since if we can design an experiment that includes all of the data required by economic analysis it may answer the questions that we want to answer in a scientifically rigorous and highly acceptable way. It would also automatically deal with many of the problems of uncertainty about data that modelling has to worry about. In practice, however, this has proved to be very difficult to do. The reasons are partly that there is reluctance by those who undertake clinical trials to include economic data and alter their trial protocol to meet economics considerations; and partly because clinical trials as normally carried out have proved unsuitable as the only source of data for economic evaluations (Buxton *et al.*, 1997; Halpern *et al.*, 1998).

This unsuitability of clinical trials mainly results from their artificial nature. To ensure replicability of results, they are conducted under the equivalent of laboratory conditions, which means that they may not be representative of actual medical practice, which is what economic evaluation is seeking to inform, and may not be widely generalisable. Even the economic data that are collected may not be typical of the wider world. It might be argued that it is possible to conduct a trial that would overcome these problems, and in fact there are trials – called pragmatic trials – that attempt to do this. But such trials have to collect a very large amount of data and collect them for a very long time; they will therefore be very expensive and take a long time to report. Decision making cannot always wait a long time, and in any case given change in health care, such a trial might be looking at an obsolete technology or problem that has changed considerably.

In addition, for financial and practical reasons, many clinical trials do not follow all the participants until they have died. If the time horizon of an economic evaluation is the final follow-up point in the trial, and this is not after the last patient has died, then the incremental costs and benefits of an intervention may not reflect the true costs and benefits that would be found if a longer time horizon was used. One solution to this problem is to extrapolate beyond the end of the trial, for example modelling lifetime costs and benefits. However, to do this requires an economic model of the kind described above.

As a result, many argue not only that it is inevitable that real-world clinical trial data will of necessity have to be supplemented by a great deal of economic modelling, but that this is in fact a superior way of conducting economic evaluation. As Halpern *et al.* (1998) put it, modelling deals with a real-world problem – decision making with imperfect knowledge under uncertainty – and provides timely information. However, it is the case that economic models can and should include data from clinical trials, and if the trial contains relevant economic data then these are a good source of such information.

12.8 Dealing with uncertainty: sensitivity analysis

We have discussed how decision analysis deals with certain types of uncertainty by assigning probabilities to events within a model. Clinical trials also incorporate uncertainty, since effectiveness results are generally provided as both a mean effect and also a confidence interval. Other aspects of uncertainty are dealt with by sensitivity analysis, which is a set of techniques that essentially seek to analyse how sensitive results are to uncertainty. In the context of modelling, it analyses how sensitive results are to changes in the model, for example changes in the structure of the decision tree or in the data that are contained within it.

Uncertainty takes various different forms, and taxonomies have been developed to classify them. Manning *et al.* (1996) distinguished between *parameter* and *modelling* uncertainty. Parameter uncertainty is 'uncertainty about the true numerical values of the parameters used as inputs' in an economic evaluation model. It can arise if the values are unknown, there is no consensus about them, they are subject to sampling variability, or it is unclear how they relate to different populations. Modelling uncertainty comprises *model structure* uncertainty, which concerns how the elements of the model are fitted together, and *modelling process* uncertainty, which results from decisions made by the analyst. All of these types of uncertainty can be addressed through sensitivity analysis.

What do we do if we find that the results are sensitive to changes in assumptions or data? Essentially, we need to improve the data that we have and to reduce the amount of uncertainty. In what follows, we refer to the model that has the best assumed structure and data as the *base case*. The assumptions and data that we wish to test are referred to as *parameters* of the model.

12.8.1 One-way sensitivity analysis

One-way sensitivity analysis means looking at how sensitive results are to changes in one parameter. Figure 12.5 illustrates this, using the example of the alternatives of surgery and drug therapy for a particular illness and the sensitivity of the results to assumptions about the appropriate discount rate. The *CER* for surgery versus drug therapy is measured as the incremental cost per QALY gained, calculated as the cost of surgery minus the cost of drug therapy divided by the QALYs associated with surgery minus the QALYs associated with drug therapy. The issue for the decision maker is whether the *CER* is below the ceiling ratio, in which case surgery is the preferred option, or above it, in which case drug therapy is preferred.

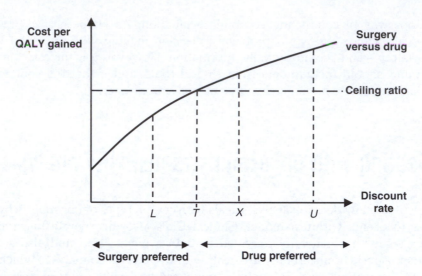

Figure 12.5 One-way sensitivity analysis

The solid line shows how *CER* changes as the discount rate changes. It increases as the discount rate increases because, although there are some longer-term follow-up and maintenance costs for surgery, most of its costs are immediate, while the drugs must be taken over a long period. As a result, the incremental cost of surgery rises as the discount rate rises because the cost of the drug option falls; hence the *CER* is increasing.

The point *X* shows the base case value of the discount rate. Drug therapy is preferred because the *CER* is higher than the ceiling ratio, shown by the horizontal dashed line.

If at every possible value of the parameter the decision to accept or reject surgery is the same, then the decision is clear cut and we can confidently state that the decision is not sensitive to the value of the uncertain parameter. In our example, this is not the case. At low levels of the discount rate, surgery is preferred, but as it increases the relative cost-effectiveness changes so that at some point drug therapy is preferred. At the point *T* the *CER* is equal to the ceiling ratio, and a change in the preferred option occurs. This kind of analysis is known as *threshold analysis.* This is not the same usage of this term as in cost-effectiveness threshold, which is another term for the ceiling ratio. *T* is the threshold value for the parameter being varied, in this case the discount rate, between accepting one option and another.

If *T* and *X* are very different, then it is reasonable to say that the results are not sensitive to the values of the parameter; if they are very similar, then they are sensitive. But what do we mean by 'very different' and 'very similar'? A simple way to understand this is to consider what may be called a *plausible range* for the parameter. This is defined by plausible upper and lower values for the parameter, shown in the figure as *U* and *L*. It could be informed by expert opinions or some other method. A popular method used to be to raise and lower the base case value by some percentage. Where possible, a better approach is to use proper statistical procedures, which will be described below. Whatever the source, given a plausible range *U* to *L* it is easy to tell whether the optimal decision is sensitive to the assumptions underlying the parameter value. If *T* lies within *U–L*, as in the example, it is sensitive; if outside, it is not.

12.8.2 Multi-way sensitivity analysis

It is possible to vary more than one parameter at the same time and view the combined impact on the outcomes. Unfortunately, for more than two or three parameters, this becomes very cumbersome, but it is quite easy to see how this works for two parameters, as in Figure 12.6. The two parameters are the discount rate, as before, and the assumed proportion of patients that experience adverse events with the drug. Obviously, the drug adverse event rate will not affect the surgical option, but the higher it is the higher the cost for the drug option and therefore the better the relative cost-effectiveness of surgery. Each point on the figure shows a different combination of the discount rate and adverse event rate. Some will favour surgery and others drug therapy; the solid line shows all of the combinations where the *CER* of surgery compared to drug therapy is equal to the ceiling ratio – in other words, a threshold line rather than a point.

Plausible ranges may also be defined, and in combination they define an area in which the results are plausible, shown as the grey box. Note that in this case, if we were to look at separate one-way analyses of the parameters, we would conclude that the results were not sensitive to the value of them. This is shown by the lines that pass through the base case *X*, which in each case cross the threshold outside of the relevant plausible range. However, in combination the results are sensitive to the assumptions, since the threshold line is partly within the plausible region. The reason is that the one-way analyses are evaluated at the base case value for all parameters, but the two analyses are evaluated at all plausible values. One-way analyses can therefore be misleading. In fact, we should investigate the impact of the plausible ranges of *all* parameters in combination.

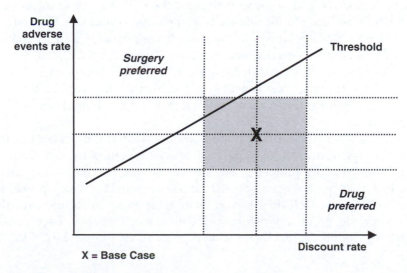

Figure 12.6 Two-way sensitivity analysis

12.8.3 Statistically-based sensitivity analysis

The problem with 'plausible range' methods is that their basis is often unclear and not testable. Statistical theory gives us a way in which we can quantify uncertainty in a consistent and easily interpretable way, by regarding the base case results as a *point estimate* of cost-effectiveness and sensitivity analysis as providing an *interval estimate*, or confidence interval. When this is done as part of a decision analysis model, it is called *probabilistic sensitivity analysis*, but when it is forms part of a trial-based analysis it is called *stochastic cost-effectiveness analysis*. Many of the analytical tools used in these contexts are very similar, but the concepts and methods underlying them are sometimes rather different.

In stochastic cost-effectiveness analysis we have patient level cost and outcome data from economic analysis alongside clinical trial from which we wish to estimate a confidence interval for the *CER*. Unfortunately, this is problematic because ratios do not have simple probability distributions, and the distribution from which confidence intervals can be calculated has to be approximated. There are a number of possible solutions to this, but the most popular is to employ a statistical technique called *bootstrapping*, where the distribution of *CERs* is generated by repeated sampling from the data.

In the context of modelling, a *CER* distribution can be created using Monte Carlo simulations. This requires a distribution to be assumed, if it is not known, for each of the model's parameters, and samples to be taken from those distributions from which the *CER* is calculated. Repeating this many times builds up an empirical distribution of *CERs* in a similar way to bootstrapping, although the sampling is not from real observations but from simulated observations derived from, in some cases, assumed distributions.

There is, however, a far worse problem with *CERs*. It is quite possible that the distribution of *CERs* may spread over more than one quadrant of the CE plane and the *CER* has discontinuities at the boundaries between different quadrants. In particular, a distribution may include both positive and negative values for the *CER* and these mean such different things that it makes no sense to include them in the same confidence interval.

There are two possible solutions to this, which we introduced in Chapter 10: the net benefits approach and the cost-effectiveness acceptability curve (CEAC), which are both based on a critical ceiling ratio or threshold defining the level of cost-effectiveness that a treatment must achieve to be acceptable. Net benefit is not subject to the problem that the *CER* has, because it is a single number rather than a ratio. It is therefore straightforward to calculate a confidence interval for it.

The CEAC deals with this in a different way, essentially by retaining the *CER* but replacing the concept of a confidence interval. It was invented by van Hout *et al.* (1994) specifically to deal with the problems with cost-effectiveness confidence intervals in the context of clinical trials but has been adapted for use in modelling using probabilistic rather than stochastic CEA. The *CER* distribution enables us to calculate the probability that a treatment is acceptable, given a particular value for the ceiling ratio. Each possible level of the ceiling ratio is plotted against its associated probability, giving the CEAC described in Chapter 10.

Summary

1. The perspective of an economic evaluation is important because it determines which method of economic evaluation is to be used, what constitutes a benefit and a cost, and how these are to be valued. Common viewpoints are that of the health service and that of society as a whole. Researchers should be explicit about the viewpoint they adopt.

2. When estimating costs, the aim is to estimate the value of the resources used in terms of their opportunity costs. The process of economic costing involves three steps: identifying and describing resource use changes; quantifying them in physical units; and valuing them.

3. Approaches to costing fall into two broad types: macro- or 'top-down' costing, and micro- or 'bottom-up' costing, distinguished largely by the level of disaggregation with which individual resources are measured and valued.

4. It is important to ensure that, where any cost data relate to different years, these be inflation-adjusted prior to analysis.

5. Quality-adjusted life years (QALYs) can be measured as the area under a curve relating HRQOL to time. Empirically, calculation of QALYs can be problematic because HRQOL is not measured continuously but at discrete points in time.

6. Healthy year equivalents (HYEs) attempt to incorporate two key features of health state values, representing utilities and placing life years and health within the same metric. A two-stage measurement procedure assesses a health state's utility, then converts it into an equivalent number of healthy life years. Proponents of HYEs claim that they are uniquely suitable for economic evaluation; critics that HYEs have theoretical shortcomings and are impractical.

7. Disability-adjusted life years (DALYs) were developed as a measure of population ill health that is easily measured in a wide variety of countries, especially those with lower incomes. This was seen as an improvement on using mortality alone, including disability, which is more easily measured than quality of life. DALYs combine information on the time that people live with a disability with the time that they lose to premature mortality.

8. Alternatives in economic evaluation may differ with respect to their timing. Most people put a lower weight on costs and outcomes that occur in the future, so these should be discounted compared to those that occur in the present. Economic evaluation weights yearly costs and benefits using a discount rate and sums them to form a present value.

9. It is generally accepted that future costs should be discounted in an economic evaluation and, in CBA, that benefits should also be discounted. There is a debate about whether or not to discount health outcomes such as QALYs, and what the appropriate discount rate is.

10. There are many calculations behind the estimates of costs and benefits, which are embodied in what is called an economic evaluation model. In practice, all economic evaluation in health care involves modelling of some kind, because economic evaluations are usually based on different sources of data, which have to be linked together, and there are many sources of uncertainty about the numerical information used in an economic evaluation, which will result in uncertainty about its results.

11. The main purpose of economic evaluation is to inform decisions about alternative uses of scarce resources. This involves using uncertain information; in practice, although uncertainty can be reduced, it is unlikely that we can remove it entirely. Decision analysis specifically looks at decision making under uncertainty, using theories of probability and of expected utility.

12. The most common decision analysis technique involves the use of a decision tree, which is a useful way of envisioning a decision analysis model. Markov models are a way in which dynamic real-world processes can be modelled.

13. Uncertainty can be dealt with in economic evaluation using sensitivity analysis. One-way sensitivity analysis looks at how sensitive results are to changes in one parameter. Multi-way sensitivity analysis varies more than one parameter at the same time and views the combined impact on the outcomes.

14. Stochastic cost-effectiveness analysis estimates a confidence interval for the *CER* from patient level cost and outcome data. One method of doing this is to use bootstrapping, where the distribution of *CER*s is generated by repeated sampling from the data. It is also possible to compute confidence intervals around net benefit measures.

15. An alternative statistical framework to the confidence interval is to use the cost-effectiveness acceptability curve.

CHAPTER 13

The use of economic evaluation in decision making

13.1 The decision-making context: why is economic evaluation used?

The methods of economic evaluation detailed in Chapters 10–12 were developed to inform resource allocation decisions about health care. We have already considered how methodological issues, such as uncertainty regarding costs and effects, can be handled in analysis and reported to users. The aim of this chapter is to consider how in practice economic evaluation evidence is used in decision making, and to highlight issues that persist in making resource allocation decisions based on value for money.

Two decades ago, studies reported that the growing enthusiasm of economists in undertaking economic evaluation was not matched by use of the resulting information in practice. Few decision makers reported using economic evidence in the process of making practical decisions (Ludbrook and Mooney, 1984; Drummond, 1987). The situation now is markedly different. Economic evaluation is widely and systematically used in many developed economies, such as Australia, the UK, New Zealand and Canada. In developing economies, aid and development agencies make extensive use of economic evaluation evidence to help target scarce resources to greatest effect (World Bank, 1993). Perhaps the most prominent example of the use of economic evaluation in decision making is the National Institute for Health and Clinical Excellence (NICE). Box 13.1 discusses its use of cost-effectiveness analysis to guide its recommendations to the NHS in England and Wales regarding the use of new and existing medicines, treatments and procedures. The following seem to be the main motivations for using economic evaluation in decision making.

BOX 13.1   Decision making using economic evaluation in the UK: the National Institute for Health and Clinical Excellence (NICE)

In England and Wales, the National Institute for Health and Clinical Excellence (NICE) was established in 1999 to address geographic variations in access ('postcode prescribing', see Box 13.2) by providing national-level guidance on the effectiveness and cost-effectiveness of new health technologies in the NHS.

Three centres produce different types of NICE guidance: the Centre for Public Health Excellence deals with the promotion of good public health and the prevention of ill health; the Centre for Clinical Practice deals with the appropriate treatment and care of people with specific diseases and conditions; and the Centre for Health Technology Evaluation deals with the use of new and existing medicines, treatments and procedures based on technology appraisals.

NICE's technology appraisal process involves consideration of both clinical and economic evidence. Two types of technology appraisal are undertaken: Multiple Technology Appraisals (MTAs) and Single Technology Appraisals (STAs). MTAs typically cover more than one technology for a single indication, or one technology for more than one indication. They are undertaken in the following stages.

1. The Department of Health (DH) produces a list of provisional appraisal topics.
2. Consultees and commentators are identified, including national organisations and groups representing patients and carers, and bodies representing health professionals, manufacturers and research groups.
3. NICE works with the DH to develop a scope document, which sets out what the appraisal will cover and the questions to be asked. Consultees and commentators can comment on the draft scope.
4. The DH formally refers technology appraisal topics to NICE.
5. NICE commissions an independent academic centre to review published clinical and economic evidence on the technology and prepare an assessment report. This usually includes an economic evaluation of the technology conducted using a set of methodological guidelines. Consultees and commentators are invited to comment on the report.
6. The assessment report and comments on it are drawn together in an evaluation report.
7. An independent appraisal committee considers the evaluation report. It hears evidence from nominated clinical experts, patients and carers before making its first recommendations in the appraisal consultation document (ACD). Consultees and commentators have four weeks to comment on the ACD. It is made available online so that health professionals and members of the public can comment on it.
8. The independent appraisal committee considers the comments on the ACD, then makes its final recommendations in the final appraisal determination (FAD). The FAD is submitted to NICE for approval. Consultees can appeal against the final recommendations in the FAD.

9. Guidance is issued: If there are no appeals, or an appeal is not upheld, the final recommendations are issued as NICE guidance.

STAs cover a single technology for a single indication, and were introduced due to concerns over the time NICE takes to produce guidance using its MTA process. The stages are similar to those described above, except that at stage 5 evidence is submitted by the manufacturer or sponsor of the technology. Rather than commissioning an academic centre to conduct an independent economic evaluation, NICE commissions an independent technical review of the manufacturer's evidence submission, which is then used to prepare an Evidence Review Group report. This is then considered in the evaluation report at stage 6.

NICE wields considerable power with respect to health technology evaluation: in 2002 the implementation of its decisions was made mandatory in the NHS in England and Wales. There are four categories of recommendations: 'recommended' – the drug or treatment is recommended for use in line with the marketing authorisation; 'optimised' – recommended for use in a smaller subset of patients than originally stated in the marketing authorisation; 'only in research' – recommended only for use in a research study such as a clinical trial; and, 'not recommended'. By October 2011 NICE had published 149 MTAs and 87 STAs, a total of 236 appraisals, containing 454 individual recommendations. Sixty-three percent of the recommendations were 'recommended', 19% were 'optimised', 5% were 'only in research' and 13% were 'not recommended' (NICE 2011).

(a) To maximise the benefits from health care spending

The health care systems in the UK and New Zealand, both of which are publicly funded, fixed-budget systems, use economic evaluation to make national-level decisions about the mix of health care services to fund. In some cases, this is also accompanied by economic evaluation at a local or regional level by budget-holders to inform their resource allocation decisions. Exactly how benefit is defined and measured differs between jurisdictions. For example, in the UK, benefit is equated with health improvement, preferably measured by QALYs gained (NICE, 2008). However, in neighbouring France, scepticism about theoretical and empirical issues regarding QALYs has led to their being *not* recommended as a basis for social choices. Instead, cost–benefit analysis (CBA) is used for decisions about reimbursement of pharmaceuticals (Collège des Èconomistes de la Santé, 2004).

(b) To overcome regional variations in access

An important motivation behind the establishment of NICE was to address 'postcode prescribing' – variations in access to health care depending on place of residence (Rawlins and Culyer, 2004; Devlin and Parkin, 2004). In the UK, this is regarded as an equity issue because in a national health care system such variations are difficult to defend. Variations in medical practice across regional and national borders have, however, long been observed and questioned (see, for example, Cooper, 1975). There is an extensive literature on variations in medical practice in the USA (Wennberg and Gittleson, 1982). In Box 13.2 we show how these variations in medical practice care are not just unfair but also inefficient.

BOX 13.2   ## The inefficiency of 'postcode lotteries' in health care

Differences in access to treatments in the NHS frequently give rise to high-profile cases – for example, in 2006 it became evident that women diagnosed with breast cancer in one region of the UK have access to the drug Herceptin^{TM}, which women in other regions with similar diagnoses were being denied. This and other cases of 'postcode lotteries' for health care gave rise to media interest, political pressure and legal challenges to local health care funders, some of which were successful and led to women being granted access to this treatment ('Woman wins battle for breast cancer treatment' *Guardian*, 13 April 2006).

Most of the assertions about postcode rationing in the UK, both by the NHS and by stakeholders, have focused on the implications for equity. Specifically, geographical variations in access violate *horizontal* equity in health care use, which we discussed in Chapter 7: 'like' individuals (clinically) are being treated in an 'unlike' manner (in terms of access to treatment technologies).

Another way of thinking about postcode rationing is that it is *inefficient*. It suggests variations in medical practice that are unjustified by clinical evidence, or by epidemiological or cost differences between regions. Imagine that the health system comprises just three regions, each of which holds different information and views about the value for money of Herceptin. Region 1 believes that, given the cost of procuring Herceptin (approximately £24 000 per patient per year) represented by the marginal cost curve, and given their view of the marginal value of this treatment (shown by MB_1), the optimum use of this drug is Q_0. In contrast, Region 3, facing the same marginal cost of procurement, believes there is considerable marginal value (MB_3) to its patients of accessing this treatment – resulting in Q' treatments being consumed.

Let us assume that Region 2 is correct in its assessment of marginal value, MB_2. Given MB_2, by denying Herceptin to its patients, Region 1 generates a welfare loss shown by area a – too little is being consumed given that the 'true' marginal value is MB_2, not MB_1. Similarly, Region 3, which has recommended Q', generates a welfare loss of area b: too much is consumed, and for each unit in excess of Q^*, $MC > MB$. The variation between regions generates a total welfare loss = $(a + b)$.

Alternatively, if the evidence ultimately suggests that Region 1's assessment of costs and benefits is most accurate, then the correct decision is that this treatment should not be made available at all. In that case, the welfare loss of Regions 2 and 3 providing this treatment = $(c + d + b)$.

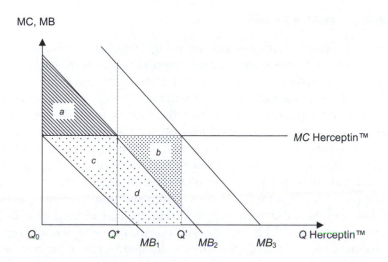

The approach described above is broadly similar to that developed by Phelps (Phelps and Parente, 1990; Phelps and Mooney, 1992; Phelps, 1995) as a means of estimating the welfare losses associated with 'small area medical variations' observed in the US, often referred to as 'Wennberg variations' (Wennberg and Gittleson, 1982). There are problems with the approach – for example, in the absence of a definitive view of clinical benefit and marginal value, the approach generally assumes the *average* intervention rate is the correct one. Nevertheless, the magnitude of welfare losses is striking: for example, Phelps and Parente (1990) estimated the annual welfare losses from variations in the use of CABG alone to be $US0.75 billion. These studies suggest that medical variations in the US are a source of considerable inefficiency.

Are there any circumstances under which such local variations might be justified? For example, what if, instead of arising from imperfect information about clinical benefit, they arise from differences in the value placed on particular kinds of health benefits in each region? Although this may seem implausible as an explanation for postcode rationing, the existence of distinctive local preferences and priorities is, arguably, precisely the point of delegating purchasing decisions to local budget-holders. However, local preferences can only be met by sacrificing national consistency: thus there is an unavoidable tension between localism and centralism.

Medical variations are evident not only within but also *between* countries. This poses particular challenges for Europe, where inconsistencies in access to health care technologies have generated legal challenges. European Court of Justice rulings have upheld the right of a citizen in one country to travel to another country to receive 'medically necessary' care and to claim this against their social insurance cover – even if that treatment is denied in their home country (Watson, 2001). The implication is that it may become increasingly difficult for any single European country effectively to make a decision to withhold a new treatment – and that decisions about what is good value for money will need to be harmonised across Europe.

(c) To contain costs and manage demand

Perhaps the most widespread motivation for using economic evaluation is to provide a defensible, systematic and consistent way of responding to new, high-cost technologies. Economic evaluation has tended to focus on new technologies – especially pharmaceuticals – and rather more rarely on assessing the value for money of older technologies or services that provide non-therapeutic support or care. In part, this may be explained both by the rationale of decision makers and by pragmatic considerations: new technologies that have satisfied the requirements for licensing have an evidence base which is more amenable to economic evaluation than services that have never been subject to randomised controlled trials.

Demand management is clearly a key issue in fixed-budget health care systems that have to reconcile fixed resources to demand. However, demand management is arguably an even *more* pressing issue in demand-driven systems, where unconstrained growth in health care spending is a cause for concern. This includes social insurance systems, such as in France and Germany. It also includes the use of economic evaluation in private-sector, demand-driven systems, where setting coverage limits for third-party funding provides a key means of avoiding moral hazard (Garber, 2001). Although it is more unusual for cost-effectiveness to be *explicitly* used to determine resource allocations in health care in the USA (Garber, 1994), examples of that can be found, as well as other means of containing costs. For example, the US Supreme Court in 2000 ruled that patients could not sue their health maintenance organisation (HMO) in Federal court for giving doctors financial incentives to cut medical costs; Justice Souter noted that 'no HMO organisation could survive without some incentive connecting physician reward with treatment rationing' (Charatan, 2000). Box 13.3 discusses Oregon's internationally well-known for its experiment with the use of cost-effectiveness to decide priorities for health care spending in its Medicaid programme.

BOX 13.3   The Oregon Health Plan

Medicaid is a publicly funded programme in the USA which aims to deliver all medically necessary care to the poor. In the late 1980s, the USA was faced with increasing demands for Medicaid coupled with cost-inflation. The inevitability of rationing prompted re-evaluation of the coverage provided by Medicaid in Oregon. This resulted in the Oregon Health Plan, the idea underpinning which is that, given a finite budget, an expansion of *who* is covered could only be achieved by a restricting *what* is covered. The Oregon Health Services Commission developed a systematic and explicit basis for deciding what health services should be included, and which excluded, from the benefit package provided by Medicaid (Kitzhaber, 1993).

The method originally used was to assign all possible treatments into 'condition-treatment' pairs, informed by clinical judgements. Each pair was then assessed in terms of its cost per QALY gained. The Commission consulted the public extensively – meeting interest groups and communities, and generating population-specific health state valuations using methods similar to those described in Chapter 10, via a telephone survey. The output of these analyses was a prioritised list of over 700 condition-treatment pairs – effectively, a giant league table. The intention was that the political process would determine the Medicaid budget, and pairs on the list would be funded down to the point at which the budget was exhausted; pairs below that are excluded from the benefit package.

Oregon's plan was hailed as a brave experiment in prioritisation. Oregon continued to make explicit use of a prioritised list updated each year, as the basis for planning Medicaid coverage. The five top and five bottom items of their 2006 list were:

Line	Diagnosis	Treatment
1	Severe/moderate head injury: haematoma/oedema with loss of consciousness	Medical and surgical treatment
2	Type I diabetes mellitus	Medical therapy
3	Peritonitis and retroperitoneal infections	Medical and surgical treatment
4	Acute glomerulonephritis: with lesion of rapidly progressive glomerulonephritis	Medical therapy including dialysis
5	Pneumothorax and haemothorax	Tube thoracostomy/thoracotomy, medical therapy
705	Mental disorders with no effective treatments or no treatment necessary	Evaluation
706	Neurological conditions with no effective treatments or no treatment necessary	Evaluation
707	Dental conditions (e.g. orthodontics)	Cosmetic dental services
708	Hepatorenal syndrome	Medical therapy
709	Spastic dysphonia	Medical therapy
710	Disorders of refraction and accommodation	Radial keratotomy

Source: egov.oregon.gov/DAS/OHPPR/HSC/docs/4-1-06_line_descriptions.txt

However, the Oregon experiment cannot be seen as a success for economic evaluation as a means of ranking health services; this was abandoned early on, before the scheme was approved or implemented. What went wrong?

The first prioritised list produced by the Commission in 1990 was widely criticised. Certainly there were aspects of the economic evaluations which could be criticised on technical or economic grounds – for example, costs were 'usual, customary and reasonable charges', that is prices, which may or may not reflect marginal cost, and do not reflect changes in resource use elsewhere in the health sector (savings) as a result of the intervention. More importantly, though, the resulting list included many priorities that seemed counterintuitive – appearing to favour minor treatments over lifesaving ones (Hadorn, 1991). For example, treatment for thumb-sucking and acute headaches received higher rankings than treatment for AIDS or Cystic Fibrosis (Maynard and Bloor, 1998). Such was the controversy that the list based on cost-effectiveness was never submitted for the Federal Waiver required for its adoption. The Commission fundamentally reconsidered the basis for its priorities, rejecting cost-effectiveness in favour of prioritisation principally with respect to five-year survival and improvement in symptoms, with priorities also determined by groups of services, and hand-adjustments to rankings. The prioritised list finally approved in 1994 was not based on ranking by cost-effectiveness.

In terms of its own objectives, the Oregon Health Plan has succeeded: by constraining the depth of coverage, the breadth of cover has been expanded so that all Oregonians below the poverty line can access the services on the list. This is clearly an important achievement. Oregon's experience demonstrates clearly, however, that the application of economic evaluation in social decision making is not just a technical exercise; nor are the issues in using economics to inform social choices merely technical in nature. By making explicit decisions on criteria other than cost-effectiveness, Oregon will be satisfying legitimate social goals – nevertheless, the package of care delivered by Medicaid will not be *efficient* (Tengs, 1996).

Garber, (1994) has suggested that considerable use has been made behind the scenes of economic evaluation to contain costs and inform health care decisions in the health care system in the USA. This may change following the enactment of the Patient Protection and Affordable Care Act in 2010, which amongst other things saw the creation of a new Patient Centered Outcomes Research Institute (PCORI), whose purpose is 'to assist patients, clinicians, purchasers, and policy-makers in making informed health decisions by advancing the quality and relevance of evidence concerning the manner in which diseases, disorders, and other health conditions can effectively and appropriately be prevented, diagnosed, treated, monitored, and managed through research and evidence synthesis that considers variations in patient subpopulations, and the dissemination of research findings with respect to the relative health outcomes, clinical effectiveness, and appropriateness of the medical treatments'. Notably, the PCORI is forbidden to use cost per QALY or similar thresholds when making its recommendations, much to the consternation of some US health economists (Neuman and Weinstein, 2010).

(d) To regulate or negotiate prices in health care markets

Garber (1994) notes that cost-effectiveness analysis is sometimes also used by US health care insurers to negotiate prices to be paid to health care providers. A similar example, but at the national level, is New Zealand's Pharmaceutical Management Agency Company (PHARMAC). PHARMAC uses economic evaluation principally to achieve the objective noted in (c). However, PHARMAC's role is not merely to make recommendations but also to purchase drugs for the country's health care system. PHARMAC therefore has considerable monopsony power. When technologies are assessed by it to have a cost-effectiveness ratio that is too high, presumably by reference to a threshold (see Section 13.7), this can be used as a bargaining tool with industry to negotiate lower prices. PHARMAC has been manifestly successful in achieving reductions in New Zealand's drugs bill – although the absence of any pharmaceutical industry in that country is probably no coincidence! Maynard *et al.* (2004)

argue that NICE should also be given similar budget-holding status, although the importance of the pharmaceutical industry in the UK economy makes it unlikely that such a strategy would ever be implemented.

More recently, the Department of Health in England is introducing Value Based Pricing (VBP) from 2014 (Department of Health, 2010). The prices that the NHS pays to drug manufacturers for new medicines will be regulated by linking pricing to the estimated value of the treatment. This might be seen as an extension of the current use of economic evaluation by NICE. Currently, NICE recommends a technology for a group or sub-group of patients, based on the incremental cost per QALY gained at a pre-determined price. Under VBP, the same evidence on incremental effectiveness will be used to establish the maximum price the NHS should be willing to pay for the technology.

While the details of VBP are still being established, two things are notable. First, the notion of 'value' is somewhat broader than health improvement, measured as QALYs gained. While the cost per QALY gained will probably continue to be the principal consideration, it seems that VBP in England will also entail the introduction of a systematic approach to taking into account other decision criteria, such as burden of disease, unmet need, innovation, and wider societal benefits.

Secondly, the introduction of VBP places considerable importance on the cost-effectiveness threshold to be used in this decision-making process. Under VBP, the cost-effectiveness of the drug is assessed before the price is set by the pharmaceutical company and a price is calculated for the drug so that its *CER* is exactly equal to the cost-effectiveness threshold. This is the maximum price that can be charged by the pharmaceutical company. Pricing to achieve the *CER* in this way means that the health benefits offered by the drug are just offset by the health benefits displaced elsewhere in the health system, that is, their opportunity costs (Claxton *et al.*, 2008). The basis for setting the cost-effectiveness threshold is a matter of considerable importance, both in decision making about cost-effectiveness and value-based pricing. We discuss this in detail in Section 13.7.

Our focus in (a)–(d) has been on the use of economic evaluation techniques to inform decisions about the right mix of services to purchase. Other, *non*-evaluative methods of economic analysis are also occasionally used to inform *other* sorts of priorities and resource allocation decisions. For example, econometric models underpin the population-based funding formulae used in the UK (Department of Health, 2008). These are used to produce algorithms that determine how the total NHS budget is allocated between the principal budget holders and purchasers of health care for local populations in England, where population size is weighted by a range of factors that act as proxies for health needs. Further, the tools developed to measure HRQOL (see Chapter 11) have also been used in New Zealand and Canada to decide clinical priorities for treatment by ranking individual patients on waiting lists in order of their need or capacity to benefit (Hadorn and Holmes, 1997; Derrett *et al.*, 2003). There is growing interest in the UK in using measures of HRQOL to manage the demand for secondary care generated by primary care providers, by incorporating them into referral guidelines for GPs. HRQOL measures are also being used to measure the quality of care delivered to patients; HRQOL data, as well as other Patient Related Outcome Measures (PROMs), are used to calculate the health gain after surgical treatment using pre-and post-operative surveys, and to measure differences in the performance of health care providers (Devlin and Appleby, 2010).

13.2 Who buys economic evaluations? Does it matter?

The previous section lists the various rationales that might motivate decision makers' use of economic evaluation evidence. Given that decision makers are increasingly concerned with evidence on value for money, an obvious additional reason why economic evaluations are undertaken is that they are commissioned by stakeholders who have an interest in the provision of a good or service. Obvious stakeholders include the pharmaceutical industry, clinicians and patients.

That many economic evaluations are often commissioned by stakeholders who profit or otherwise benefit directly from the result may suggest that caution is required in the use of this evidence in decision making: 'He who pays the piper calls the tune'! We might expect industry-commissioned evaluations to be more likely to conclude that a technology is acceptable value for money than independent evidence (see Freemantle and Maynard, 1994, and the response by Jönsson, 1994). Miners *et al.* (2005) show exactly that, finding a statistically significant difference between cost-effectiveness ratios in evidence submitted to NICE by manufacturers and that by independent assessments, and in the expected direction. This is important, because as agencies such as NICE come under pressure to speed up their decision-making processes (see Box 13.1), it is generally achieved by forgoing independent evidence and relying to a greater extent on industry submissions.

Decision makers can respond to the issue of bias in a number of ways: at the simplest level, the incentives facing industry are entirely transparent, so caveat emptor applies to the use, in decision making, of evidence provided by industry. Further, decision makers have introduced increasingly strong directives about the methods required to be used in evidence to be submitted. This builds on a more general move initiated by academic health economists to make consistent the methods used in appraisal (Weinstein *et al.*, 1996; Drummond *et al.*, 2005) so that valid comparisons of value for money may be made across studies. The best-known examples of this include, in the USA, the Washington Panel (Gold *et al.*, 1996) and, in the UK and Canada, the work of Drummond and others (Drummond *et al.*, 2005). Further, decision makers in some health economies (England – in contrast to Scotland) commission their own, independent analysis, and the availability of that exerts some discipline on industry not to over-inflate benefit or under-estimate *CER*s. Recent moves to speed up the evaluation and to 'fast track' the decision process for new drugs in the UK involve a greater reliance on manufacturer-sponsored evidence, with the role of independent analysts being critically to review that evidence.

13.3 Is economic efficiency all that matters?

Economic evaluation is concerned with efficiency and indeed, depending on the exact methods selected, on specific views of efficiency (see Chapter 10). If, from a given budget, the objective is to maximise health improvement or, alternatively, to maximise welfare, then a resource allocation determined solely by evidence on cost-effectiveness or cost benefit analysis will achieve that. But that begs the question: is efficiency all that matters? Is it the only objective? What other considerations or criteria might be or are being used to guide resource allocation in the health sector?

13.3.1 Need

The most obvious contender for an alternative, systematic and explicit but non-economics approach to resource allocation is to decide priorities on the basis of need, defined by the presence of illness, or the burden of disease, rather than those with the greatest capacity to benefit or the greatest capacity for benefit per pound spent. Needs-based approaches are used in the allocation of public health system funds between regions in the UK and New Zealand. For example, as already noted, a population-based funding formula determines what share of the total health care budget each receives and this is driven largely by measures of population need.

However, perhaps the best-known example of priorities being influenced by measures of need is the Global Burden of Disease study (Lopez *et al.*, 2006), an extensive international set of studies which aimed to influence and inform priorities by generating data on the magnitude of health problems of various kinds in various populations. A major concern of the project is the development of measures that could capture the extent of problems with diseases and injuries in terms of both mortality and morbidity, and in a way that would facilitate comparison of the size of a given problem across disease areas and between countries. The principal measure developed was the disability-adjusted life year (DALY) (see Chapter 11). Measures of DALYs by disease area and by country are widely used by the World Bank and by WHO to inform priorities for health care in developing countries. Examples of the approach may also be found in developed countries; for example, in Bowie *et al.* (1997), who report these data for the south and west regions of England.

Many economists are highly critical of priority setting based on burden of disease. Williams (1999, 2000) and Mooney and Wiseman (2000) argue that information on the size of the problem is irrelevant for priority setting unless it is accompanied by, or a precursor to, data on the effectiveness of interventions available for the treatment of each disease and on their costs. Williams (1999) sums up these arguments succinctly: 'What we need to know is what impact different interventions will have, not what impact different diseases have.' Given that position, Mooney and Wiseman (2000) argue that the use of burden of disease information in setting priorities 'is likely to lead to inefficient and inequitable resource use'. Thus, although 'giving health care to those who need it' seems a laudable goal, the outcome will be less improvement in health, overall, than is possible from the available budget. As Maynard (1996) has pointed out, such inefficiency is unethical since it means potential patients are deprived of care from which they could benefit. An example of the way in which burden of disease information can mislead decision making is provided in Box 13.4.

BOX 13.4   **Needs and costs – and why obvious conclusions are sometimes wrong**

In the same way that Bowie *et al.* (1997) report DALYs by disease area for England, evidence on the global burden of disease was generated in New Zealand in 1998. The New Zealand government was interested in using these data to help analyse its priorities for health care. Initial analysis suggested that a useful way of presenting the data was to show the percentage of total DALYs by disease area, represented by the shaded bars in the figure below. Because the vertical axis measures percentages, it is possible also to display the percentage of total health care spending in each disease area – this is represented by the lines.

The result is quite striking. Some areas (such as maternity) account for a high percentage of spending, but barely *any* morbidity and mortality. In contrast, other areas, such as cancers, account for a large share of the ill health but receive a relatively small proportion of spending. *Prima facie*, the conclusion seems obvious: too much is being spent on maternity and too little on cancer. Spending should be reallocated between disease areas. Do you agree?

Costs and DALYs by clinical/disease area in New Zealand

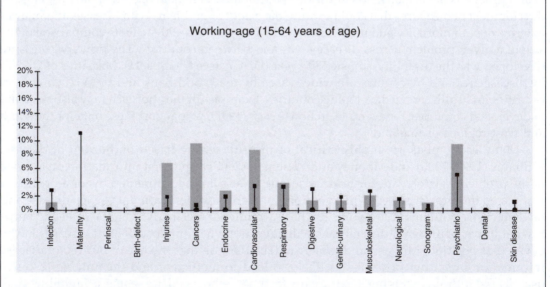

Source: Devlin. N, and Parkin. D, *Does NICE have a cost effectiveness threshold and what other factors influence its decisions?* **Health Economics, 2004; 437–452**. Reproduced with permission from the NZ Treasury Discussion Paper 00/4

Although the evidence seems compelling, this graph is misleading (Devlin and Hansen, 2000). It shows a static picture of existing distributions of ill health and spending. What is unknown is (for example) how a given reduction in spending on maternity would increase morbidity and mortality in that clinical/disease area, compared to how an increase in spending by that same amount on cancer would decrease morbidity and mortality. The reason why morbidity and mortality in maternity is so low is likely to be related in at least some way to the resources devoted to it; how a reduction in spending would affect that cannot be discerned from these data. Similarly, although the spending on cancer seems too low relative to the DALYs in that area, it is not obvious from these data how an increase in spending would affect health. For example, although many new drugs are available for treating cancer, these tend to be relatively expensive and to produce relatively small gains in survival or quality of life. Spending more money on prevention, rather than cures, may be the best strategy, but changes to lifestyle and health behaviour are difficult to effect, and the health gains are produced far into the future and would not be evident on the current distribution of DALYs shown in the figure.

Data on *total* needs by disease area, even if accompanied by data on *total* costs, are, of themselves, of little relevance to priority setting. Costs and consequences are, we would argue as economists, always most usefully represented as *marginal* or incremental costs and effects.

13.3.2 Equity

The efficient use of scarce health care resources, defined as the maximisation of health, is unlikely to be the sole objective of a society. For example, it may be that society is interested both in increasing health overall and in reducing inequalities in health between population sub-groups. Society may be prepared to forgo some improvement in health in order to achieve fairness. But what is meant by equity? How is it to be measured? Exactly what sacrifices are we willing to make in its pursuit?

We discussed concepts of equity in the distribution of health care in Chapter 7. For example, one definition of fairness in health care that has been suggested is to achieve equality (or at least to reduce inequalities) in people's lifetime experience of health. This view is evident in Williams' (1997) idea of the 'fair innings': he suggests that there are strong normative grounds for resources to be transferred from the elderly, who have already enjoyed their 'three score and ten', to the young. The focus of equity concerns could, however, alternatively or simultaneously be expressed in terms of wealth, income, geography, ethnicity or gender, rather than age; and equity could be construed in terms of fairness in access to health care, or utilisation of health care, rather than health outcomes.

One way of thinking about the efficiency–equity trade-off is that it exists only because of the approach selected to measure efficiency. If QALYs gained is used as the measure of benefit and cost per QALY gained is the measure of efficiency, then preferences about the distribution of the QALYs gained becomes a separate issue requiring separate analysis and consideration. Ideas about equity tend not to be built into the analysis so that, by default, cost–utility analysis (CUA) is utilitarian: 'a QALY is a QALY is a QALY', and no distinction is made about who obtains these health gains. Dolan *et al.* (2005) have provided empirical evidence which fundamentally questions this as a defensible basis for resource allocation. They contend that there is good evidence to suggest both that society has a diminishing marginal valuation for improvements and that society is not indifferent as to who gains them. In particular, there is evidence that the social value of health improvements is higher if the person has worse lifetime health prospects and if the person has dependants; there is also value attached to reducing inequalities in health.

Similarly, in CBA the focus is on weighing up benefits and costs, in monetary terms, based on Kaldor–Hicks compensation tests discussed in Chapter 9, which requires only the possibility of compensation and redistribution. CBA rarely includes explicit weights to address equity. If, however, decision makers could refer to a fully specified social welfare function, then decisions would address both the magnitude of net benefits and their distribution – and the maximisation of social welfare, subject to resource constraints, would incorporate equity considerations, as reflected in the characteristics and properties of the social welfare function, directly into the analysis. Under these circumstances, there is no trade-off between efficiency and equity.

13.3.3 Process-of-care considerations

In CUA, the benefits of health care are restricted to improvements in length and quality of life. A problem with this approach is that it is neutral to, or excludes from consideration, characteristics of health care products, services or delivery modes that may, in themselves, be the subject of patients' preferences, independently of their effects on health. Patients may, for example, prefer health care services that respect privacy and autonomy, that preserve their dignity, that fully inform them of their options, that allow them at least some choice, that avoid unnecessary waiting and delays, that are provided by friendly health care professionals, that minimise time away from dependents, and so on. None of these characteristics will be reflected in a CUA, other than where they have a measurable effect on survival and quality of life.

There are three ways in which this can be justified. First, there may be a trade-off between better process of care and increased health, so that if resources are devoted to improved process, this reduces the amount that can be devoted to health improvement. It is possible that people's preferences are so strongly in favour of health that improved process of care would have to be enormously important to outweigh improved outcomes of care – their preferences may be what is called lexicographic. As an extreme example, it is likely that few would be willing to trade off even a few cancer cures for an improvement in the quality of hospital food – assuming that the latter has no impact on health.

Secondly, it may be that the trade-off is small or even non-existent but that the utility from health care is very large compared to that from process of care. Since process of care improvements may be even harder to quantify than health gain, it may be justifiable to ignore them. The problem with this is that the balance of importance between process and outcome will differ between types of health care, and indeed some health care services, such as cosmetic care and fertility services, may have very little health output at all. Of course, this may not matter if the purpose of the health service is to improve health rather than to just provide health care.

Thirdly, it may be that it is simply a mistake to consider these two aspects together, and that they should be considered at different levels of decision making. For example, the question of what should be provided by health services, and the priority that different types of care should have, should be decided on the basis of health, since that is the objective of a health service. However, the question of how it should be provided could take into account these wider process attributes. Ultimately, of course, these have to be reconciled if there is indeed a potential trade-off between them, but that is arguably yet again a different level of decision making.

The latter, even though it is really just a way of denying or concealing the trade-off, is probably the most widespread response. For example, in England and Wales, NICE makes decisions about the availability of treatments mainly on the basis of health improvements, but a key policy goal of the Department of Health (see Box 2.1 in Chapter 2) is to improve the choices available to NHS patients. The opportunity cost of offering choice of location and timing of care in terms of reduced availability of care does not seem to be explicitly considered. Shah *et al.* (2011) examine the broad range of benefits taken into account in Department of Health decision making in England, and note the apparent discrepancy between these and the decision criteria used by NICE. Different parts of the health care system seem to be pursuing different maximands – with obvious implications for allocative efficiency.

13.3.4 Ethical imperatives

In addition to the considerations set out above, it has been argued that even the most carefully considered health care prioritisation process will buckle when confronted with certain ethical imperatives. For example, Hadorn (1991) argued that the so-called 'rule of rescue' will almost inevitably dominate cost-effectiveness in decision making. The *CER* of an intervention may be unfavourable, but if an identified life is at stake, and if survival depends on treatment, then survival will override all other factors, including the duration of survival, quality of life, and cost-effectiveness. Although compelling, the rule of rescue does not provide a systematic or fully articulated ethical framework for understanding choices. Is it equally important in cases where a life is saved for 20 years, 20 days, 20 minutes or 20 seconds? It seems implausible that there is no limit to the preparedness to devote resources to rescuing life – especially when the life that is saved may be of unacceptably poor quality. McKie and Richardson (2003) argued that the rule can be defended on utilitarian grounds, to the extent that rescues provide value by reinforcing people's beliefs that they live in a community that values life highly. However, they also point out that the rule discriminates in favour of saving lives where those lives belong to identifiable people, but in effect discriminates against lives that are saved by reducing a population's risk of death.

Ethical issues might be relevant in other ways. For example, instances of differential access to treatment for obese and non-obese people, and between smokers and non-smokers for smoking-related diseases, are becoming more common – usually on the grounds of differences in the probability of success of treatment but occasionally, one suspects, influenced by notions of individual culpability and desert. Further, decisions about the availability of assisted death, abortion, infertility treatments, and the selection of genetic characteristics in foetuses, among other things, may consider cost-effectiveness. But it is unlikely to be the only, or even the principal, consideration in deciding what health services to make available.

13.4 How is economic evaluation used to make decisions in practice?

Consider the following: a decision maker is presented with information on a new health care intervention. A CUA demonstrates that, compared to the treatment widely used at present, the new treatment saves money and results in better health outcomes; that is, the new treatment dominates the one that is currently used. The decision maker has all the information required, from this one piece of analysis, in order to recommend in favour of the new treatment.

That scenario is relatively rare. Most new technologies improve health, but at additional cost. In such cases, whether the decision maker deems the technology to be good value for money or not depends on a comparison of the cost per QALY gained against something else. That something else may be the cost per QALY gained for other treatments that are competing for resources; or it may be some 'benchmark' cost per QALY that is considered to be the cut-off for what is acceptable to society – the ceiling ratio or cost-effectiveness threshold. Either way, decisions rely on comparisons. What should these comparators be, and how are they selected? There are three main approaches to making such comparisons in decision making using economic evaluation evidence. They are: cost-effectiveness league tables; programme budgeting and marginal analysis (PBMA); and cost-effectiveness thresholds.

13.5 Cost-effectiveness league tables

One approach which is often used to help decision makers put the results of an economic evaluation into context is to show the incremental cost per QALY gained alongside results from other evaluations of other interventions. Ranking these from lowest cost per QALY gained to highest cost per QALY gained creates a 'league table' of value for money. For early examples, see Williams (1985) and Maynard (1991).

Table 13.1 shows a cost-effectiveness league table for the USA, based on information reported in Garber and Phelps (1997). Each line in the league table shows the *CER* produced for a given health care product or service by a cost-effectiveness study. Many of the *CERs* reported in these tables will have been superseded by medical innovations, or more up-to-date economic appraisals – and of course they are reported in terms of 1993 dollars, so cannot be taken to represent the costs today. Nevertheless, this provides a good example of the kind of side-by-side comparisons of economic evaluation results that can be used in order to give

| TABLE 13.1 | **Example of a cost-effectiveness league table** |

Intervention	Cost per QALY gained US$ (1993)
Low-dose lovastatin for high cholesterol: male heart attack survivors, aged 55–64 years, cholesterol > 250	2 158
Low-dose lovastatin for high cholesterol: male heart attack survivors, aged 55–64 years, cholesterol < 250	2 293
Physician advice about smoking cessation, 1% quit rate, males aged 45–50	3 777
CABG, left main coronary artery disease	8 768
Neonatal intensive care units: infants 1 000–1 500 gms	10 927
Pap smear starting at age 20, continuing to age 74, every 3 years, compared to no screening	24 011
Hypertension screening, 40-year-old males	27 519
Breast cancer screening, annual examination and mammography, females 55–65	41 008
Hypertension screening, 40-year-old females	42 222
Neonatal intensive care units: infants 500–999gms	77 161
CABG, single vessel disease with moderate angina	88 087
Exercise electrocardiogram as a screening test, 40-year-old males	124 374
Exercise electrocardiogram as a screening test, 40-year-old females	335 217
Low-dose lovastatin for high cholesterol: female non-smokers	2 023 440

Source: Reprinted from Journal of Health Economics, 16:1, Garber & Phelps, Economic Foundations of cost-effectiveness analysis, 1–31, © 1997, with permission from Elsevier

decision makers some idea of how the results of a given economic evaluation compare with those for other treatments.

Unfortunately, there are many problems with the use of league tables. First, problems arise from the lack of consistency in the methods used by each of the research teams who produced each reported *CER*. Differences in method include: what perspective is taken in estimating costs; what discount rate was used, and whether it was applied equally to costs and

QALYs; what instrument was used to measure HRQOL; what and whose valuations were used to estimate QALYs; whether results are reported as average or incremental cost-effectiveness ratios, and so on. Differences in any of these will render the *CERs* produced from various economic evaluation studies non-comparable. This issue is particularly important where league tables comprise results from a range of studies, as is the case in Table 13.1. However, if cost-effectiveness analysis is undertaken with the express purpose of facilitating between-treatment comparisons, using standardised methodologies, then this criticism can be overcome. This was attempted by the Oregon Health Services Commission – see Box 13.3. Effectively, Oregon commissioned bespoke economic evaluations of all health care services provided under the auspices of Medicaid, and used this to construct a comprehensive league table or prioritised list.

Secondly, the use of league tables assumes that the original context of the study in each case is transferable to the specific context within which decisions are currently being made (Gerard and Mooney, 1993). There may be factors specific to each decision-making context which limit the appropriateness of generalising from league table results.

Thirdly, the reporting of economic evaluation results as a single *CER* in league tables suggests a degree of certainty over results, and therefore rankings between health care services, that may be quite misleading; the confidence intervals around each *CER* may alter, or considerably blur, the rankings apparent between them.

Fourthly, league tables treat each line as being an independent alternative from the others, so that interactions between costs and benefits of programmes are not addressed.

Finally, although league tables aim to help the decision maker to consider cost-effectiveness results in context, it is not entirely clear how decision makers are intended to use the information. For example, should they recommend in favour of funding a therapy if there are treatments farther down the league table, that is treatments that are *less* cost-effective, that have already been funded? What if previous decisions were made without access to evidence? Or if a treatment was funded despite being poor value for money, because of *other* characteristics or criteria?

How, then, do decision makers *actually* use these league tables to inform their decisions? Garber and Phelps (1997) suggest that 'most practitioners of cost-effectiveness analysis discard interventions with cost-effectiveness values at the bottom range of a table such as this one, and conclude that interventions in the realm of $50 000 per QALY are "OK" but that more expensive technologies become more and more "out of bounds"; the $50 000 criterion is arbitrary and owes more to being a round number than to being a well-formulated justification for a specific dollar value'. This provides a rather sobering prospect for economists; despite the development of ever more sophisticated means of estimating and reporting cost-effectiveness, the results are being used in a fairly crude way, where they are being used at all. Garber and Phelps (1997) conclude that the league table approach to comparisons of *CERs*, although common, 'provides little guidance regarding the optimal cost-effectiveness ratio – that is, the willingness to pay for a health effect'.

Instead of comparing the *CERs* from various studies with each other, if decision makers know what value society placed on each QALY gained, this could serve as the benchmark for decision makers. If the cost per QALY gained of any given therapy is higher than the societal value per QALY, the therapy should be rejected. We return to this idea of a societal cost-effectiveness 'threshold' in Section 13.7.

13.6 Programme budgeting and marginal analysis

Programme budgeting and marginal analysis (PBMA) is a pragmatic approach to resource allocation which has become widely used internationally. It is intended as a planning tool for rationing resources in the context of the public sector, in the absence of a market that would do that. Its aim is to make manageable the impossible remit of a central planner. PBMA comprises two distinct elements: programme budgeting (PB) and marginal analysis (MA).

13.6.1 Programme budgeting

Programme budgeting (PB) refers to a form of output-based budgeting, which focuses the budgetary process on the outputs of health services (Craig *et al.*, 1995). Costs are linked to the production of health outputs, rather than to the purchase of health care inputs as in standard accounting systems. The PB part of PBMA therefore involves assigning costs to programmes, defined in terms of the types of output produced, so that current resource allocations are described. PB focuses the budgetary process on the *output* of the health service rather than the inputs required to produce that output. Box 13.5 shows a typical PB approach, using data published by the Department of Health in England (see also Chapter 6, Box 6.6). PB makes it clear what budgets are currently being used *for*, rather than simply the services purchased. This offers a clearer indication of the different needs that a purchaser is trying to meet.

BOX 13.5   Programme budgeting in the NHS in England

Programme budgeting data derived from HRGs (see Chapter 6, Box 6.6) are used in the NHS to examine current patterns of spending matched with outcomes. Although as cross-sectional data they are subject to the same interpretation problems discussed in Box 13.4, they offer information useful to commissioners of health care by enabling comparisons across geographical areas and over time.

The following chart shows NHS spending per head of population in the 23 programme budgets for one Primary Care Trust (PCT) in 2009–10 compared with its 'ONS cluster'. This is a classification of areas by the UK Office of National Statistics according to socio-demographic characteristics. This PCT, Haringey, is in the London Cosmopolitan cluster. Other comparisons can be made, but this illustrates the method.

Spending on mental health is everywhere the largest item, followed by GMS/PMS, which means General and Personal Medical services, that is General Practitioner care. Haringey spends less than its cluster on the first of these and more on the second. 'Miscellaneous' is not a real Programme Budget; it means unclassified.

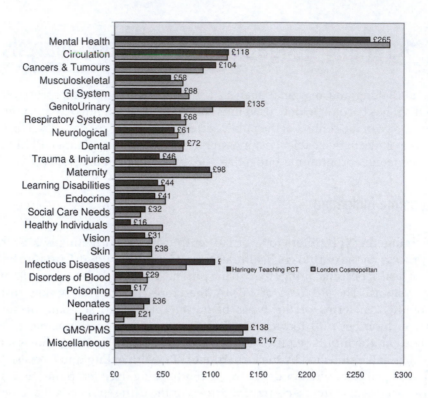

It is also possible to compare spending and outcome, as in the following chart, which compares Haringey with all other PCTs in England:

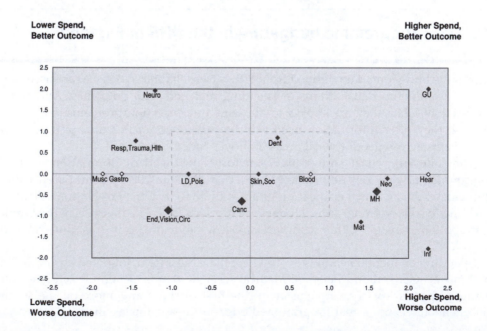

The spend and outcome figures are *z-scores*, which measure how far the PCT is from the mean. The suggestion is that areas that fall into the Higher Spend, Worse Outcome quadrant should be priorities for investigation. This is especially the case for those falling outside the inner box, which means a *z*-score greater than or less than 2.

Source: NHS Spending and Outcome Tool (SPOT), used by permission of the Yorkshire and Humber Public Health Observatory http://www.yhpho.org.uk/ sue.baughan@york.ac.uk

PB may be undertaken at this macro level, looking at the whole of expenditure, divided into large programmes, for example disease groups. It may also be undertaken at the micro level, looking at expenditure within these programmes, for example different care settings for a particular disease group. The latter involves a finer level of detail of information about services. Some sub-categories are available within the English programme budgets, for example Cancers are categorised by site, and Mental Health is divided into Substance Misuse, Organic Mental Disorders, Psychotic Disorders, Child & Adolescent and other.

If programme budgets are established, the next step is economic evaluation of health service provision within those programme budgets. Its aim is to make sure that the programme goals are maximised within the allocated budget. This is the marginal analysis element.

13.6.2 Marginal analysis

Marginal analysis (MA) is the appraisal of the added benefits and added costs of a proposed investment (or the lost benefits and lower costs of a proposed disinvestment). MA establishes whether the current expenditure pattern is appropriate and how it might be changed to increase health gain. Its basis is not a comparison of the costs and benefits of all uses of resources but, more pragmatically, an evaluation *at the margin* of different ways of using resources. MA can take place within programmes or between programmes. The cost and benefit or effectiveness implications of shifting resources within programmes or from one programme to another can be examined, with the goal of maximising health gain within available resources.

The MA part really, therefore, simply refers to the application of standard approaches to economic evaluation and could include any of the approaches described in Chapter 11. Examples of PBMA can be found in decision-making processes at the national level (for example, Ashton *et al.*, 2000) and at the local level (for example, Miller *et al.*, 1997) across a variety of countries; Mitton and Donaldson (2001) provide a comprehensive review of international experience in using PBMA.

13.7 Cost-effectiveness thresholds

CUA and CEA are the most commonly used methods in the economic evaluation of health care. Yet, as we have already noted, whether the decision maker deems the technology to be good value for money depends on a comparison of the *CER*s against some 'benchmark' *CER* – the ceiling ratio or cost-effectiveness threshold. Further, as noted earlier, the introduction of value-based pricing requires explicit decision rules about what is considered acceptable value for money, so that this can be used to determine maximum prices.

What might the basis for such a threshold be? Two broad approaches can be identified. The first is to establish society's willingness to pay for health gain, for example for an additional QALY. This implies that once the threshold has been set the health system should undertake all activities that produce a lower *CER* than the threshold. It also implies that, according to society's preferences, the identified threshold ought to be used to set the health budget.

The second approach is where the health budget is set exogenously and the cost-effectiveness threshold is set to the level that will maximise the health benefit from that budget. In theory this value could be found if we knew the size of the budget and the cost-effectiveness of all technologies to be funded from that budget. A cost-effectiveness league table could be constructed. The health budget is then spent on items at the top of the league table, moving down it and providing those services that are needed, until the budget is exhausted (see Appleby *et al.*, 2009). The *CER* of the last technology provided before the budget runs out is the threshold because this is the first technology that would be displaced if a more cost-effective technology came along.

The notion of a single, optimal cost-effectiveness threshold is represented in Figure 13.1. The vertical axis shows the probability of rejection, from 0 to 1, and the cost per QALY gained is shown on the horizontal axis. If we can confidently identify the threshold, the probability of rejecting a treatment is 0 at any cost per QALY gained below the threshold, and 1 above it.

In practice, the world is much more complicated. Imperfections in information, political processes and decision making may make it difficult to infer much, in any precise way, about what the cost-effectiveness threshold ought to be. Additionally, even if we knew with certainty the value society places on a QALY, or the opportunity cost of a QALY to the health care system, cost-effectiveness is unlikely to be the only criterion influencing decisions. For example, Rawlins and Culyer (2004) describe the normative basis of NICE's decisions and state that other criteria it considers include wider social costs and benefits, such as the effects of treatment on productivity and patients' ability to return to work, the innovative nature of

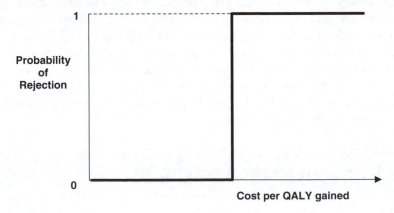

Figure 13.1 The cost-effectiveness threshold as a point

Source: Devlin, N. & Parkin, D. (2004). Does NICE have a cost effectiveness threshold and what other factors influence its decisions? A binary choice analysis. Health Economics, 13, 437–452 © 2004 John Wiley & Sons Limited. Reproduced with Permission

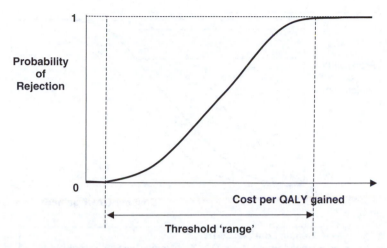

Figure 13.2 The cost-effectiveness threshold as a range, reflecting trade-offs against efficiency
Source: Devlin, N. & Parkin, D. (2004). Does NICE have a cost effectiveness threshold and what other factors influence its decisions? A binary choice analysis. Health Economics, 13, 437–452 © 2004 John Wiley & Sons Limited. Reproduced with Permission

the treatment, and consistency with its previous judgements. They rule out other criteria, such as affordability, differential treatment on the grounds of orphan drug status, and the characteristics of those gaining QALYs, including age, other than where it is an indicator of risk or benefit. In New Zealand, the prioritisation framework, which used CUA, also included considerations of equity, acceptability and Treaty of Waitangi obligations (an agreement of 1840 between the British Crown and the indigenous people of New Zealand), in addition to cost-effectiveness (Ashton *et al.*, 2000). If cost-effectiveness is not all that matters, this suggests that decision makers are prepared to sacrifice some efficiency in the pursuit of these other desired outcomes. This suggests that there is no single cost-effectiveness threshold, but rather a lower and upper threshold, as shown in Figure 13.2. Within the range between the two, cost-effectiveness is being traded off against other objectives.

A further complicating factor is that there is uncertainty regarding the *CER*s; decision makers' response to uncertainty will therefore be important in understanding the way evidence on cost-effectiveness is used in decisions. For example, in Figure 13.3, the probability of rejection for any given *CER*, with which there is associated uncertainty, will depend on whether the decision maker is risk averse (prefers proven therapies) or a risk lover (prepared to give the benefit of the doubt). NICE has stated that its decisions take into account the degree of uncertainty surrounding estimates of cost-effectiveness, although it has not stated how it is taken into account.

Finally, another complicating factor is that the decision response to a given *CER* may depend on whether the decision is for a new or a currently used therapy – that is, whether the decision involves investing in a new technology or disinvesting in an old one. O'Brien *et al.* (2002) provide evidence that the willingness to accept (WTA) values for giving up QALYs by reducing or removing existing health services, may be different from the willingness to pay (WTP) to obtain QALYs from new services. If this is the case, this suggests the probability of rejection is lower at every *CER* for extant as opposed to new therapies, as shown in Figure 13.4.

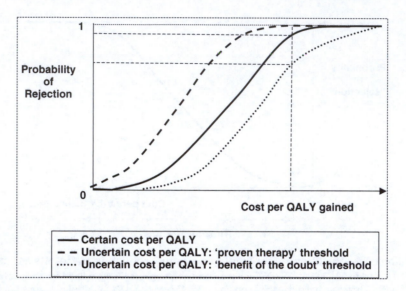

Figure 13.3 The cost-effectiveness threshold under uncertainty
Source: Devlin, N. & Parkin, D. (2004). Does NICE have a cost effectiveness threshold and what other factors influence its decisions? A binary choice analysis. Health Economics, 13, 437–452 © 2004 John Wiley & Sons Limited. Reproduced with Permission

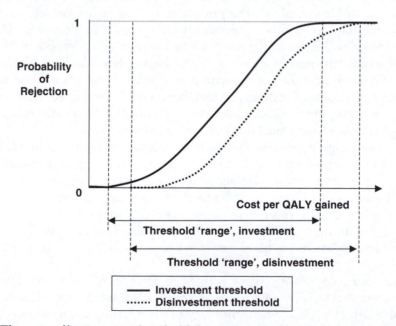

Figure 13.4 The cost-effectiveness threshold for investments and disinvestments
Source: Devlin, N. & Parkin, D. (2004). Does NICE have a cost effectiveness threshold and what other factors influence its decisions? A binary choice analysis. Health Economics, 13, 437–452 © 2004 John Wiley & Sons Limited. Reproduced with Permission

What is the value of the cost-effectiveness threshold in different countries? There is emerging evidence, but the basis for such thresholds seems to be arbitrary, and they are difficult to link either to society's valuation of health gain or to the value that will maximise the health benefit from a given budget. Eichler *et al.* (2004) distinguish four approaches that have been used to identify cost-effectiveness thresholds: values proposed by individual authors or institutions (i.e., rules of thumb); values estimated using willingness to pay (WTP) methods; values obtained from other non-medical programs; and values inferred from past decisions.

The thresholds stated by NICE in England and Wales are an example of the first approach. The stated basis of the cost-effectiveness threshold is to identify the value that will maximise the health benefit from a given budget:

> Given the fixed budget of the NHS, the appropriate threshold to be considered is that of the opportunity cost of programmes displaced by new, more costly technologies. (NICE, 2008)

The difficulty with this approach is that the cost-effectiveness of many health care programmes is unknown. This, coupled with the competing criteria influencing decisions, is why NICE's cost-effectiveness threshold is expressed as a range (NICE, 2008), as in Figure 13.2:

> The Appraisal Committee does not use a precise ICER threshold above which a technology would automatically be defined as not cost-effective or below which it would . . . . [T]he Institute considers that it is most appropriate to use a threshold range.
>
> Below a most plausible ICER of £20,000 per QALY gained, the decision to recommend the use of a technology is normally based on the cost-effectiveness estimate and the acceptability of a technology as an effective use of NHS resources.
>
> Above a most plausible ICER of £20,000 per QALY gained, judgements about the acceptability of the technology as an effective use of NHS resources will specifically take account of the following factors
>
> > The degree of certainty around the ICER. . . .
> > Whether there are strong reasons to indicate that the assessment of the change in HRQL has been inadequately captured. . . .
> > The innovative nature of the technology. . . .
>
> As the ICER of an intervention increases in the £20,000 to £30,000 range, the Committee's judgement about the acceptability of the technology as an effective use of NHS resources will make explicit reference to the relevant factors listed above.
>
> Above a most plausible ICER of £30,000 per QALY gained, the Committee will need to identify an increasingly stronger case for supporting the technology as an effective use of NHS resources, with regard to the factors listed above.

In order to gauge the role of these competing criteria, Devlin and Parkin (2004) constructed a league table of NICE decisions and used logistic regression techniques to model the effect of cost-effectiveness and other factors on the probability of a recommendation for or against use. Their results suggest that NICE decisions could be predicted on the basis of cost-effectiveness, uncertainty, burden of disease, and whether or not the therapy was the only treatment available for the condition. Decisions appeared to be neutral to the budget impact, the net effect on NHS costs if the therapy was accepted. Dakin *et al.* (2006) used similar techniques, but instead of reporting each decision as a binary yes/no decision, three decision outcomes were considered: recommended for, recommended against, and recommended for restricted use. Their results suggest that the quantity and quality of clinical evidence has a distinctive role in the decision-making process independent of evidence on cost-effectiveness. Cost-effectiveness evidence seems to explain decisions to recommend for or against a therapy; whereas clinical evidence is the more important consideration in decisions to recommend restricted or unrestricted use.

A 'rule of thumb' in Canada is that evidence of value for money is thought to be strong with a *CER* less than Can$20 000 per QALY gained and weak with a *CER* in excess of Can$100 000 (Laupacis *et al.*, 1992). The WHO's CHoosing Interventions that are Cost Effective (CHOICE) project is based on the average national income per person, where interventions with an incremental cost per DALY averted less than the gross domestic product (GDP) per person are deemed to be highly cost-effective. Those with a *CER* from 1 to 3 times GDP per person are cost-effective, and those more than 3 times GDP per person are not cost-effective. In the USA, US$50 000 per QALY gained has often been quoted as the cost-effectiveness threshold (Hirth *et al.*, 2000), though the restrictions on the use of *CER*s imposed on PCORI, referred to above, may mean that this is less likely to be applied in the future.

By contrast to these 'rules of thumb', a project estimating a WTP-based value of a QALY, using techniques of the kind discussed in Section 11.8, is the Social Value of a QALY (SVQ) project (Baker *et al.*, 2010).

The cost-effectiveness of interventions that affect health is also relevant in sectors outside of health care such as transportation, occupational health and safety, and fire prevention. A number of reviews have been undertaken to assemble *CER*s for lifesaving interventions in these different sectors (see, for example, Tengs *et al.*, 1995, and Ramsberg and Sjöberg, 1997).

A further example of research to infer the cost-effectiveness threshold from previous decisions is George *et al.* (2001), who constructed a league table from Australia's Pharmaceutical Benefits Advisory Committee (PBAC) decisions, and tested for statistically significant differences between the *CER*s of accepted and rejected therapies. The findings suggested that the PBAC 'has been broadly consistent with the use of economic efficiency as a criterion for decision making'. They could not establish a single threshold, but found evidence that the PBAC appears to have been unlikely to recommend in favour of a drug if the *CER* exceeded AU$76 000 (1998/9 values) and was unlikely to reject a drug for which the *CER* was less than AU$42 000.

13.8 Evaluating economic evaluation

Our focus in this chapter has been on the use of economic evaluation in countries or contexts where it has been adopted as an integral part of systematic decision-making processes about health technologies and health care resource allocation at the national or state-wide level.

Because these decision-making processes are well documented, it facilitates consideration of their strengths and weaknesses.

However, and notwithstanding the increase in use of economic evaluation, there is still considerable scope for extending its use in decision making in health care. Von der Schulenburg (2000) conducted a survey of decision makers in Austria, France, Finland, The Netherlands, Norway, Portugal, Spain and the UK which revealed that only one-third said they considered the results of a health economics study when making a decision. The authors suggested that an important factor hindering greater use was lack of knowledge about the techniques of economic evaluation. Similarly, the work of Garber (1994) and others in the USA suggests considerable scope for improving efficiency in the US health care system by use of economic evaluation. We commenced this book by arguing that health care is an economic good. Given that this is the case, and the importance of health both to individuals and to societies, economic analysis offers a powerful – and still largely untapped – means of helping decision makers ensure that health care resources have the greatest impact possible.

It is also clear from our discussion of decision making in health care that there is some degree of mismatch between the science of evaluation and the art of decision making. The advances in economic evaluation during the last decade have occurred in the development of statistical and modelling techniques. Exciting developments in the methods and tools of economic evaluation have not been matched by development of decision-making processes they seek to support. For example, the use of cost-effectiveness evidence relies ultimately on at least some notion of the value society places on health gain; yet, despite two decades of research applying CUA, research on the value of a QALY is only in its infancy. Further, as we noted in Chapter 12, although cost-effectiveness acceptability curves have now become the gold standard for handling and reporting uncertainty in economic evaluation, to our knowledge there has been no research to examine the way in which decision makers actually interpret and use such evidence, or whether or not they find it helpful and informative.

Still further, although cost-effectiveness may be considered important, it is not the only thing that matters to decision makers. The incorporation of equity issues into evaluation, via the development and use of explicit weights, is feasible and could strengthen the normative legitimacy of evaluation; but research on this issue has yet to have an impact on the practice of economic evaluation. We have been unable to find a single example of a published CUA which uses weights to address distributional issues.

Finally, the methods of economic evaluation have tended to assume that the methods for priority setting should be independent of the financing system. However, clearly decisions about what health services are prioritised interacts with the financing regime; Hauck et al. (2004) argued that 'the rules for setting priorities may vary legitimately between systems with different approaches to the financing of health care'. The interaction between the assessment of value for money and alternative means of raising revenue and sharing costs remains undeveloped. There remains considerable scope to improve the methods of evaluation, to develop decision-aids and to strengthen decision processes – and ultimately, therefore, to improve outcomes.

There are those, of course, who would argue that priorities cannot or should not be set in an explicit, rational manner, and that rather than seeking technical solutions it would be better to 'muddle along' (see, for example Mechanic, 1997) by making implicit judgements. Further, and as we have noted at various points throughout this chapter, the evidence generated from economic evaluation may not be ideal and may not fully address all the issues of relevance to decision makers, and it may be unclear exactly how it should be used to make a decision. However, as Dowie (1995) points out, many of the criticisms of explicit priority setting focus on problems with the use of CUA compared to some unspecified theoretical ideal method of deciding on the resource allocation. For example, he argues that, notwithstanding the problems and limitations associated with cost-effectiveness league tables, it is likely that simply making this information available will in itself improve decision making, compared to the decisions that would be made if that information were not available.

Ultimately, resource allocation decisions cannot be avoided. Therefore, the relevant question – indeed the *key* issue – is whether the use of economic evaluation, even in an imperfect way, leads to better decisions than those that would have been made otherwise.

Summary

1. Economic evaluation is used in health care generally for one or more of the following reasons: to maximise the benefits possible from health care spending; to overcome regional variations in access (for example, 'postcode prescribing'); to contain costs/manage demand; and to regulate or negotiate prices in health care markets.
2. Economic evaluations are commissioned by stakeholders who have an interest in the provision of a good or service. Obvious stakeholders include the pharmaceutical industry; clinicians; and patients. There is evidence that the type of stakeholder may affect the outcome of the economic analysis.
3. There are factors other than cost-effectiveness that might legitimately or illegitimately be used in deciding whether to provide a particular health care programme. Other considerations include: the need for health care measured by, for example DALYs; equity; process of care; and ethical imperatives, such as the rule of rescue. Needs-based priority setting can be criticised on the grounds that it does not account for the impact that different interventions will have.
4. Economic evaluation can be used in a variety of ways in practice as an aid to decision making. The three main approaches are cost-effectiveness league tables; programme budgeting and marginal analysis (PBMA); and cost-effectiveness thresholds.
5. Cost-effectiveness league tables involve ranking programmes from the lowest cost per QALY gained to the highest cost per QALY gained. There are many problems associated with the construction of league tables. The main one is the lack of consistency in the methods used to compute the *ICER*s of the different interventions compiled in the table.
6. PBMA is a pragmatic approach to resource allocation which has become widely used internationally. PB involves assigning costs to programmes, defined in terms of the types of output produced, so that current resource allocations are described. MA refers to the application of standard approaches to economic evaluation.

7. Cost-effectiveness thresholds can be used in decision making, reflecting the maximum amount of money that the decision maker is willing to pay for an additional QALY, for example. They could be based on society's willingness to pay for health gain, or to maximise the health benefit from a given budget.

8. The cost-effectiveness threshold may be a point estimate, with a binary decision to accept or reject an intervention. It may also be represented by a range of values if there are criteria other than cost-effectiveness that are important. The threshold may also include in it consideration of the uncertainty surrounding the value of the *ICER*, and that the decision to accept or reject an intervention might depend on whether the decision is for a new versus a currently used therapy.

9. Four approaches have been used to identify cost-effectiveness thresholds: values proposed by individual authors or institutions; values estimated using willingness to pay methods; values obtained from other non-medical programs; and values inferred from past decisions. The basis for such thresholds seems to be arbitrary, and they are difficult to link either to society's valuation of health gain or to the value that will maximise the health benefit from a given budget.

10. While there has in recent years been an increase in use of economic evaluation, there is still considerable scope for extending its use in decision making in health care. Resource allocation decisions cannot be avoided. Therefore, the key issue is whether or not the use of economic evaluation, even in an imperfect way, leads to better decisions than those that would have been made otherwise.

REFERENCES

Abasolo, I., Manning, R. and Jones, A. (2001) Equity in utilization of and access to public-sector GPs in Spain. *Applied Economics*, **33**, 349–364.

Anderson, P., Butcher, K. and Levine, P. (2003) Maternal employment and overweight children. *Journal of Health Economics*, **22**, 477–504.

Anonychuk, A., Bauch, C., Fikre Merid, M. *et al.* (2009) A cost-utility analysis of cervical cancer vaccination in preadolescent Canadian females. *BMC Public Health*, **9**, 401.

Antonazzo, E., Scott, A., Skatun, D. and Elliott, R. (2003) The labour market for nursing: a review of the labour supply literature. *Health Economics*, **12**, 465–478.

Appleby, J., Devlin, N., Parkin, D. *et al.* (2009) Searching for cost effectiveness thresholds in the NHS. *Health Policy*, **9**, 239–245.

Aronson, J., Johnson, P. and Lambert, P. (1994) Redistributive effect and unequal tax treatment. *Economic Journal*, **104**, 262–270.

Arrow, K.J. (1951) *Social Choice and Individual Values*. New York: John Wiley & Sons Inc.

Arrow, K.J. (1963) Uncertainty and the welfare economics of medical care. *The American Economic Review*, **53**, 941–973.

Arrow, K.J. (1972) *General Economic Equilibrium: Purpose, Analytic Techniques, Collective Choice*. Nobel memorial lecture, December 12. http://nobelprize.org/nobel_prizes/economics/laureates/1972/arrow-lecture.pdf (accessed 1 December 2011).

Ashton, T., Devlin, N. and Cumming, J. (2000) Priority setting in New Zealand – translating principles into practice. *Journal of Health Services Policy and Research*, **5**(3), 170–175.

Bach, S. (2007) Going global? The regulation of nurse migration in the UK. *British Journal of Industrial Relations*, **45**, 383–403.

Baker, C., Messmer, P., Gyurko, D. *et al.* (2000) Hospital ownership, performance, and outcomes: assessing the state-of-the-science. *Journal of Nursing Administration*, **30**, 227–240.

Baker, R., Bateman, I., Donaldson, C. *et al.* (2010) Weighting and valuing quality-adjusted life-years using stated preference methods: preliminary results from the Social Value of a QALY Project. *Health Technology Assessment*, **14**(27).

Baumol, W., Panzar, J. and Willig, R. (1982) *Contestable Markets and the Theory of Industry Structure*. San Diego: Harcourt Brace Jovanovich.

Beazoglou, T., Brown, L.J. and Heffley, D. (1993) Dental care utilization over time. *Social Science and Medicine*, **37**, 1461–1472.

Becker, G.S. (1964) *Human Capital*. New York: Columbia University Press for the National Bureau of Economic Research.

Becker, G.S. (1965) A theory of the allocation of time. *Economic Journal*, **75**, 493–517.

Becker, G.S and Murphy, K.M. (1988) A theory of rational addiction. *Journal of Political Economy*, **96**, 675–700.

Beech, R., Rudd, A.G., Tilling, K. and Wolfe, C.D.A. (1999) Economic consequences of early inpatient discharge to community-based rehabilitation for stroke in an inner-London teaching hospital. *Stroke*, **30**, 729–735.

Bentham, J. (1780) An introduction to the principles of morals and legislation. In: Burns, J.H. and Hart, L.H.A. (1970) *Collected Works of Jeremy Bentham*. London: Athlone Press.

Bergner, M., Bobbitt, R.A., Carter, W.B. and Gilson, B.S. (1981) The Sickness Impact Profile: development and final revision of a health status measure. *Medical Care*, **19**, 787–805.

Berndt, E., Bui, L., Reiley, D. and Urban, G. (1995) Information, marketing, and pricing in the US antiulcer drug market. *American Economic Review*, **85**, 100–105.

Besley, T., Hall, J. and Preston, I. (1999) The demand for private health insurance: do waiting lists matter? *Journal of Public Economics*, **72**, 155–181.

Bhatia, M.R. and Fox-Rushby, J.A. (2003) Validity of willingness to pay: hypothetical versus actual payment. *Applied Economics Letters*, **10**, 737–740.

Birch, S. and Donaldson, C. (2003) Valuing the benefits and costs in health care programmes: where's the extra in extra-welfarism. *Social Science and Medicine*, **56**, 1121–1133.

Birch, S., Jerrett, M. and Eyles, J. (2000) Heterogeneity in the determinants of health and illness: the example of socioeconomic status and smoking. *Social Science and Medicine*, **51**, 307–317.

Black, W.C. (1990) The cost-effectiveness plane: a graphic representation of cost-effectiveness. *Medical Decision Making*, **10**, 212–215.

Blendon, R., Schoen, C., DesRoches, C. *et al.* (2003) Common concerns amid diverse systems: health care experiences in five countries. *Health Affairs*, **22**, 106–121.

Blinder, A. (1973) Wage discrimination: reduced form and structural estimates. *Journal of Human Resources*, **8**, 436–455.

Blomqvist, A. and Carter, R.A.L. (1997) Is health care really a luxury? *Journal of Health Economics*, **16**, 207–229.

Bloor, K. and Maynard, A. (1993) Cost-effective prescribing of pharmaceuticals: the search for the holy grail? In Drummond, M. and Maynard, A. (eds), *Purchasing and Providing Cost-Effective Health Care*. London: Churchill-Livingstone.

Boadway, R. and Bruce, N. (1984) *Welfare Economics*. Oxford: Blackwell.

Bowie, C., Beck, S., Bevan, G. *et al.* (1997) Estimating the burden of disease in an English region. *Journal of Public Health Medicine*, **19**, 87–92.

Bradshaw, J.R. (1972) A taxonomy of social need. In: McLachlan, G. (ed) *Problems and Progress in Medical Care: Essays on Current Research*. Oxford: Nuffield Provincial Hospital Trust.

Brazier, J., Akehurst, R., Brennan, A. *et al.* (2005) Should patients have a greater role in valuing health states? *Applied Health Economics and Health Policy*, **4**, 201–208.

Brook, R.H., Ware, J.E., Davies-Avery, A. *et al.* (1979) Overview of adult health status measures fielded in Rand's health insurance study. *Medical Care*, **17**, 1–131.

Brooks, R. (1996) Euroqol: the current state of play. *Health Policy*, **37**, 53–72.

Brouwer, W., Culyer, A., van Exel, N. and Rutten, F. (2008) Welfarism vs. extra-welfarism. *Journal of Health Economics*, **27**, 325–338.

Brouwer, W., Niesson, L., Postma, M. and Rutten, F. (2006a) Need for differential discounting of costs and health effects in cost effectiveness analysis. *British Medical Journal*, **331**, 446–448.

Brouwer, W.B., van Exel, N., Baltussen, R. and Rutten, F. (2006b) A dollar is a dollar is a dollar – or is it? *Value in Health*, **9**, 341–347.

Brown, D. (1988) Do physicians utilize aides? *Journal of Human Resources*, **23**, 342–355.

Buchmueller, T. and DiNardo, J. (2002) Did community rating induce an adverse selection death spiral? Evidence from New York, Pennsylvania and Connecticut. *American Economic Review*, **92**, 280–294.

Buckingham, K. (1993) A note on HYE (Healthy Years Equivalent). *Journal of Health Economics*, **11**, 301–309.

Burge, P., Devlin, N., Appleby, J. *et al.* (2005) Do patients always prefer quicker treatment? A discrete choice experiment of patients' preferences in the London Patient Choice Project. *Applied Health Economics and Health Policy*, **3**, 183–194.

Busino, G. (1987) Pareto, Vilfredo. In: *The New Palgrave Dictionary of Economics*, vol. **3**. London: Palgrave.

Buxton, M.J., Drummond, M.F., van Hout, B. *et al.* (1997) Modelling in economic evaluation: an unavoidable fact of life. *Health Economics*, **6**, 217–227.

Byford, S. and Raftery, J. (1998) Perspectives in economic evaluation. *British Medical Journal*, **316**, 1529–1530.

Charatan, F. (2000) US Supreme Court bans federal law suits against health maintenance organisations. *British Medical Journal*, **320**, 1688.

Chou, S., Grossman, M. and Saffer, H. (2004) An economic analysis of adult obesity: results from the Behavioral Risk Factor Surveillance System. *Journal of Health Economics*, **23**, 565–587.

Claxton, K., Briggs, A., Buxton, M. *et al.* (2008) Value based pricing for drugs: an opportunity not to be missed? *British Medical Journal*, **336**, 251–254.

Coase, R. (1960) The problem of social cost. *Journal of Law and Economics*, **3**, 1–44.

CMS, Centers for Medicare and Medicaid Services (2011) *National Health Expenditure Projections 2010-2020*. http://www.cms.gov (accessed 5 December 2011).

Collège des Économistes de la Santé (2004) *French guidelines for the economic evaluation of health care technologies*. http://www.ces-asso.org (accessed 4 December 2011).

Cooper, M.H. (1975) *Rationing Health Care*. London: Croom Helm.

Cooper, M.H. and Culyer, A.J. (1968) *The Price of Blood*. London: Institute of Economic Affairs.

Craig, N., Parkin, D. and Gerard, K. (1995) Clearing the fog on the Tyne: programme budgeting in Newcastle and North Tyneside Health Authority. *Health Policy*, **33**, 107–125.

CSDH, Commission on Social Determinants of Health (2008). *Closing the Gap in a Generation: Health Equity Through Action on the Social Determinants of Health. Final Report of the Commission on Social Determinants of Health*. Geneva: World Health Organization.

Culyer, A.J. (1971) Merit goods and the welfare economics of coercion. *Public Finance*, **26**, 546–572.

Culyer, A.J. (1976) *Need and the National Health Service*. Oxford: Martin Robertson.

Culyer, A.J. (1983) *The Political Economy of Social Policy*. Oxford: Martin Robertson.

Culyer, A.J. (1989) The normative economics of health care finance and provision. *Oxford Review of Economic Policy*, **5**, 34–68. (Reprinted in McGuire, A., Fenn, P. and Mayhew, K. (eds), *Providing Health Care*. Oxford: Oxford University Press, 1991.)

Culyer, A.J. and Wagstaff, A. (1993) QALYs versus HYEs. *Journal of Health Economics*, **11**, 311–323.

Culyer, A.J., Williams, A. and Lavers, R.J. (1971) Social indicators: health. *Social Trends*, **2**, 31–42. (Reprinted in Culyer, A.J., Williams, A. and Lavers, R.J. (1972) Health indicators. In: Shonfield, A. and Shaw, S. (eds) *Social Indicators and Social Policy*. London: Heinemann).

Cutler, D., Glaeser, E. and Shapiro, J. (2003) Why have Americans become more obese? *Journal of Economic Perspectives*, **17**, 93–118.

Cutler, D., Lincoln, B. and Zeckhauser, R. (2010) Selection stories: understanding movement across health plans. *Journal of Health Economics* **29**, 821–838.

Cyert, R.M. and March, J.G. (1963) *A Behavioural Theory of the Firm*. New York: Prentice-Hall.

Dafny, L. (2010) Are health insurance markets competitive? *American Economic Review*, **100**, 1399–1431.

Dakin, H., Devlin, N. and Odeyemi, I. (2006) "Yes", "No" or "Yes, but"? Multinomial modelling of NICE decision-making. *Health Policy*, **77**, 352–367.

Dasgupta, A.K. and Pearce, D.N. (1972) *Cost Benefit Analysis: Theory and Practice*. London: Macmillan Books.

Department of Health (2008) *Resource Allocation: Weighted Capitation Formula*, 6th edition. http://www.dh.gov.uk/PublicationsAndStatistics (accessed 4 December 2011).

Department of Health (2010) *A New Value-Based Approach to the Pricing of Branded Medicines – a Consultation*. London: Department of Health.

Derrett, S., Devlin, N., Hansen, P. and Herbison, P. (2003) Prioritising patients for elective surgery. A prospective study of clinical priority assessment criteria (CPAC) in New Zealand. *International Journal of Health Technology Assessment*, **19**, 91–105.

Devlin, N. and Appleby, J. (2010) *Getting the Most out of PROMs: Putting Health Outcomes at the Heart of NHS Decision-Making*. London: King's Fund/Office of Health Economics.

Devlin, N. and Hansen, P. (2000) *Allocating Vote: Health – 'Needs Assessment' and an Economics-Based Approach. New Zealand Treasury Working Paper 00/4*. Wellington: The Treasury. http://www.treasury.govt.nz/publications/research-policy/wp/2000/00-04/twp/00-04.pdf (accessed 4 December 2011).

Devlin, N. and Parkin, D. (2003) Funding fertility: issues in the allocation and distribution of resources to assisted reproduction technologies. *Human Fertility*, **6**, S2–S6.

Devlin, N. and Parkin, D. (2004) Does NICE have a cost effectiveness threshold and what other factors influence its decisions? A binary choice analysis. *Health Economics*, **13**, 437–452.

Devlin, N., Appleby, J. and Parkin, D. (2003) Patients' views on explicit rationing: what are the implications for health service decision-making? *Journal of Health Services Research and Policy*, **8**, 183–186.

Devlin, N., Parkin, D. and Browne, J. (2010) Patient-reported outcome measures in the NHS: new methods for analysing and reporting EQ-5D data. *Health Economics*, **19**, 886–905.

Dolan, P. (1999) US and UK health economics: a reply to Joe Newhouse's paper. *Health Economics*, **8**, 177.

Dolan, P. and Edlin, R. (2002) Is it really possible to build a bridge between cost benefit and cost effectiveness analysis? *Journal of Health Economics*, **21**, 827–843.

Dolan, P., Shaw, R., Tsuchiya, A. and Williams, A. (2005) QALY maximization and peoples' preferences: a methodological review. *Health Economics*, **14**, 197–208.

Donaldson, C., Thomas, R. and Torgerson, D.J. (1997) Validity of open-ended and payment scale approaches to eliciting willingness to pay. *Applied Economics*, **29**, 79–84.

Dougherty, E., Soderstrom, L. and Schiffrin, A. (1998) An economic evaluation of home care for children with newly diagnosed diabetes: results from a randomized controlled trial. *Medical Care*, **36**, 586–598.

Dowie, J. (1995) The danger of partial evaluation. *Health Care Analysis*, **3**, 232–234.

Drummond, M.F. (1980) *Principles of Economic Appraisal in Health Care*. Oxford: Oxford University Press.

Drummond, M.F. (1987) Economic evaluation and the rational diffusion and use of health technology. *Health Policy*, **7**, 309–324.

Drummond, M.F., Sculpher, M.J., Torrance, G.W. *et al.* (2005) *Methods for the Economic Evaluation of Health Care Programmes*, 3rd edition. Oxford: Oxford University Press.

Eichler, H., Kong, S., Gerth, W. *et al.* (2004) Use of cost-effectiveness analysis in healthcare resource allocation decision-making: how are cost-effectiveness thresholds expected to emerge? *Value in Health*, **7**, 518–528.

Enthoven, A. and Kronick, R. (1989) A consumer-choice health plan for the 1990s: universal health insurance in a system designed to promote quality and economy. *New England Journal of Medicine*, **320**, 29–37.

Erbsland, M., Ried, W. and Ulrich, V. (1995) Health, health care and the environment; econometric evidence from the German micro data. *Health Economics*, **4**, 169–182.

Evans, R. (1974) Supplier-induced demand: some empirical evidence and implications. In: Perlman, M. (ed) *The Economics of Health and Medical Care*. London: Macmillan.

Evans, R. (1984) *Strained Mercy: The Economics of Canadian Health Care*. Toronto: Butterworths.

Evans, R. G., Barer, M.L. and Marmor, T.R. (1994) *Why are some people healthy and others not?* New York: Aldine de Gruter.

Farley, P. (1986) Theories of the price and quantity of physician services – a synthesis and critique. *Journal of Health Economics*, **5**, 315–333.

Farrell, M.J. (1957) The measurement of productive efficiency. *Journal of the Royal Statistical Society Series A*, **120**, 253–281.

Finlayson, B., Dixon, J., Meadows, S. and Blair, G. (2002) Mind the gap: the policy response to the nursing shortage. *British Medical Journal*, **325**, 541–544.

Fournier, G.M. and Mitchell, J.M. (1992) Hospital costs and competition for services: a multiproduct analysis. *Review of Economics and Statistics*, **74**, 627–634.

Fox-Rushby, J. (2002) *Disability Adjusted Life Years (DALYs) for Decision Making?* London: Office of Health Economics.

Freemantle, N. and Maynard, A. (1994) Something rotten in the state of clinical and economic evaluations? *Health Economics*, **3**, 63–67.

Friedman, M. (1953) The methodology of positive economics. In: Friedman, M. *Essays in Positive Economics*. Chicago: University of Chicago Press.

Friedman, M. and Savage, L. (1948) The utility analysis of choice. *Journal of Political Economy*, **56**, 279–304.

Fries, J.F. (1980) Ageing, natural death, and the compression of morbidity. *New England Journal of Medicine*, **303**, 130–135.

Fuchs, V.R. (1978) The supply of surgeons and the demand for operations. *Journal of Human Resources*, **13**, 35–56.

Fuchs, V.R. (1998) *Who Shall Live? Health, Economics and Social Choice (expanded edition)*. River Edge, New Jersey: World Scientific.

Gafni, A. (1991) Willingness-to-pay as a measure of benefits. Relevant questions in the context of public decision making about health care programs. *Medical Care*, **29**, 1246–1252.

Gafni, A. and Birch, S. (1993) Economics, health and health economics: HYEs versus QALYS. *Journal of Health Economics*, **11**, 301–339.

Garber, A.M. (1994) Can technology assessment control health spending? *Health Affairs*, **13**, 115–126.

Garber, A.M. (2001) Evidence-based coverage policy. *Health Affairs*, **20**, 62–82.

Garber, A.M. and Phelps, C.E. (1997) Economic foundations of cost-effectiveness analysis. *Journal of Health Economics*, **16**, 1–31.

George, B., Harris, A. and Mitchell, A. (2001) Cost-effectiveness analysis and the consistency of decision making: evidence from pharmaceutical reimbursement in Australia (1991 to 1996). *Pharmacoeconomics*, **19**, 1103–1109.

Gerard, K. and Mooney, G. (1993) Cost effectiveness league tables: handle with care. *Health Economics*, **3**, 57–58.

Gerdtham, U. and Jönsson, B. (2001) International comparisons of health care expenditure. In: Culyer, A.J. and Newhouse, J.P. (eds) *Handbook of Health Economics*, vol. 1A. Amsterdam: North Holland.

Gerdtham, U., Sögaard, J., Andersson, F. and Jönsson, B. (1992a) *Econometric Analysis of Health Expenditure: A Cross Section Study of OECD Countries*. Linköping: Centre for medical Technology Assessment (CMT), University of Linköping.

Gerdtham, U., Sögaard, J., Jönsson, B. and Andersson, F. (1992b) A pooled cross-section analysis of health care expenditure of the OECD countries. In: Zweifel P. and Frech H. (eds), *Health Economics Worldwide*. Dordrecht: Kluwer.

Gerdtham, U.G., Sögaard, J., MacFarlan, M. and Oxley, H. (1998) The determinants of health expenditure in the OECD countries. In Zweifel, P. (ed), *Health, the Medical Profession and Regulation*. Dordrecht: Kluwer Academic Publications.

Gold, M.R., Siegel, J.E., Russell, L.B. and Weinstein, M.C. (1996) *Cost-effectiveness in Health and Medicine*. New York: Oxford University Press.

Goldberg, D., Gater, T., Sartorious, N. *et al.* (1997) The validity of two versions of the GHQ in the WHO study of mental illness in general health care. *Psychological Medicine*, **27**, 191–197.

Goodman, C., Kachur, P., Abdulla, S. *et al.* (2009) Concentration and drug prices in the retail market for malaria treatment in rural Tanzania. *Health Economics*, **18**, 727–742.

Gravelle, H. and Smith, D. (2001) Discounting for health effects in cost-benefit and cost-effectiveness analysis. *Health Economics*, **10**, 587–600.

Gravelle, H., Hole, A. and Santos, R. (2011) Measuring and testing for gender discrimination in physician pay: English family doctors. *Journal of Health Economics*, **30**, 660–674.

Gravelle, H., Simpson, P.R. and Chamberlain, J. (1982) Breast cancer screening and health service costs. *Journal of Health Economics*, **1**, 185–207.

Griffin, S.O., Jones, K. and Tomar, S.L. (2001) An economic evaluation of community water fluoridation. *Journal of Public Health Dentistry*, **61**, 78–86.

Grossman, M. (1972) On the concept of health capital and the demand for health. *Journal of Political Economy*, **82**, 223–255.

Grossman, M. (2000) The human capital model. In: Culyer, A.J. and Newhouse, J.P. (eds), *Handbook of Health Economics*, vol. 1a. Amsterdam: North-Holland.

Gruenberg, E.M. (1977) The failure of success. *Millbank Memorial Fund Quarterly*, **55**, 3–24.

Grytten, J. and Skau, I. (2009). Specialisation and competition in dental health services. *Health Economics*, **18**, 457–466.

Hadorn, D. (1991) Setting health care priorities in Oregon: cost effectiveness meets the rule of rescue. *Journal of the American Medical Association*, **265**, 2218–2225.

Hadorn, D. and Holmes, A. (1997) The New Zealand priority criteria project. Part 1: overview. *British Medical Journal*, **314**, 1130–1131.

Hall, R.E. and Jones, C.I. (2007) The value of life and the rise in health spending. *Quarterly Journal of Economics*, **122**, 39–72.

Hallinen, T.A., Soini, E.J.O., Eklund, K. and Puolakka, K. (2010) Cost-utility of different treatment strategies after the failure of tumour necrosis factor inhibitor in rheumatoid arthritis in the Finnish setting. *Rheumatology*, **49**, 767–777.

Halpern, M.T., McKenna, M. and Hutton, J. (1998) Modelling in economic evaluation: An unavoidable fact of life. *Health Economics*, **7**, 741–742.

Ham, C. (1996) Contestability: a middle path for health care. *British Medical Journal*, **312**, 70–71.

Hammond, P.J. (1996) Interpersonal comparisons of utility: why and how they are and should be made. In: Hamlin, A.P. (ed) *Ethics and Economics*, vol. I. Cheltenham: Edward Elgar.

Hansen, P. and King, A. (1996) The determinants of health care expenditure: a cointegration approach. *Journal of Health Economics*, **15**, 127–137.

Hansen, P. and Scuffham, P.A. (1995) The cost-effectiveness of compulsory bicycle helmets in New Zealand. *Australian Journal of Public Health*, **19**, 450–454.

Harris, J. (1985) *The Value of Life*. London: Routledge and Kegan Paul.

Harris, J.E. (1977) The internal organization of hospitals: some economic implications. *Bell Journal of Economics*, **8**, 467–482.

Harvey, C.M. (1995) Proportional discounting of future costs and benefits. *Mathematics of Operations Research*, **20**, 381–399.

Hauck, K., Smith, P.C. and Goddard, M. (2004) *The economics of priority setting for health care: a literature review. Health, Nutrition and Population (HNP) Discussion paper*. Washington: The World Bank.

Hawthorne, G., Richardson, J. and Osborn, R. (1999) The Assessment of Quality of Life (AQoL) instrument: a psychometric measure of health-related quality of life. *Quality of Life Research*, **8**, 209–224.

Heckman, J. (1979) Sample selection bias as a specification error. *Econometrica*, **47**, 153–1561.

Henderson, N. and Bateman, I. (1995) Empirical and public choice evidence for hyperbolic social discount rates and the implications for intergenerational discounting. *Environmental and Resource Economics*, **5**, 413–423.

Hicks, J.R. (1939) The foundations of welfare economics. *Economic Journal*, **49**, 694–712.

Hirsch, B. and Schumacher, E. (2005) Classic or new monopsony? Searching for evidence in nursing labor markets. *Journal of Health Economics*, **24**, 969–989.

Hirth, R., Chernew, M., Miller, E. *et al.* (2000) Willingness to pay for a quality-adjusted life-year: in search of a standard. *Medical Decision Making*, **20**, 332–342.

HM Treasury (2003) *The Green Book. Appraisal and Evaluation in Central Government*. London: HMSO. http://www.hm-treasury.gov.uk/data_greenbook_index.htm (accessed 9 December 2011).

HM Treasury (2011) *Public Expenditure Statistical Analyses 2011, Cm 8104*. London: Her Majesty's Stationery Office.

Hochman, H.M. and Rodgers, J.D. (1969) Pareto optimal redistribution. *American Economic Review*, **59**, 542–557.

Hollingsworth, B. and Peacock, S. (2008) *Efficiency Measurement in Health and Heath Care*. Oxford: Routledge.

Hollingsworth, B. and Wildman, J. (2003) The efficiency of health production: re-estimating the WHO panel data using parametric and non-parametric approaches to provide additional information. *Health Economics*, **12**, 493–504.

Horsman, J., Furlong, W., Feeny, D. and Torrance, G. (2003) The Health Utilities Index (HUI®): concepts, measurement properties and applications. *Health and Quality of Life Outcomes*, **1**, 54.

Horwitz, J. and Nichols, A. (2009) Hospital ownership and medical services: market mix, spillover effects, and nonprofit objectives. *Journal of Health Economics*, **28**, 924–937.

Jacobsson, F., Carstensen, J. and Borgquist, L. (2005) Caring externalities in health economic evaluation: how are they related to severity of illness? *Health Policy*, **73**, 172–182.

Jarahi, L., Karbakhsh, M. and Rashidian, A. (2011) Parental willingness to pay for child safety seats in Mashad, Iran. *BMC Public Health*, **11**, 281.

Johannesson, M. (1995) A note on the depreciation of the societal perspective in economic evaluation of health care. *Health Policy*, **33**, 59–66.

Johansson, P.-O. (1991) *An Introduction to Modern Welfare Economics*. Cambridge: Cambridge University Press.

Johansson, P.-O. (1995) *Evaluating Health Risks: An Economics Approach*. Cambridge: Cambridge University Press.

Jönsson, B. (1994) Economic evaluation and clinical uncertainty: response to Freemantle and Maynard. *Health Economics*, **3**, 305–307.

Juniper, E.F, Guyatt, G.H., Ferrie, P.J. and Griffith, L.E. (1993) Measuring quality of life in asthma. *American Review of Respiratory Disease*, **147**, 832–838.

Kakwani, N. (1977) Measurement of tax progressivity: an international comparison. *Economic Journal*, **87**, 71–80.

Kaldor, N. (1939) Welfare propositions and interpersonal comparisons of utility. *Economic Journal*, **49**, 549–552.

Katouzian, H. (1980) *Ideology and Method in Economics*. New York: Macmillan.

Keeler, E. and Cretin, S. (1983) Discounting of life savings and other non-monetary effects. *Management Science*, **29**, 300–306.

Kinge, J. and Morris, S. (2010) Socioeconomic variation in the impact of obesity on health related quality of life. *Social Science and Medicine*, **71**, 1864–1871.

Kitzhaber, J.A. (1993) Prioritising health services in an era of limits: the Oregon experience. *British Medical Journal*, **307**, 373–377.

Klevorick, A. and McGuire, T. (1987) Monopolistic competition and consumer information: pricing in the market for psychologists' services. *Advances in Health Economics and Health Services Research*, **8**, 235–253.

Knapp, M. (1984) *The Economics of Social Care*. London: Macmillan.

Knapp, M. and Beecham, J. (1993) Reduced list costings: examination of an informed short cut in mental health research. *Health Economics*, **2**, 313–322.

Lakdawalla, D., Philipson, T. and Bhattacharya, J. (2005) Welfare-enhancing technological change and the growth of obesity. *American Economic Review*, **95**, 253–257.

Lancaster, K. (1971) *Consumer Demand: A New Approach*, New York: Columbia University Press.

Laupacis, A., Feeny, D., Detsky. A. and Tugwell, P. (1992) How attractive does a new technology have to be to warrant adoption and utilization? Tentative guidelines for using clinical and economic evaluations. *Canadian Medical Association Journal*, **146**, 473–481.

Laver, K., Ratcliffe, J., George, S. *et al.* (2011) Early rehabilitation management after stroke: what do stroke patients prefer? *Journal of Rehabilitation Medicine*, **43**, 354–358.

Layard, R. (2005) *Happiness. Lessons from a New Science*. London: Penguin.

Leu, R.E. (1986) The public-private mix and international health care costs. In Culyer, A.J. and Jönsson, B. (eds), *Public and Private Health Services*. Oxford: Basil Blackwell.

Levaggi, R., Orizio, G., Domenighini, S. *et al.* (2009) Marketing and pricing strategies of online pharmacies. *Health Policy*, **92**, 187–196.

Linna, M. (1998) Measuring hospital cost efficiency with panel data models. *Health Economics*, **7**, 415–427.

Little, I.M.D. (1957) *A Critique of Welfare Economics*. Second edition. Oxford: Oxford University Press.

Loewenstein, G. and Prelec, D. (1993) Preferences for sequences of outcomes. *Psychological Review*, **100**, 91–108.

Lopez, A., Mathers, C., Ezati, M. *et al.* (eds) (2006) *Global Burden of Disease and Risk Factors*. New York: Oxford University Press.

Ludbrook, A. (2004) *Effective and cost-effective measures to reduce alcohol misuse in Scotland: an update*. Edinburgh: Scottish Executive.

Ludbrook, A. and Mooney, G. (1984) *Economic Appraisal in the NHS: Problems and Challenges*. Aberdeen: Health Economics Research Unit, University of Aberdeen.

Ludbrook, A., Godfrey, C., Wyness, L. *et al.* (2001) *Effective and cost-effective measures to reduce alcohol misuse in Scotland: a literature review.* Edinburgh: Scottish Executive.

Lyden, F.J. and Miller, E.G. (1972) *Planning Programming Budgeting. A Systems Approach to Management.* Chicago: Markham Publishing Company.

Madden, D., Nolan, A. and Nolan, B. (2005) GP reimbursement and visiting behaviour in Ireland. *Health Economics*, **14**: 1047–1060.

Maniadakis, N. and Gray, A. (2000) The economic burden of back pain in the UK. *Pain*, **84**, 95–103.

Manning, W., Fryback, D. and Weinstein, M.C (1996) Reflecting uncertainty in cost-effectiveness analysis. In: Gold, M.R., Siegel, J.E., Russell, L.B. and Weinstein, M.C. (eds) *Cost-effectiveness in Health and Medicine.* New York: Oxford University Press.

Manning, W.G., Newhouse, J.P., Duan, N. *et al.* (1987) Health insurance and the demand for medical care: evidence from a randomized experiment. *American Economic Review*, **77**, 251–277.

Manski, C.F. (1977) The structure of random utility models. *Theory and Decision*, **8**, 229–254.

Marris, R. (1963) A model of 'managerial' enterprise. *Quarterly Journal of Economics*, **77**, 185–209.

Masiye, F. and Rehnberg, C. (2005) The economic value of an improved malaria treatment programme in Zambia: results from a contingent valuation survey. *Malaria Journal*, **4**, 60–68.

Maynard, A. (1991) Developing the health care market. *Economic Journal*, **101**, 1277–1286.

Maynard, A. (1996) Rationing health care. *British Medical Journal*, **313**, 1499.

Maynard, A. and Bloor, K. (1998) *Our Certain Fate: Rationing in Health Care.* London: Office for Health Economics.

Maynard A., Bloor K., and Freemantle N. (2004) Challenges for the National Institute for Clinical Excellence. *British Medical Journal*, **329**, 227–229.

McCoskey, S. and Selden, T.M. (1998) Health care expenditure and GDP: panel data unit root tests results. *Journal of Health Economics*, **17**, 369–376.

McGuire, A., Parkin, D., Hughes, D. and Gerard, K. (1993) Econometric analyses of national health expenditures: can positive economics help to answer normative questions? *Health Economics*, **2**, 113–126.

McGuire, T. (2001) Physician agency. In: Culyer, A.J. and Newhouse, J.P. (eds), *Handbook of Health Economics*, vol. 1A. Amsterdam: North Holland.

McKie, J. and Richardson, J. (2003) The rule of rescue. *Social Science and Medicine*, **56**, 2407–2419.

Mechanic, D. (1997) Muddling through elegantly: finding the proper balance in rationing. *Health Affairs*, **16**, 83–92.

Mehrez, A. and Gafni, A. (1989) Quality adjusted life years, utility theory, and healthy-years equivalents. *Medical Decision Making*, **9**, 142–149.

Merrison, A. (Chairman) (1979) *Report of the Royal Commission on the National Health Service.* London: HMSO, London.

Miller, P., Parkin, D., Craig, N. *et al.* (1997) Less fog on the Tyne? Programme budgeting in Newcastle and North Tyneside. *Health Policy*, **40**, 217–229.

Miller, R. and Luft, H. (2002) HMO plan performance update: an analysis of the literature, 1997–2001. *Health Affairs*, **21**, 63–86.

Miners, A., Garau, M., Fidan, D. and Fischer, A.J. (2005) Comparing estimates of cost effectiveness submitted to NICE by different organisations: retrospective study. *British Medical Journal*, **330**, 65–68.

Mishan, E.J. (1971) *Cost Benefit Analysis*. London: Macmillan Books.

Mitton, C. and Donaldson, C. (2001) Twenty-five years of programme budgeting and marginal analysis in the health sector, 1974–1999. *Journal of Health Services Research and Policy*, **6**, 239–248.

Mooney, G. (1983) Equity in health care: confronting the confusion. *Effective Health Care*, **1**, 179–185.

Mooney, G. (1994) *Key Issues in Health Economics*. New York: Harvester Wheatsheaf.

Mooney, G. and Russell, E. (2003) Equity in health care: the need for a new economics paradigm? In: Scott, A., Maynard, A. and Elliott B. (eds), *Advances in Health Economics*. London: John Wiley & Sons Ltd.

Mooney, G. and Wiseman, V. (2000) Burden of disease and priority setting. *Health Economics*, **9**, 369–372.

Mooney, G., Hall, J., Donaldson, C. and Gerard, K. (1991) Utilisation as a measure of equity: weighing heat? *Journal of Health Economics*, **10**, 475–480.

Moreno-Serra, R. and Wagstaff, A. (2010) System-wide impacts of hospital payment reforms: evidence from Central and Eastern Europe and Central Asia. *Journal of Health Economics*, **29**, 585–602.

Morris, S., Sutton, M. and Gravelle, H. (2005) Inequity and inequality in the use of health care in England: an empirical investigation. *Social Science and Medicine*, **60**, 1251–1266.

Moskowitz, M. (1987) Costs of screening for breast cancer. *Radiologic Clinics of North America*, **25**, 1031–1037.

Mossialos, E., Dixon, A., Figueras, J. and Kutzin, J. (2002) *Funding Health Care: Options for Europe. Policy Brief No. 4*. London: European Observatory on Health Care Systems.

Mullahy J. (2010) Understanding the production of population health and the role of paying for population health. *Preventing Chronic Disease*, **7**(5).

Müller-Riemenschneider, F., Reinhold, T., Berghofer, A. and Willich, S. (2008) Health-economic burden of obesity in Europe. *European Journal of Epidemiology*, **23**, 499–509.

Muurinen, J.M. and Le Grand, J. (1985) The economic analysis of inequalities in health. *Social Science and Medicine*, **20**, 1029–1035.

National Institute for Clinical Excellence (2004) Fertility: Assessment and Treatment for People with Fertility Problems. *Clinical Guideline 11*. London: RCOG Press.

NICE, National Institute for Health and Clinical Excellence (2008) *Guide to the methods of technology appraisal*. London: National Institute for Health and Clinical Excellence.

NICE, National Institute for Health and Clinical Excellence (2009) *Methods for the development of NICE public health guidance*. London: National Institute for Health and Clinical Excellence.

NICE, National Institute for Health and Clinical Excellence (2011) *Technology Appraisal Recommendation Summary*. London: National Institute for Health and Clinical Excellence.

Neumann, P. and Weinstein, M. (2010) Legislating against use of cost-effectiveness information. *New England Journal of Medicine*, **363**, 1495–1497.

Newhouse, J.P. (1970) Toward a theory of non-profit institutions: an economic model of a hospital. *American Economic Review*, **60**, 64–74.

Newhouse, J.P. (1977) Medical care expenditures: a cross-national survey. *Journal of Human Resources*, **12**, 115–124.

Newhouse, J.P. (1998) US and UK health economics: two disciplines separated by a common language? *Health Economics*, **7**, S79–S92.

NHS Information Centre (2010) *NHS maternity statistics, England: 2008–09*. London: Department of Health. http://www.ic.nhs.uk/pubs/maternity0910 (accessed 5 December 2011).

Nozick, R. (1974) *Anarchy, State and Utopia*. New York: Basic Books.

Nuffield Council on Bioethics (2011) *Human Bodies: donation for medicine and research* London: Nuffield Council on Bioethics.

Nyman, J.A. and Bricker, D.L. (1989) Profit incentives and technical efficiency in the production of nursing home care. *The Review of Economics and Statistics*, **71**, 586–593.

Oaxaca, R. (1973) Male-female wage differentials in urban labor markets. *International Economic Review*, **14**, 693–709.

O'Brien, B., Gersten, K., Willan, A. and Faulkner, L. (2002) Is there a kink in consumers' threshold value for cost effectiveness in health care? *Health Economics*, **11**, 175–180.

O'Donnell, O., van Doorslaer, E., Wagstaff, A. and Lindelow, M. (2008) *Analyzing health equity using household survey data: a guide to techniques and their implementation*. Washington DC: The World Bank.

OECD, Organisation for Economic Co-operation and Development (2008) *The looming crisis in the health workforce: how can OECD countries respond?* Paris: Organisation for Economic Co-operation and Development.

Olson, E. and Rodgers, D. (1991) The welfare economics of equal access. *Journal of Public Economics*, **45**, 91–106.

Oswald, A. and Powdthavee, N. (2007) Obesity, unhappiness and the challenge of affluence: theory and evidence. *Economic Journal*, **117**, F441–F454.

Parkin D., and Devlin, N. (2003) Measuring efficiency in dental care. In: Scott, A., Maynard, A., and Elliott, R. (eds) *Advances in Health Economics*. London: John Wiley and Sons Ltd.

Parkin, D. and Devlin, N. (2006) Is there a case for using visual analogue scale valuations in cost utility analysis? *Health Economics*, **15**, 653–664.

Parkin, D. and Yule, B. (1988) Patient charges and the demand for dental care in Scotland, 1962-1981. JT *Applied Economics*, **20**, 229–242.

Parkin, D., McGuire, A. and Yule, B. (1987) Aggregate health care expenditures and national income: is health care a luxury good? *Journal of Health Economics*, **6**, 109–127.

Parsonage, M. and Neuberger, H. (1992) Discounting and health benefits. *Health Economics*, **1**, 71–76.

Patrick, D. L. and Erickson, P. (1993) *Health Status and Health Policy: Quality of Life in Health Care Evaluation and Resource Allocation*. New York: Oxford University Press.

Paul, S.M., Mytelka, D.S., Dunwiddie, C.T. *et al.* (2010) How to improve R&D productivity: the pharmaceutical industry's grand challenge. *Nature Reviews Drug Discovery*, **9**, 203–214.

Pauly, M. and Satterthwaite, M. (1981) The pricing of primary care physicians services – a test of the role of consumer information. *Bell Journal of Economics*, **12**, 488–506.

Pauly, M.V. (1978) Is medical care different? In Greenberg, A. (ed) *Competition in the Health Care Sector: Past, Present and Future*. Colorado: Aspen Systems.

Pauly, M.V. and Redisch, M. (1973) The not-for-profit hospital as a physician's cooperative. *American Economic Review*, **63**, 87–100.

Pearce, D. and Özdemiroglu, E. (2002) *Economic Valuation with Stated Preference Techniques*. London: Department for Transport, Local Government and the Regions.

Peeters, A., Barendregt, J., Willekens, F. *et al.* (2003) Obesity in adulthood and its consequences for life expectancy: a life-table analysis. *Annals of Internal Medicine*, **138**, 24–32.

Phelps, C.E. (1995) Welfare loss from variations. *Journal of Health Economics*, **14**, 253–260.

Phelps, C.E. and Mooney, C. (1992) Correction and update on priority setting in medical technology assessment in medical care. *Medical Care*, **30**, 744–751.

Phelps, C.E. and Parente, S. (1990) Priority setting in medical technology and medical practice assessment. *Medical Care*, **29**, 703–723.

Pozen, A. and Cutler, D.M. (2010) Medical spending differences in the United States and Canada: the role of prices, procedures, and administrative expenses. *Inquiry*, **47**, 124–134.

Propper, C., Rees, H. and Green, K. (2001) The demand for private medical insurance in the UK. A cohort analysis. *Economic Journal*, **111**, 180–200.

Ramsberg, J. and Sjöberg, L. (1997) The cost-effectiveness of lifesaving interventions in Sweden. *Risk Analysis*, **17**, 467–478.

Ramsey, S., Willke, R., Briggs, A. *et al.* (2005) Good research practices for cost-effectiveness analysis alongside clinical trial: The ISPOR RCT-CEA task force report. *Value in Health*, **8**, 521–533.

Rawlins, M.D. and Culyer, A.J. (2004) National Institute of Clinical Excellence and its value judgements. *British Medical Journal*, **329**, 224–227.

Rawls, J. (1971) *A Theory of Justice*. Cambridge, MA: Harvard University Press.

Rees, R. (1989) Uncertainty, information and insurance. In: Hey, J. (ed) *Current Issues in Microeconomics*. London: MacMillan.

Reinhardt, U. (1972) A production function for physician services. *Review of Economics and Statistics*, **54**, 55–66.

Rice, T. (1998) *The Economics of Health Reconsidered*. Chicago: Health Administration Press.

Roberts, J. (1998) Spurious regression problems in the determinants of health care expenditure: a comment on Hitiris. *Applied Economics Letters*, **7**, 279–283.

Robinson, J. (1980) *Collected Economic Papers, 1951–1980*, vol. II. Cambridge, MA: MIT Press.

Roemer, J. (1998) *Equality of Opportunity*. Cambridge, MA: Harvard University Press.

Rost, K.T. (2000) Policing the 'wild west' world of internet pharmacies. *Food and Drug Law Journal*, **55**, 619–640.

Rothschild, M. and Stiglitz, J. (1976) Equilibrium in competitive insurance markets – essay on economics of imperfect information. *Quarterly Journal of Economics*, **90**, 629–649.

Ruark, J.E., Raffin, T.A. and the Stanford University Medical Center Committee on Ethics (1988) Initiating and withdrawing life support: principles and practice in adult medicine. *New England Journal of Medicine*, **318**, 25–30.

Ryan, M. (1997) Should government fund assisted reproductive techniques? A study using willingness to pay. *Applied Economics*, **29**, 841–849.

Ryan, M. and Farrar, S. (2000) Using conjoint analysis to elicit preferences for health care. *British Medical Journal*, **320**, 1530–1533.

Samuelson, P.A. (1937) A note on the measurement of utility. *The Review of Economic Studies*, **4**, 155–161.

Scherer, F. (2000) The pharmaceutical industry. In: Culyer, A. and Newhouse, J.P. (eds) *Handbook of Health Economics: 1B*. Amsterdam: North Holland.

Scitovsky, T. (1941) A note on welfare propositions in economics. *Review of Economic Studies*, **9**, 77–88.

Sen, A. (1970) *Collective Choice and Social Welfare*. Amsterdam: North Holland.

Sen, A. (1977) Social choice theory: a re-examination. *Econometrica*, **45**, 53–90.

Sen, A. (1985) *Commodities and Capabilities*. Amsterdam: North Holland.

Sen, A. (2002) Health: perception versus observation. *British Medical Journal*, **324**, 860–861.

Seshamani, M. and Gray, A. (2002) The impact of ageing on expenditures in the National Health Service. *Age and Ageing*, **31**, 287–294.

Seshamani, M. and Gray, A. (2004) A longitudinal study of the effects of age and time to death on hospital costs. *Journal of Health Economics*, **23**, 217–235.

Shah, K., Praet, C., Devlin, N. *et al.* (2011) *Is the aim of the health care system to maximise QALYs? An investigation of 'what else matters' in the NHS. OHE Research Paper 11/03*. London: Office of Health Economics.

Shields, M. and Ward, M. (2001) Improving nurse retention in the National Health Service in England: the impact of job satisfaction on intentions to quit. *Journal of Health Economics*, **20**, 677–701.

Simoens, S., Villeneuve, M. and Hurst, J. (2005) *Tackling Nurse Shortages in OECD Countries: OECD Health Working Paper 19*. Paris: Organisation for Economic Co-operation and Development.

Sintonen, H. (1981) An approach to measuring and valuing health states. *Social Science and Medicine*, **15C**, 55–65.

Stahlnacke, K., Soderfeldt, B., Unell, L. *et al.* (2005). Changes over 5 years in utilization of dental care by a Swedish age cohort. *Community Dental and Oral Epidemiology*, **33**, 64–73.

Stinnett, A.A. and Mullahy, J. (1998) Net health benefits: a new framework for the analysis of uncertainty in cost-effectiveness analysis. *Medical Decision Making*, **19**, S68–S80.

Sugden, R. and Williams, A. (1978) *The Principles of Practical Cost-Benefit Analysis*. Oxford: Oxford University Press.

Suraratdecha, C. and Okunade, A.A. (2006) Measuring operational efficiency in a health care system: a case study from Thailand. *Health Policy*, **77**, 2–23.

Sutton, M. (2002) Vertical and horizontal aspects of socio-economic inequity in general practitioner contacts in Scotland. *Health Economics*, **11**, 537–549.

Szende, A., Oppe, M. and Devlin, N. (eds) (2007) *EQ5D Valuation Sets: An Inventory, Competitive Review and Users' Guide. EuroQol Group Monographs*, vol. 2. Springer.

Szeto, K.L. and Devlin, N. (1996) The cost-effectiveness of mammography screening: evidence from a microsimulation model for New Zealand. *Health Policy*, **38**, 101–115.

Tengs, T. (1996) An evaluation of Oregon's Medicaid rationing algorithms. *Health Economics*, **5**, 171–181.

Tengs, T., Adams, M., Pliskin, J. *et al.* (1995) Five hundred life-saving interventions and their cost effectiveness. *Risk Analysis*, **15**, 369–390.

Thurston, N. and Libby, A. (2002) A production function for physician services revisited. *Review of Economics and Statistics*, **84**, 184–191.

Titmuss, R.M. (1972) *The Gift Relationship*. London: Allen and Unwin.

Torgerson, D. and Spencer, A. (1995) Marginal costs and benefits. *British Medical Journal*, **312**, 35.

Tsuchiya, A. and Williams, A. (2001) Welfare economics and economic evaluation. In McGuire, A. and Drummond, M.F. (eds), *Economic Evaluation in Health Care: Merging Theory with Practice*. Oxford: Oxford University Press.

Tsuchiya, A., Dolan, P. and Shaw, R. (2003) Measuring people's preferences regarding ageism in health: some methodological issues and some fresh evidence. *Social Science and Medicine*, **57**, 687–696.

Turner, K., Adams, E., Grant, A. *et al.* (2011). Costs and cost effectiveness of different strategies for chlamydia screening and partner notification: an economic and mathematical modelling study. *British Medical Journal*, **341**, c7250.

Tussing, A.D. and Wojtowycz, M.A. (1986) Physican-induced demand by Irish GPs. *Social Science and Medicine*, **23**, 851–860.

US Census Bureau (2010) *Historical Health Insurance Tables*. New York: US Census Bureau.

US Congressional Budget Office (2007) *The Long-Term Outlook for Health Care Spending*. http://www.cbo.gov/ftpdocs/87xx/doc8758/11-13-LT-Health.pdf (accessed 5 December 2011).

van der Pol, M. and McKenzie, L. (2010) Costs and benefits of tele-endoscopy clinics in a remote location. *Journal of Telemedicine and Telecare*, **16**, 89–94.

van Doorslaer, E. and Jones, A. (2003) Inequalities in self-reported health: validation of a new approach to measurement. *Journal of Health Economics*, **22**, 61–87.

van Doorslaer, E. and Koolman, X. (2004). Explaining the differences in income-related health inequalities across European countries. *Health Economics*, **13**, 609–628.

van Doorslaer, E., Koolman, X. and Jones, A. (2004) Explaining income-related inequalities in doctor utilisation in Europe. *Health Economics*, **13**, 629–647.

van Doorslaer, E., Wagstaff, A., van der Burg, H. *et al.* (1999) The redistributive effect of health care finance in twelve OECD countries. *Journal of Health Economics*, **18**, 291–313.

van Doorslaer, E., Wagstaff, A., van der Burg, H. *et al.* (2000) Equity in the distribution of health care in Europe and the US. *Journal of Health Economics*, **19**, 553–583.

van Hout, B. (1998) Discounting costs and effects: a reconsideration. *Health Economics*, **7**, 581–594.

van Hout, B.A., Al, M.J., Gordon, G.S. and Rutten, F.F.H. (1994) Costs, effects and C/E ratios alongside a clinical trial. *Health Economics*, **3**, 309–319.

von der Schulenburg, J.M. (ed) (2000) *The Influence of Economic Evaluation Studies on Health Care Decision-Making*. Amsterdam: IOS Press.

Vickrey, B.G., Hays, R.D., Harooni, R. *et al.* (1995) A health-related quality of life measure for multiple sclerosis. *Quality of Life Research*, **4**, 187–206.

Viscusi, W.K. (2004) The value of life: estimates with risks by occupation and industry. *Economic Inquiry*, **42**, 29–48.

Wagstaff, A. (1986a) The demand for health: theory and applications. *Journal of Epidemiology and Community Health*, **40**, 1–11.

Wagstaff, A. (1986b) The demand for health: some new empirical evidence. *Journal of Health Economics*, **5**, 195–233.

Wagstaff, A. (1993) The demand for health: an empirical formulation of the Grossman model. *Health Economics*, **2**, 189–198.

Wagstaff, A. (2002) Inequality aversion, health inequalities and health achievement. *Journal of Health Economics*, **21**, 627–641.

Wagstaff, A. and van Doorslaer, E. (1997) Progressivity, horizontal equity and reranking in health care finance: a decomposition analysis for the Netherlands. *Journal of Health Economics*, **16**, 499–516.

Wagstaff, A. and van Doorslaer, E. (2000a) Measuring and testing for inequity in the delivery of health care. *Journal of Human Resources*, **35**, 716–733.

Wagstaff, A. and van Doorslaer, E. (2000b) Equity in health care finance and delivery. In: Culyer, A. and Newhouse, J.P. (eds) *Handbook of Health Economics: 1B*. Amsterdam: North Holland.

Wagstaff, A., van Doorslaer, E., van der Burg, H. *et al.* (1999) Equity in the finance of health care: some further international comparisons. *Journal of Health Economics*, **18**, 263–290.

Wagstaff, A., van Doorslaer, E. and Watanabe, N. (2003) On decomposing the causes of health sector inequalities, with an application to malnutrition inequalities in Vietnam. *Journal of Econometrics*, **112**, 219–227.

Watson, R. (2001) European Court's ruling paves way for cross-border treatment. *British Medical Journal*, **323**, 128.

Weaver, M. and Deolalikar, A. (2004) Economies of scale and scope in Vietnamese hospitals. *Social Science and Medicine*, **59**, 199–208.

Weinstein, M.C. and Stason, W.B. (1977) Foundations of cost effectiveness analysis for health and medical practices. *New England Journal of Medicine*, **296**, 716–721.

Weinstein, M.C., Siegel, J.E., Gold, M.R., Kamlet, S. and Russell, L.B. (1996) Recommendations of the panel on cost-effectiveness in health and medicine. *Journal of the American Medical Association*, **276**, 1253–1258.

Weitzman, M.L. (1994) On the 'environmental' discount rate. *Journal of Environmental Economics and Management*, **26**, 200–209.

Weitzman, M.L. (1999) Just keep discounting, but . . . . In: Portnet, P.R. and Weyant, J.P. (eds) *Discounting and Intergenerational Equity*. Washington DC: Resources for the Future.

Wennberg, J. and Gittleson, A. (1982) Variations in medical care among small areas. *Scientific American*, **246**, 1255–1260.

Whitehead, M. (1994) Equity issues in the NHS: who cares about equity in the NHS? *British Medical Journal*, **308**, 1284–1287.

Whynes, D.K. and Walker, A.R. (1995) On approximations in treatment costing. *Health Economics*, **4**, 31–39.

Williams, A. (1985) Economics of coronary artery bypass grafting. *British Medical Journal*, **291**, 326–329.

Williams, A. (1997) Intergenerational equity: an exploration of the fair innings argument. *Health Economics*, **6**, 117–132.

Williams, A. (1999) Calculating the global burden of disease: time for a strategic reappraisal? *Health Economics*, **8**, 1–8.

Williams, A. (2000) Comments on the response by Murray and Lopez. *Health Economics*, **9**, 83–86.

Williams, A. and Cookson, R. (2000) Equity in Health. In: Culyer, A., Newhouse, J.P. (eds). *Handbook of Health Economics: 1B*. Amsterdam: North Holland.

Williamson, O.E. (1963) Managerial discretion and business behaviour. *American Economic Review*, **53**, 1032–1057.

Woolhandler, S., Campbell, T. and Himmelstein, D. (2003) Costs of health care administration in the United States and Canada. *New England Journal of Medicine*, **349**, 768–775.

World Bank (1993) *World Development Report. Investing in Health*. Oxford: Oxford University Press.

WHO, World Health Organisation (2006) *World Health Report: Working Together for Health*. Geneva: World Health Organisation.

Yett, D. (1973) The nursing shortage. In Cooper, M. and Culyer, A. (eds) *Health Economics*. Middlesex: Penguin. Reprinted from Yett, D. (1970) The chronic "shortage" of nurses: a public policy dilemma. In: Klarman, H. (ed) *Empirical Studies in Health Economics*. Baltimore: The Johns Hopkins Press.

Yildiz, Z., Ayhan, S. and Erdogmus, S. (2009) The impact of nurses' motivation to work, job satisfaction, and sociodemographic characteristics on intention to quit their current job: An empirical study in Turkey. *Applied Nursing Research*, **22**, 113–118.

Zere, E., Mbeeli, T., Shangula, K. *et al.* (2006) Technical efficiency of district hospitals: evidence from Namibia using Data Envelopment Analysis. *Cost Effectiveness and Resource Allocation*, **4**, 5.

Zweifel, P., Felder, S., and Meier, M. (1999) Ageing of population and health care expenditure: a red herring? *Health Economics*, **8**, 485–496.

AUTHOR INDEX

SUBJECT INDEX